Neurosurgery Research Progress

nova
Medicine & Health
New York

Neurosurgery Research Progress

The Handbook of Neuromodulation (2 Volume Set)
Albert J. Fenoy, MD, Georgios Matis, MD, PhD,
Pritam Majumdar, PhD,
Sait Ozturk, MD (Editors)
2022. ISBN: 978-1-68507-617-7 (Hardcover)
2022. ISBN: 978-1-68507-789-1 (eBook)

Neuroendoscopic Procedures and Challenges
Soner Duru, MD (Editor)
2021. ISBN: 978-1-68507-092-2 (Softcover)
2021. ISBN: 978-1-68507-155-4 (eBook)

Craniospinal Vascular Diseases and Endovascular Neurosurgery
Xianli Lv MD
Guihuai Wang MD
James Wang MD (Editors)
2021. ISBN: 978-1-53619-342-8 (Hardcover)
2021. ISBN: 978-1-53619-357-2 (eBook)

More information about this series can be found at
https://novapublishers.com/product-category/series/neurosurgery-research-progress/

Amit Agrawal, Pradeep Chouksey,
Adesh Shrivastava, Sumit Raj
and Rakesh Mishra
Editors

Advances in Neurosurgery Research

nova
Medicine & Health
New York

DOI: https://doi.org/10.52305/HXFW4771

Library of Congress Cataloging-in-Publication Data

ISBN: 978-1-68507-859-1

Published by Nova Science Publishers, Inc. † New York

Contents

Preface

Neurosurgery has witnessed technological advances since its inception as a separate speciality. As with other medical specialities, it is constantly evolving and changing, making it essential for the concerned practitioners to update and change. Globally, individual societies have played the role of formulating and disseminating these changes, for example, WHO on classification and diagnostics of the tumour, brain trauma foundation guidelines for the management of trauma etc. However, as these critical pieces of information are often scattered, it is cumbersome and time consuming for readers to locate them in one place. We designed this book to help the practitioners in the field of neurosurgery and allied neurosciences discipline access the exciting and updated changes in neurosurgical topics in recent years. Our motivation behind this work was to lead the readers to the point where they can understand, recognize, and translate the recent changes into their practice.

We have segregated recent neurosurgery advances among topics pertinent to individual pathologies of subspecialties in two volumes to facilitate this process. Other similar texts and textbooks of neurosurgery provide details on each topic; however, due to the sheer volume of information, other texts fail to provide detailed information on the recent advances. We believe that the recent advances of today are the basics of tomorrow. Therefore, the idea was to present these recent advances together in a single collection with this book. The idea of this book is not to be a stand-alone book for neurosurgery readers.

On the other hand, this book will provide complementary information to the other texts and act as a valuable addition to bookshelves. Relevant references are provided with each chapter for a more detailed discussion on the topics covered. Special mention is given to topics often not covered in other similar texts. This book presents updated information on general neurosurgery, neurosurgical oncology, functional neurosurgery, CSF disorders, neuroimaging, techniques, advances in ICP monitoring and innovation in neurosurgery. We hope that this book will be a helpful reference resource for trainees, researchers, and anyone practising neurosurgery.

The authors of the chapters are well-renowned neurosurgeons active in their respective fields of clinical care and research.

Editors

Chapter 1

Recent Research in CSF Dynamics

Naveen Mehrotra[1], Dilip K. Macharla[1] and Manas Panigrahi[2]

[1]Department of Neurosurgery, Sunshine Hospitals, Secunderabad, Telangana, India
[2]Department of Neurosurgery, KIMS Hospitals, Secunderabad, Telangana, India

Abstract

The complex dynamics of Cerebrospinal fluid (CSF) formation, circulation, and absorption are still debatable and poorly understood. The traditional concept of CSF dynamics was based on the active CSF secretion in the ventricular system, unidirectional flow, and passive absorption through the arachnoid villi. However, recent research suggests that water ultrafiltration across the capillary walls results in the formation of CSF and ISF throughout the CNS. A secondary route of CSF circulation along the Virchow-robin spaces, known as the "glymphatic system," is responsible for clearing wastes and solutes. Aquaporin (AQP) channels aid in the bi-directional transport of water, ions, and solutes across the cell membrane. Impaired functioning of the glymphatic system and AQP channels causes disruption of normal CSF dynamics, which is seen in neurological diseases like dementia and idiopathic intracranial hypertension.

In: Advances in Neurosurgery Research
Editors: Amit Agrawal, Pradeep Chouksey, Adesh Shrivastava et al.
ISBN: 978-1-68507-859-1

Abbreviations

ASV	Aqueduct stroke volume,
AQP	Aquaporin,
CSF	Cerebrospinal fluid,
CP	Choroid plexus,
ICP	Intra-cranial pressure,
iNPH	Idiopathic normal pressure hydrocephalus,
ISF	Interstitial fluid,
PC-MRI	Phase-contrast magnetic resonance imaging,
SAS	Subarachnoid space,
VP Shunt	Ventriculoperitoneal shunt,
VRS	Virchow robin space

Introduction

The cerebrospinal fluid (CSF) is a clear, colorless fluid surrounding the brain and spinal cord. The CSF spaces include the ventricles and the subarachnoid spaces of the brain and spine, along with the central canal of the spinal cord. Apart from being protective, CSF aids in maintaining the homeostasis of interstitial fluid of brain parenchyma and regulating its neuronal functioning, supply of nutrients, and regulation of intracranial pressure. Disruptions in the composition and hydrodynamics of CSF impact cerebral physiology and functioning, observed in hydrocephalus and other neurological conditions, reflecting the importance of exchanges between CSF and neuronal environment (Sakka, Coll, and Chazal, 2011).

CSF Functions and Its Physiology

CSF plays a vital role in providing buoyancy for the approximately 1.2kg human brain, which is suspended in CSF is equivalent to a mass of 45 grams, allowing the brain to maintain its density without being impaired by its weight (Cushing, 1925). The metabolic functions of the CSF include the supply of nutrients to the neuronal and glial cells with the removal of degradation products of cellular metabolism. The CSF serves as a "sink" wherein the substances formed after cerebral metabolic activity diffuse into the CSF and pass into the vascular system (Davson, 1966). Moreover, CSF has also been implicated in immunologic aspects and regularisation of the sleep-wake cycle (Tumani, Huss, and Bachhuber, 2017; Hayaishi, 2000).

At a rate of 0.3-0.4mL/min, the amount of CSF produced is approximately 400-600mL/day (Sakka, Coll, and Chazal, 2011; Khasawneh, Garling, and Harris, 2018). The CSF volume is estimated to be around 150mL in adults, distributed as 25mL in ventricles, 50mL in cranial, and 75mL in spinal subarachnoid spaces. The rate of CSF turnover is approximately four times in 24 hours and is directly proportional to CSF formation rate and inversely related to CSF volume. Clearance of brain metabolites depends on a CSF renewal of 0.3-0.4% per minute, with brain catabolites building up when its turnover falls by > 50% (Johanson et al., 2008).

The CSF pressure is 10-15cm H_2O in normal adults and varies with posture, carotid pulsation, respiration, abdominal pressure, jugular venous pressure, state of arousal, and physical activity (Dreha-Kulaczewski et al., 2015). With more than a century over, the CSF physiology and dynamics are still presented as a hypothesis rather than a proven fact (Orešković, Radoš, and Klarica, 2017).

CSF Secretion

The traditional hypothesis about the secretion, circulation, and absorption of CSF is based on three basic premises; i.e., CSF secreted actively by the choroid plexus(CP) within the ventricles, arachnoid villi-mediated passive CSF absorption into the dural venous sinuses, and CSF circulation is unidirectional from the site of production to the site of absorption (Orešković, Radoš, and Klarica, 2017). According to the traditional hypothesis, CSF is mostly formed in the choroid plexus, and a biological pump actively secretes it. In fact, CSF circulation and reabsorption are only the consequence of CSF active secretion.

Milhorat removed the choroid plexus from both lateral ventricles in humans and monkeys, found no substantial difference in the CSF secretion and composition, and challenged the traditional hypothesis (Milhorat, 1976). Tamburrini et al. reported that about 1 L of CSF/day was secreted even after total choroid plexectomy (Tamburrini et al., 2006).

A recent hypothesis named after Bulat-Klarica-Oreskovic' is based on experiments in which they inserted a cannula with a stopcock for the occlusion and drainage of CSF in the cat's aqueduct of Sylvius. They blocked the aqueduct for 120-190 minutes and observed ventricular size and CSF pressure in the cat's ventricle and cisterna magna. As per the traditional hypothesis, they should have observed ventricular dilatation with an increase in pressure, but in reality, there was no increase in pressure or dilatation of ventricles noted in the X-ray ventriculography (done before and 2 hours after aqueduct occlusion) (Bulat and Klarica, 2011; Orešković, Radoš, and Klarica, 2017).

The recent theory presumes that CSF and interstitial fluid (ISF) are formed due to water filtration across arterial capillary walls throughout the CNS (Orešković, Radoš, and Klarica, 2017). The ISF, the fluid in the cerebral parenchyma, the CSF, and the fluid in the subarachnoid spaces form a functional unit, and the volumes of these fluid compartments are typically controlled by modifications in the osmotic and hydrostatic pressure gradients across the capillaries and the ISF-CSF unit (Chikly and Quaghebeur, 2013). Moreover, the choroid plexus weighs only two to three grams. In contrast, cerebral capillaries provide an extensive contact surface ($250cm^2/g$ of the tissue), about 5,000 times larger than the capillary surface area of the choroid plexus. The vast surface area of the microvasculature in the craniospinal space assumes more significance than the smaller surface area of the choroid plexus and the venous sinuses involved in the production and absorption of CSF (Chikly and Quaghebeur, 2013).

Thus, CSF is formed and absorbed everywhere in the CSF system rather than being formed in a particular portion of the brain (CP of ventricles) and being absorbed (arachnoid villi) in another with no unidirectional circulation as traditionally believed (Oresković et al., 2010; Orešković, 2015; Bering, 1952).

CSF Circulation

The traditional concept is that the CSF produced by the CP in the ventricles flows unidirectionally out of the ventricular system (lateral ventricles to the third ventricle and the fourth ventricle via aqueduct and out of the fourth ventricle via the foramen of Magendie and Lushka) into the craniospinal subarachnoid spaces, to be finally absorbed via the arachnoid villi into the cerebral venous sinuses.

Oreskovic and Klarica et al. challenged this concept. They inserted a cannula with a stopcock in the aqueduct of Sylvius of cats and monitored CSF flow but did not retrieve any CSF via the cannula even after 3 hours of aqueductal occlusion. Similar results (no outflow of CSF) were obtained in control cats without aqueduct occlusion. They noticed that CSF continuously pulsated, but no fluid was drained during these experiments (Oreskovic, Klarica, and Vukic, 2001). The CSF movement is influenced by blood vessel pulsation in a to and fro craniocaudal direction. The strongest pulsatile CSF movements are seen at the base of the brain, interhemispheric region, and cerebral gyri (Orešković, Radoš, and Klarica, 2017). So, during systole, blood flow into the brain causes its inward expansion, compressing the ventricles and outward expansion, causing compression of the cortical veins and subarachnoid spaces. The inward expansion of the brain leads to pulsatile outflow of CSF through the aqueduct and the ventricular system. The brain volume decreases during diastole, and the CSF flow reverses through the foramen magnum and the aqueduct (Shapey, Toma, and Saeed, 2019). A recent MRI study has found that more than cardiac pulsations, inspiration affected CSF flow by causing to and fro movement across the aqueduct and facilitating mixing in the ventricles (Dreha-Kulaczewski et al., 2015). In addition, CSF movements inside the spinal subarachnoid spaces are also influenced by gravity in different body positions (Yamada, 2014; Yamada and Kelly, 2016; Klarica et al., 2014).

The pial artery becomes an arteriole as it enters the brain parenchyma from the CSF-filled subarachnoid space. Virchow – Robin spaces are the perivascular fluid-filled spaces around the arterioles of the cerebral parenchyma, which are surrounded by a layer of pia, arteriolar basement membrane, and astrocytic foot process (Kulik et al., 2008; Zhou et al., 2021). Approximately 11% of CSF enters the perivascular Virchow- Robin spaces, facilitating the exchange of water and solutes between the CSF and ISF (Jessen et al., 2015).

A secondary CSF circulation pathway exists along these Virchow-Robin spaces, which resemble the lymphatics in other body parts. Since it involves the astroglia, it is called the "glymphatic system" (Shapey, Toma, and Saeed, 2019). The Virchow-Robin space's outer wall is formed by the glial membrane, consisting of continuous astrocytic end-feet. This glymphatic system is responsible for clearing wastes and solutes, and its impairment is believed to result in many pathologies, such as Alzheimer's disease in which the β-amyloid is removed insufficiently (Iliff et al., 2012).

CSF Reabsorption

In 1914, Weed demonstrated that the arachnoid villi and granulations are the major sites of CSF reabsorption, supporting the traditional hypothesis. Arachnoid villi are microscopic, while arachnoid granulations are visible to the naked eye (Weed, 1914). The recent theory suggests that a significant portion of CSF is reabsorbed via extra-arachnoidal pathways (Iliff et al., 2012; Johanson et al., 2008; Bradley, 2015). These pathways include lymphatics near the cribriform plate and the perineural sheath of cranial nerves, especially the optic, trigeminal, facial, and vestibulocochlear nerves. These accessory pathways are particularly active in neonates because arachnoid villi are not completely functional until 18 months of age. Similarly, in the elderly, the accessory pathways become more prominent because of fibrous changes in the arachnoid granulations (Sakka, Coll, and Chazal, 2011).

Aquaporins and Water Transport

Aquaporin (AQP) water channels play an essential role in water movement in the central nervous system. They aid in the bi-directional transport of water, solutes, and ions across the cell membrane. Water transport can happen via diffusion or AQP mediated; the diffusional transport is nonspecific and low capacity, whereas AQP mediated is rapid and has high capacity and remarkable selectivity (Brinker et al., 2014). At least 14 different types of aquaporins have been identified by reverse transcription-polymerase chain reaction (RT-PCR), and at least six have been found in the brain AQP 1,4,5 have specific water permeability, AQP 3 and 9 permeate water and solutes, and AQP8 facilitates ion transport (Zelenina, 2010). AQP4 is the most abundant form and is primarily located in the astrocyte processes and end-feet at critical interfaces between the brain and major water-containing compartments like the blood-brain barrier and blood-CSF barrier, signifying its importance in regulating brain fluid homeostasis (Bothwell, Janigro, and Patabendige, 2019; Speake, Freeman, and Brown, 2003; Rash et al., 1998). AQP4 is postulated to have a role in the pathogenesis and resolution of brain edema, clearing K+ ions released during neuronal activity, and is strongly upregulated in brain tumors and injured brain tissue (Chai et al., 2013). AQP 1 is expressed on membranes of the apical surface of choroid plexus epithelium, facilitating a CSF secretion. AQP 9 is believed to have a role in energy metabolism and removing excess lactate from the ischemic focus (Brinker et al., 2014; Nakada and Kwee, 2019).

Imaging of CSF Circulation

Phase-contrast MRI is a primary, non-invasive technique used to visualize moving fluid, providing qualitative and quantitative evaluation. CSF circulation happens because of two types of motions- a bulk flow and a pulsatile flow. The bulk flow is slow, discrete, dependent hydrostatic pressure gradient and cannot be measured by imaging. In contrast, pulsatile CSF flow is based on the Monroe-Kellie doctrine and can be visualized using PC-MRI. The mean CSF flow velocity is about 5-8cm/s (Korbecki et al., 2019).

The CSF shows bidirectional motion both at the foramen of Monro and the aqueduct during cardiac and respiratory movements. The CSF moves caudally during systole and in the cephalic direction during diastole; CSF moves superiorly into the ventricles in the inspiration phase, and the flow is reversed during the expiration (Matsumae et al., 2019).

Clinical Implications

Any increase in intracranial pressure (ICP) due to the disruption of CSF flow can be life-threatening and implicated in various neurological pathologies like hydrocephalus, intracranial hypertension, dementia, traumatic brain injury, brain tumors, stroke, etc... Still, surprisingly, the exact cellular mechanisms leading to these manifestations are either poorly understood or researched.

Idiopathic Normal Pressure Hydrocephalus (iNPH)

Idiopathic NPH is a surgically reversible most common neurodegenerative disorder characterized by gait apraxia, urinary incontinence, and cognitive decline. The exact pathogenesis is elusive, but alterations in CSF hydrodynamics have been postulated to be the initiating factor for iNPH. The CSF flow has both bulk and pulsatile components under normal physiological conditions. The bulk flow is maintained by continuous production of CSF and follows the traditional route of the lateral ventricle to the third ventricle and fourth ventricle via aqueduct. The pulsatile flow of CSF is driven by arterial pulsatility and intracranial blood inflow. Disturbances in CSF pulsatility have been implicated in the pathogenesis of iNPH (Wang et al., 2020). The CSF pulsatility is represented by Aqueduct stroke volume (ASV), defined as the mean CSF flow volume across the aqueduct during systole and diastole (Marmarou et al., 2005; Vivas-Buitrago et al., 2019). Bradley et al. found that iNPH patients with an aqueductal stroke volume above 42μL were benefited from ventriculoperitoneal shunt placement (Bradley et al., 1996). Reduced CSF drainage has also been implicated in the development of iNPH. Over 83% of iNPH patients had CSF outflow of 12mmHg/mL/min, compared to a healthy cohort where it never exceeded 10mmHg/mL/min, and it had a role in predicting shunt responsiveness (Kim et al., 2015; Boon et al., 1998). The glymphatic system mediated by Aquaporin 4 (AQP4) is involved in the clearance of excess fluid and waste metabolites from CNS, and it is impaired in patients with iNPH. The following mechanisms about iNPH were postulated after delayed clearance of intrathecal CSF tracer (gadobutrol) was noted in contrast-enhanced MRI. The CSF stagnates in the dilated perivascular spaces, which compress the penetrating arteries and reduce their pulsatility. The density of AQP4 is decreased in the astrocytic perivascular end-feet in patients with iNPH resulting in CSF accumulation (Reeves et al., 2020; Wang et al., 2020). Accumulation of toxic metabolites like β-amyloid and hyperphosphorylated tau linked to disturbances in glymphatic flow, leading to astrogliosis and neuroinflammation, causing the cognitive decline in iNPH (Kondziella et al., 2008; Eide and Ringstad, 2019; Angelucci et al., 2019; Chen et al., 2017). CSF diversion either by VP shunt or ETV attempts to reverse the CSF dynamics and provides therapeutic relief to patients with iNPH.

Subarachnoid Hemorrhage

Aneurysmal SAH is a catastrophic hemorrhagic cerebrovascular disease associated with significant morbidity. The RBCs can be seen in CSF as early as 30 mins post ictus. With the rupture of an aneurysm into the subarachnoid space, the ICP increases with a resultant decrease in cerebral perfusion pressure (Zhou et al., 2021).

SAH can alter the dynamics of CSF in the following ways: 1) The blood cells and related products can enter the ventricles and block the flow of CSF and similarly block the arachnoid villi (Goulay et al., 2017; Golanov et al., 2018; Ishi,i 1979). 2) Autopsy has revealed meningeal, especially arachnoidal thickening and haemosiderin deposition, which later leads to arachnoidal fibrosis, hindering communication between CSF and venous sinuses (Ishii, 1979; Zhou et al., 2021).

Post-Traumatic Hydrocephalus

The collection of CSF along the cerebral convexities, either uni or bilaterally, is called "external hydrocephalus". It happens in a subset of patients post decompressive craniectomy for traumatic brain injury. It does not fit into the classical definition of hydrocephalus characterized by the dilatation of cerebral ventricles and is possibly due to altered CSF hydrodynamics. The effects of brain pulsatility on CSF circulation can be studied using gated spin-echo MRI sequences. Akins and Guppy et al. proposed the following mechanisms causing abnormal CSF collections after decompressive craniectomy - 1) Cranial defect and durotomy lead to reduced inward expansion of the brain tissue, squeezing of ventricles and eventual reduction in the pulsatile flow of CSF, 2) Impaired CSF flow in the subarachnoid and perivascular Virchow-Robin spaces, 3) glymphatic system dysfunction causing decreased clearance of the interstitial fluid, and 4 CSF redistribution from the subarachnoid space into the ventricles, as well as subdural and subgaleal spaces (figure 1).

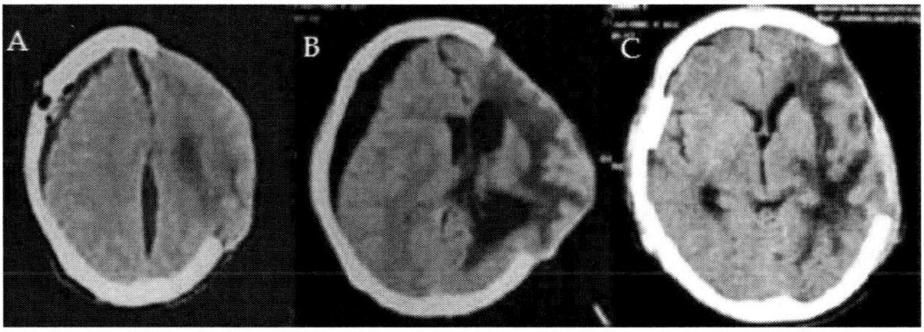

Figure 1. A) Post decompressive hemicraniectomy, subdural effusion persisting after burr-hole evacuation B) Increase in the subdural effusion and mass effect C) Post-subdural-peritoneal shunt, complete resolution of effusion suggestive of a defect in the absorption of CSF (Courtesy Dr. Swetha Pendyala, Neurosurgeon, Sunshine Hospitals, Karimnagar).

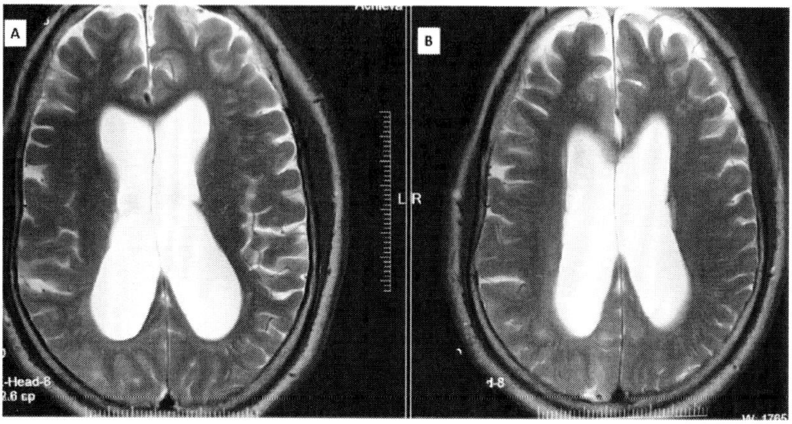

Figure 2. Axial T2W images showing ventriculomegaly with dilated sulcal spaces.

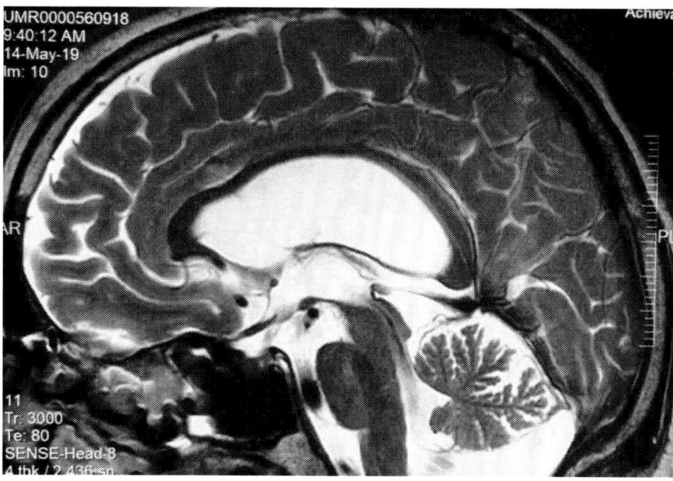

Figure 3. Flow void through the aqueduct suggestive of hyperdynamic circulation in iNPH.

In addition, they have observed improvement in the cerebral blood flow, CSF pulsatility, and hydrodynamics after cranioplasty, adequate to resolve the external hydrocephalus (Akins and Guppy, 2019). Scollato et al. confirmed the above hypothesis using phase-contrast cine MRI study that the aqueduct CSF stroke volume was unmeasurable in a patient who had undergone decompressive craniectomy for traumatic subdural hematoma; however, post cranioplasty aqueductal CSF flow was restored with systolic and diastolic fluxes of 211 μL and 190 μL per heartbeat, respectively (Scollato et al., 2015).

Idiopathic Intracranial Hypertension (IIH)

IIH is the most common cause of papilledema, typically affecting young obese females. It's a diagnosis of exclusion when other secondary causes of raised ICP have been ruled out, like intracranial space-occupying lesions, sinus thrombosis, infections of the CNS, and hydrocephalus. CSF hydrodynamics between the orbital and intracranial subarachnoid spaces are essential in the pathophysiology of disc edema. The translaminar cribrosa pressure difference (TLPD), defined as the difference between the intraocular pressure (IOP) and ICP, has been implicated in the pathogenesis of papilledema, and it can explain the presence of disc edema in patients with normal ICP (Liu et al., 2020). The orbital subarachnoid space is a complex structure with fine arachnoidal trabecular and septa, and it receives bulk CSF flow from the chiasmatic cistern. The presence of arachnoid trabeculae suggests that CSF cannot exchange freely between the intracranial and the orbital subarachnoid compartments. In the retrobulbar region, peri-optic subarachnoid space (SAS) has a typical 'cul-de-sac' configuration, preventing CSF flow reversal from the orbital SAS back into the intracranial SAS. This unique anatomy of peri-optic subarachnoid space is presumed to be responsible for the development of disc edema(Battal et al., 2011). One of the probable factors for visual loss in papilledema is reduced local CSF turnover leading to toxic changes in the microenvironment of the optic nerve (Jaggi et al., 2010; Whedon and Glassey, 2009).

Conclusion

Recent research suggests that a CSF is formed by the water filtration across the capillary walls throughout the CNS rather than just in the ventricular system (choroid plexus). The CSF and ISF constitute a functional unit, and their volumes are regulated by the osmotic and hydrostatic pressure gradients across the capillary walls. Impairment of glymphatic system, AQP channels results alters normal CSF dynamics, resulting in accumulation of CSF and metabolites as seen in several neurological conditions.

References

Akins Paul T and Guppy Kern H. 2019. "Are Hygromas and Hydrocephalus after Decompressive Craniectomy Caused by Impaired Brain Pulsatility, Cerebrospinal Fluid Hydrodynamics, and Glymphatic Drainage? Literature Overview and Illustrative Cases". *World Neurosurgery,* 130 (October). United States: e941-52. doi:10.1016/j.wneu.2019.07.041.

Angelucci Francesco, Čechová Kateřina, Průša Richard and Hort Jakub. 2019. "Amyloid Beta Soluble Forms and Plasminogen Activation System in Alzheimer's Disease: Consequences on Extracellular Maturation of Brain-Derived Neurotrophic Factor and Therapeutic Implications". *CNS Neuroscience & Therapeutics,* 25 (3): 303-13. doi:10.1111/cns.13082.

Battal B, Kocaoglu M, Bulakbasi N, Husmen G, Tuba Sanal H and Tayfun C. 2011. "Cerebrospinal Fluid Flow Imaging by Using Phase-Contrast MR Technique". *The British Journal of Radiology,* 84 (1004): 758-65. doi:10.1259/bjr/66206791.

Bering EA. 1952. "Water Exchange of Central Nervous System and Cerebrospinal Fluid". *Journal of Neurosurgery,* 9 (3). United States: 275-87. doi:10.3171/ jns.1952.9.3. 0275.

Boon AJ, Tans JT, Delwel EJ, Egeler-Peerdeman SM, Hanlo PW, Wurzer HA, Avezaat CJ, de Jong DA, Gooskens RH and Hermans J. 1998. "Dutch Normal-Pressure Hydrocephalus Study: Randomized Comparison of Low- and Medium-Pressure Shunts". *Journal of Neurosurgery,* 88 (3). United States: 490-95. doi:10.3171/ jns.1998.88.3.0490.

Bothwell Steven William, Janigro Damir and Patabendige Adjanie. 2019. "Cerebrospinal Fluid Dynamics and Intracranial Pressure Elevation in Neurological Diseases". *Fluids and Barriers of the CNS,* 16 (1). BioMed Central: 1-18. doi:10.1186/s12987-019-0129-6.

Bradley WG Jr. 2015. "CSF Flow in the Brain in the Context of Normal Pressure Hydrocephalus". *AJNR. American Journal of Neuroradiology,* 36 (5). United States: 831-38. doi:10.3174/ajnr.A4124.

Bradley WG Jr, Scalzo D, Queralt J, Nitz WN, Atkinson DJ and Wong P. 1996. "Normal-Pressure Hydrocephalus: Evaluation with Cerebrospinal Fluid Flow Measurements at MR Imaging". *Radiology,* 198 (2). United States: 523-29. doi:10.1148/radiology. 198.2.8596861.

Brinker Thomas, Stopa Edward, Morrison John and KlingePetra. 2014. "A New Look at Cerebrospinal Fluid Circulation". *Fluids and Barriers of the CNS,* 11 (1): 1-16. doi:10.1186/2045-8118-11-10.

Bulat Marin and Klarica Marijan. 2011. "Recent Insights into a New Hydrodynamics of the Cerebrospinal Fluid". *Brain Research Reviews,* 65 (2). Netherlands: 99-112. doi:10. 1016/j.brainresrev.2010.08.002.

Chai Rui Chao, Jiao Hua Jiang, Ann Yuen Kwan Wong, Feng Jiang, Kai Gao, Vatcher Greg and Cheung Hoi Yu Albert. 2013. "AQP5 Is Differentially Regulated in Astrocytes during Metabolic and Traumatic Injuries". *Glia,* 61 (10). United States: 1748-65. doi:10.1002/glia.22555.

Chen Zhongyun, Chunyan Liu, Jie Zhang, Norman Relkin, Yan Xing and Yanfeng Li. 2017. "Cerebrospinal Fluid Aβ42, t-Tau, and p-Tau Levels in the Differential Diagnosis of Idiopathic Normal-Pressure Hydrocephalus: A Systematic Review and Meta-Analysis". *Fluids and Barriers of the CNS,* 14 (1): 13. doi:10.1186/ s12987-017-0062-5.

Chikly Bruno, and Quaghebeur Jörgen. 2013. "Reassessing Cerebrospinal Fluid (CSF) Hydrodynamics: A Literature Review Presenting a Novel Hypothesis for CSF Physiology". *Journal of Bodywork and Movement Therapies,* 17 (3): 344-54. doi:10.1016/j.jbmt.2013.02.002.

Cushing Harvey. 1925. "Cameron Lectures". *The Lancet,* 206 (5332): 956-62. doi:https://doi.org/10.1016/S0140-6736(01)69060-3.

Davson, H. 1966. "Formation and Drainage of the Cerebrospinal Fluid". *The Scientific Basis of Medicine Annual Reviews*. England, 238-59.

Day Rebecca E, Kitchen Philip, Owen David S, Bland Charlotte, Marshall Lindsay, Conner Alex C, Bill Roslyn M and Conner Matthew T. 2014. "Human Aquaporins: Regulators of Transcellular Water Flow". *Biochimica et Biophysica Acta (BBA) - General Subjects,* 1840 (5): 1492-1506. doi:https://doi.org/ 10.1016/j.bbagen.2013.09.033.

Dreha-Kulaczewski Steffi, Joseph Arun A, Merboldt Klaus-Dietmar, Ludwig Hans-Christoph, Gärtner Jutta and Frahm Jens. 2015. "Inspiration Is the Major Regulator of Human CSF Flow". *Journal of Neuroscience,* 35 (6). Society for Neuroscience: 2485-91. doi:10.1523/JNEUROSCI.3246-14.2015.

Eide Per K and Ringstad Geir. 2019. "Delayed Clearance of Cerebrospinal Fluid Tracer from Entorhinal Cortex in Idiopathic Normal Pressure Hydrocephalus: A Glymphatic Magnetic Resonance Imaging Study". *Journal of Cerebral Blood Flow and Metabolism : Official Journal of the International Society of Cerebral Blood Flow and Metabolism,* 39 (7): 1355-68. doi:10.1177/0271678X18760974.

Golanov Eugene V, Bovshik Evgeniy I, Wong Kelvin K, Pautler Robia G, Foster Chase H, Federley Richard G, Zhang Jonathan Y, Mancuso James, Tc Wong Stephen and Britz Gavin W. 2018. "Subarachnoid Hemorrhage - Induced Block of Cerebrospinal Fluid Flow: Role of Brain Coagulation Factor III (Tissue Factor)". *Journal of Cerebral Blood Flow and Metabolism : Official Journal of the International Society of Cerebral Blood Flow and Metabolism,* 38 (5): 793-808. doi:10.1177/0271678x17701157.

Goulay Romain, Flament Julien, Gauberti Maxime, Naveau Michael, Pasquet Nolwenn, Gakuba Clement, Emery Evelyne et al. 2017. "Subarachnoid Hemorrhage Severely Impairs Brain Parenchymal Cerebrospinal Fluid Circulation in Nonhuman Primate". *Stroke,* 48 (8). United States: 2301-5. doi:10.1161/STROKEAHA.117.017014.

Hayaishi O. 2000. "Molecular Mechanisms of Sleep-Wake Regulation: A Role of Prostaglandin D2". *Philosophical Transactions of the Royal Society of London. Series B, Biological Sciences,* 355 (1394): 275-80. doi:10.1098/rstb.2000.0564.

Igarashi Hironaka, Tsujita Mika, Kwee Ingrid L and Nakada Tsutomu. 2014. "Water Influx into Cerebrospinal Fluid Is Primarily Controlled by Aquaporin-4, Not by Aquaporin-1: 17O JJVCPE MRI Study in Knockout Mice". *Neuroreport,* 25 (1): 39-43. doi:10.1097/WNR.0000000000000042.

Iliff Jeffrey J, Minghuan Wang, Yonghong Liao, Plogg Benjamin A, Weiguo Peng, Gundersen Georg A, Benveniste Helene et al. 2012. "A Paravascular Pathway

Facilitates CSF Flow through the Brain Parenchyma and the Clearance of Interstitial Solutes, Including Amyloid β". *Science Translational Medicine,* 4 (147): 147ra111. doi:10.1126/scitranslmed.3003748.

Ishii M. 1979. "[Subarachnoid hemorrhage and circulatory disturbance of cerebrospinal fluid--scanning electron microscopic study in clinical and autopsy cases (author's transl)]". No shinkei geka. *Neurological surgery,* 7 (6). Japan: 579-88.

Jaggi Gregor P, Harlev Mickey, Ziegler Urs, Dotan Shlomo, Miller Neil R and Killer Hanspeter E. 2010. "Cerebrospinal Fluid Segregation Optic Neuropathy: An Experimental Model and a Hypothesis". *The British Journal of Ophthalmology,* 94 (8). England: 1088-93. doi:10.1136/bjo.2009.171660.

Jessen Nadia Aalling, Finmann Munk Anne Sofie, Lundgaard Iben and Nedergaard Maiken. 2015. "The Glymphatic System: A Beginner's Guide". *Neurochemical Research,* 40 (12): 2583-99. doi:10.1007/s11064-015-1581-6.

Johanson Conrad E, Duncan John A 3rd, Klinge Petra M, Brinker Thomas, Stopa Edward G and Silverberg Gerald D. 2008. "Multiplicity of Cerebrospinal Fluid Functions: New Challenges in Health and Disease". *Cerebrospinal Fluid Research,* 5 (May): 10. doi:10.1186/1743-8454-5-10.

Khasawneh Ahmad H, Garling Richard J and Harris Carolyn A. 2018. *"Cerebrospinal Fluid Circulation: What Do We Know and How Do We Know It?"* doi:10.4103/bc.bc_3_18.

Kim Dong-Joo, Hakseung Kim, Young-Tak Kim, Byung C Yoon, Czosnyka Zofia, Kun-Woo Park and Czosnyka Marek. 2015. "Thresholds of Resistance to CSF Outflow in Predicting Shunt Responsiveness". *Neurological Research,* 37 (4). England: 332-40. doi:10.1179/1743132814Y.0000000454.

Klarica Marijan, Radoš Milan, Erceg Gorislav, Petošić Antonio, Jurjević Ivana, and Orešković Darko. 2014. "The Influence of Body Position on Cerebrospinal Fluid Pressure Gradient and Movement in Cats with Normal and Impaired Craniospinal Communication". *PloS One,* 9 (4): e95229. doi:10.1371/journal.pone.0095229.

Kondziella Daniel, Sonnewald Ursula, Tullberg Mats and Wikkelso Carsten. 2008. "Brain Metabolism in Adult Chronic Hydrocephalus". *Journal of Neurochemistry,* 106 (4). England: 1515-24. doi:10.1111/j.1471-4159.2008.05422.x.

Korbecki Adrian, Zimny Anna, Podgórski Przemysław, Sąsiadek Marek and Bladowska Joanna. 2019. "Imaging of Cerebrospinal Fluid Flow: Fundamentals, Techniques, and Clinical Applications of Phase-Contrast Magnetic Resonance Imaging". *Polish Journal of Radiology,* 84: 240-50. doi:10.5114/pjr.2019.86881.

Kulik Tobias, Kusano Yoshikazu, Aronhime Shimon, Sandler Adam L and Winn H Richard. 2008. "Regulation of Cerebral Vasculature in Normal and Ischemic Brain". *Neuropharmacology,* 55 (3): 281-88. doi:10.1016/ j.neuropharm.2008.04.017.

Liu Katy C, Fleischman David, Lee Andrew G, Killer Hanspeter E, Chen John J and Tariq Bhatti M. 2020. "Current Concepts of Cerebrospinal Fluid Dynamics and the Translaminar Cribrosa Pressure Gradient: A Paradigm of Optic Disk Disease". *Survey of Ophthalmology,* 65 (1). United States: 48-66. doi:10.1016/ j.survophthal.2019.08.005.

MacAulay N and Zeuthen T. 2010. "Water Transport between CNS Compartments: Contributions of Aquaporins and Cotransporters". *Neuroscience,* 168 (4). United States: 941-56. doi:10.1016/j.neuroscience.2009.09.016.

Marmarou Anthony, Bergsneider Marvin, Klinge Petra, Relkin Norman and McL Black Peter. 2005. "The Value of Supplemental Prognostic Tests for the Preoperative Assessment of Idiopathic Normal-Pressure Hydrocephalus". *Neurosurgery,* 57 (3 Suppl). United States: S17-28; discussion ii-v. doi:10.1227/01.neu.0000168184.01002.60.

Matsumae Mitsunori, Kagayaki Kuroda, Satoshi Yatsushiro, Akihiro Hirayama, Naokazu Hayashi, Ken Takizawa, Hideki Atsumi and Takatoshi Sorimachi. 2019. "Changing the Currently Held Concept of Cerebrospinal Fluid Dynamics Based on Shared Findings of Cerebrospinal Fluid Motion in the Cranial Cavity Using Various Types of Magnetic Resonance Imaging Techniques". *Neurologia Medico-Chirurgica,* 59 (4): 133-46. doi:10.2176/nmc.ra.2018-0272.

Milhorat TH. 1976. "Structure and Function of the Choroid Plexus and Other Sites of Cerebrospinal Fluid Formation". *International Review of Cytology,* 47. United States: 225-88. doi:10.1016/s0074-7696(08)60090-x.

Nakada Tsutomu and Kwee Ingrid L. 2019. "Fluid Dynamics Inside the Brain Barrier: Current Concept of Interstitial Flow, Glymphatic Flow, and Cerebrospinal Fluid Circulation in the Brain". *Neuroscientist,* 25 (2): 155-66. doi:10.1177/ 1073858 418775027.

Orešković D and Klarica M. 2010. "The Formation of Cerebrospinal Fluid: Nearly a Hundred Years of Interpretations and Misinterpretations". *Brain Research Reviews,* 64 (2). Netherlands: 241-62. doi:10.1016/j.brainresrev.2010.04.006.

Oreskovic D, Klarica M and Vukic M. 2001. "Does the Secretion and Circulation of the Cerebrospinal Fluid Really Exist?" *Medical Hypotheses,* 56 (5). United States: 622-24. doi:10.1054/mehy.2000.1178.

Orešković Darko. 2015. "The Controversy on Choroid Plexus Function in Cerebrospinal Fluid Production in Humans: How Long Different Views Could Be Neglected?" *Croatian Medical Journal,* 56 (3): 306-10. doi:10.3325/ cmj.2015.56.306.

Orešković Darko, Radoš Milan and Klarica Marijan. 2017. "New Concepts of Cerebrospinal Fluid Physiology and Development of Hydrocephalus". *Pediatric Neurosurgery,* 52 (6): 417-25. doi:10.1159/000452169.

Rash JE, Yasumura T, Hudson CS, Agre P and Nielsen S. 1998. "Direct Immunogold Labeling of Aquaporin-4 in Square Arrays of Astrocyte and Ependymocyte Plasma Membranes in Rat Brain and Spinal Cord". *Proceedings of the National Academy of Sciences of the United States of America,* 95 (20): 11981-86. doi:10.1073/pnas.95.20.11981.

Reeves Benjamin C, Karimy Jason K, Kundishora Adam J, Mestre Humberto, Cerci H Mert, Matouk Charles, Alper Seth L, Lundgaard Iben, Nedergaard Maiken and Kahle Kristopher T. 2020. "Glymphatic System Impairment in Alzheimer's Disease and Idiopathic Normal Pressure Hydrocephalus". *Trends in Molecular Medicine,* 26 (3): 285-95. doi:10.1016/j.molmed.2019.11.008.

Sakka L, Coll G and Chazal J. 2011. "Anatomy and Physiology of Cerebrospinal Fluid". *European Annals of Otorhinolaryngology, Head and Neck Diseases,* 128 (6). France: 309-16. doi:10.1016/j.anorl.2011.03.002.

Scollato Antonio, Gallina Pasquale, Bahl Gautam and Di Lorenzo Nicola. 2015. "Decompressive Craniectomy Arrests Pulsatile Aqueductal CSF Flux: An in Vivo Demonstration Using Phase-Contrast MRI. Case Report". *British Journal of Neurosurgery,* 29 (3). England: 440-42. doi:10.3109/02688697.2014.997671.

Shapey Jonathan, Toma A and Saeed SR. 2019. "Physiology of Cerebrospinal Fluid Circulation". *Current Opinion in Otolaryngology and Head and Neck Surgery,* 27 (5): 326-33. doi:10.1097/MOO.0000000000000576.

Speake Tracey, Freeman Lyle J and Brown Peter D. 2003. "Expression of Aquaporin 1 and Aquaporin 4 Water Channels in Rat Choroid Plexus". *Biochimica et Biophysica Acta,* 1609 (1). Netherlands: 80-86. doi:10.1016/s0005-2736(02)00658-2.

Tamburrini Gianpiero, Caldarelli Massimo, Di Rocco Federico, Massimi Luca, D'Angelo Luca, Fasano Teresa and Di Rocco Concezio. 2006. "The Role of Endoscopic Choroid Plexus Coagulation in the Surgical Management of Bilateral Choroid Plexuses Hyperplasia". *Child's Nervous System : ChNS : Official Journal of the International Society for Pediatric Neurosurgery,* 22 (6). Germany: 605-8. doi:10.1007/s00381-006-0070-2.

Tumani Hayrettin, Huss André and Bachhuber Franziska. 2017. "The Cerebrospinal Fluid and Barriers – Anatomic and Physiologic Considerations". *Handbook of Clinical Neurology,* 146: 3-20. doi:10.1016/B978-0-12-804279-3.00002-2.

Vivas-Buitrago Tito, Lokossou Armelle, Jusué-Torres Ignacio, Pinilla-Monsalve Gabriel, Blitz Ari M, Herzka Daniel A, Robison Jamie et al. 2019. "Aqueductal Cerebrospinal Fluid Stroke Volume Flow in a Rodent Model of Chronic Communicating Hydrocephalus: Establishing a Homogeneous Study Population for Cerebrospinal Fluid Dynamics Exploration". *World Neurosurgery,* 128: e1118-25. doi:https://doi.org/10.1016/j.wneu.2019.05.093.

Wang Zhangyang, Yiying Zhang, Fan Hu, Jing Ding and Xin Wang. 2020. "Pathogenesis and Pathophysiology of Idiopathic Normal Pressure Hydrocephalus". *CNS Neuroscience & Therapeutics,* 26 (12): 1230-40. doi:10.1111/cns.13526.

Weed LH. 1914. "Studies on Cerebro-Spinal Fluid. No. IV : The Dual Source of Cerebro-Spinal Fluid". *The Journal of Medical Research,* 31 (1): 93-118.11.

Whedon James M and Glassey Donald. 2009. "Cerebrospinal Fluid Stasis and Its Clinical Significance". *Alternative Therapies in Health and Medicine,* 15 (3): 54-60.

Yamada Shinya. 2014. "Cerebrospinal Fluid Physiology: Visualization of Cerebrospinal Fluid Dynamics Using the Magnetic Resonance Imaging Time-Spatial Inversion Pulse Method". *Croatian Medical Journal,* 55 (4): 337-46. doi:10.3325/cmj.2014.55.337.

Yamada Shinya and Kelly Erin. 2016. "Cerebrospinal Fluid Dynamics and the Pathophysiology of Hydrocephalus: New Concepts". *Seminars in Ultrasound, CT, and MR,* 37 (2). United States: 84-91. doi:10.1053/j.sult.2016.01.001.

Zelenina Marina. 2010. "Regulation of Brain Aquaporins". *Neurochemistry International,* 57 (4). England: 468-88. doi:10.1016/j.neuint.2010.03.022.

Zhou Jiru, Peiwen Guo, Zongduo Guo, Xiaochuan Sun, Yujie Chen and Hua Feng. 2021. "Fluid Metabolic Pathways after Subarachnoid Hemorrhage". *Journal of Neurochemistry*, June. England. doi:10.1111/jnc.15458.

Chapter 2

Blood-Brain Barrier and Cerebral Edema

Laura Marcela Acevedo-Aguilar,
Laura Marcela Mass-Hernandez
and Ivan David Lozada-Martínez*

School of Medicine, Universidad de Cartagena, Cartagena, Colombia and
Colombian Clinical Research Group in Neurocritical Care,
Latin American Council of Neurocritical Care, Cartagena, Colombia

Abstract

Adequate brain fluid regulation requires that the barriers between the different brain compartments maintain adequate integrity. In this chapter, we will specifically study the blood-brain barrier (BBB), which, among other functions, is responsible for preventing neurotoxic plasma components, blood cells and pathogens from entering the brain in order to maintain central nervous system (CNS) homeostasis. However, this barrier is susceptible to disruption, resulting in the formation of permeability pores that allow extravasation of water and plasma proteins to develop in the interstitial compartment of the brain, favoring the formation of vasogenic cerebral edema. On the other hand, we will point out the usefulness of clinical and imaging tools, such as cranial tomography (CT) and magnetic resonance imaging (MRI), in the diagnosis of cerebral edema. We will also discuss the appropriate and timely therapeutic management of this condition, where a systemic approach from general measures to specific therapeutic interventions is required to achieve a satisfactory result.

---

* Corresponding Author's Email: ilozadam@unicartagena.edu.co.

In: Advances in Neurosurgery Research
Editors: Amit Agrawal, Pradeep Chouksey, Adesh Shrivastava et al.
ISBN: 978-1-68507-859-1

Introduction

The BBB is a highly complex structure and important in maintaining normal CNS function (Kadry et al., 2020). It consists of a network of endothelial cells and perivascular cells that are responsible for maintaining its various functions (Stamatovic et al., 2016). This structure is responsible for preventing the indiscriminate passage of substances from the blood circulation to the CNS, regulating brain homeostasis and conferring protection to the brain (Obermeier et al., 2013). However, in the face of CNS injury, this structure may suffer alterations in its structural integrity and changes in its permeability due to a cascade of mechanical and molecular situations that are generated in this context (Sorby-Adams et al., 2017). This disruption of the BBB is going to allow the development of important pathological conditions such as the formation of vasogenic edema, which corresponds to the abnormal accumulation of fluid and plasma proteins in the interstitial compartment of the brain and represents a clinical condition of great importance (Michinaga and Koyama 2015). In this chapter, the structure of the BBB will be pointed out in order to obtain a better knowledge about it and, in the same way, the different mechanisms by which alterations in its integrity can occur will be discussed. Thus, the understanding of how vasogenic edema occurs in this clinical context will be facilitated and the basis and importance of diagnosis and timely treatment of this pathological condition will be detailed.

Blood-Brain Barrier

The BBB corresponds to a vascular structure with multiple cells in charge of isolating the CNS from the peripheral blood circulation (Obermeier et al., 2013; Xu et al., 2018) This complex structure protects the brain parenchyma from neurotoxic compounds, drugs and other exogenous elements through multiple membrane transporters, ATP-dependent transporters also known as ABC transporters (Kadry et al., 2020) and by forming interendothelial junctions that limit the free passage of compounds between two neighboring cells (Wilhelm et al., 2011). Likewise, it controls the input of nutrients and output of molecules from the CNS for the maintenance of an optimal neuronal milieu and subsequent brain tissue homeostasis (Erdő et al., 2017).

Neurovascular Unit

The main element of the BBB is the microvascular endothelial cells with their tight junctions, but the interaction of these with other elements such as, pericytes, astrocytes, astrocytes, microglia, neurons, immune cells and a basement membrane (Abdullahi et al., 2018) are key to the development of the BBB during the embryonic stage and to the maintenance of its integrity over time (Keaney and Campbell 2015). These components together form the anatomical and functional unit of the BBB, the so-called neurovascular unit (NVU), which manifests the relationship between the components of the BBB and the brain parenchymal cells (Stokum et al., 2016).

Endothelial Cells: First Line of Defense

The main barrier to NVU are the endothelial cells lining the walls of brain capillaries; these cells possess particular characteristics that distinguish them from endothelial cells of other tissues, such as the presence of a large number of mitochondria (Costea et al., 2019; Kadry et al., 2020), the lack of fenestrations, and the expression of reduced amounts of leukocyte adhesion molecules to limit the entry of immune cells into the brain (Ayloo and Gu 2019; Zhao et al., 2015). However, its fundamental characteristic is its limited permeability as a result of the formation of specialized tight and adherent junctions that reduce the levels of paracellular transport, thus selectively restricting molecular exchange in the BBB (Baeten and Akassoglou 2011; Castro-Dias et al., 2019).

Tight Junctions

Tight junctions are the structures primarily responsible for the impermeable paracellular barrier properties of brain endothelial cells and for the integrity of the barrier as such, as they limit the free passage of water and solutes by sealing the spaces in the apical region between endothelial cells (Liebner et al., 2018). This restriction is possible due to the integral transmembrane proteins that make up the tight junctions, these being occludin, claudin family proteins, and junctional adhesion molecules (JAMs) (Komarova et al., 2017). These proteins are bound to the cytoskeleton by cytoplasmic anchoring proteins, ZO-1, ZO-2 and ZO-3 (Sweeney et al., 2019), which are part of the

MAGUK (membrane-associated guanylate kinase) family of proteins, composed of one or multiple PDZ domains, an SH3 domain and a GUK domain (Beutel et al., 2019). These anchor proteins play a key role in the development of tight junctions and in maintaining the paracellular permeability of the barrier due to the interactions of their domains with the C-terminal end of claudins, occludins and JAMs (Bauer et al., 2014).

Thus, claudins are the most important components of the tight junction as they participate both in its formation and in the maintenance of the selective permeability of the BBB, with claudin-5 being the most predominant in it (Sorby-Adams et al., 2017). The structure of this protein family consists of four transmembrane domains, a short N-terminal end, two extracellular loops, a short intracellular loop and a long C-terminal end containing the PDZ binding motif, indispensable for interaction with cytosolic anchor proteins (Greene 2019). The first extracellular loop, ECL1, regulates paracellular movement of ions, while the second, ECL2, controls protein folding and maintains tightness of the junction (Stamatovic et al., 2016).

The occludins are integral membrane proteins with four transmembrane domains, two extracellular loops and three cytoplasmic domains: an N-terminal domain, a long C-terminal domain and a short intracellular loop (Lochhead et al., 2020). The C-terminal end interacts directly with ZO-1 and has binding sites for regulatory molecules such as kinases or connexin 26, and together with extracellular loops control paracellular permeability by assembly of occludin into dimers and oligomers (Abdullahi et al., 2018; Yuan et al., 2020).

And finally, the entry of leukocytes into the BBB will be limited due to the action of JAMs, which are integral membrane proteins that are part of the immunoglobulin superfamily (Greene at al 2016) composed of a transmembrane domain and two extracellular domains, one of them with a C-terminal end containing a PDZ binding motif that allows its connection with cytoplasmic proteins, linking the JAMs to the cytoskeleton (Castro-Dias et al., 2019).

Adherent Joints

Adherens junctions (AJs) are composed of integral calcium-dependent membrane proteins, called cadherins; these proteins interact indirectly with the actin cytoskeleton by binding to cytoplasmic proteins, called catenins, mostly alpha- and beta-catenins (Hatte et al., 2018; Keep et al., 2018).

The initiation and maintenance of cell-cell adhesion at the BBB, as well as the regulation of signaling processes and gene transcription, is carried out by adherens junctions (Garcia et al., 2018). Likewise, these junctions play an important role in the formation and support of tight junctions, since the disruption of these junctions in the absence of beta-catenin has been demonstrated in cerebral endothelial cells (Komarova et al., 2017).

GAP Joints

A third category of junctions found in the cerebral microvasculature are the so-called GAP junctions (GJs), which correspond to two hemichannels located on opposite cell membranes made up of six transmembrane proteins called connexins (Cxs), where Cx30 and Cx43 are the ones mainly expressed by astrocytes (Zhao et al., 2018). Gjs allow the passage of ions and small molecules and signal transduction between neighboring cells, favoring intercellular communication (Stamatovic et al., 2016). On the other hand, they can also work as specialized communication channels in glia and especially in astrocytes (Sun et al., 2012).

Astrocytes and Pericytes: Second Line of Defense

Astrocytes correspond to the most numerous cells in the CNS and is the most important glial cell type with multiple prolongations deriving from the cell body (Yamazaki and Kanekiyo 2017). The terminal feet of these prolongations establish a link between the vascular and neuroglial compartment in the NVU and interact with cerebral endothelial cells, maintaining not only the barrier function of the NVU microvasculature, but also allowing the regulation of cerebral blood flow in response to neural signals (Kadry et al., 2020). On the other hand, these endfeet also express aquaporins (AQPs), water channel proteins that have the function of transporting fluids across membranes in order to maintain an adequate water balance between the vascular and extracellular space, with AQP-4 being the most important isoform in the CNS (Michinaga and Koyama 2015).

In addition, astrocytes maintain the homeostasis of the neuronal microenvironment, as they control synaptic transmissions and immune reactions by regulating ion and neurotransmitter concentrations, which manifests their protective role on neurons (Keaney and Campbell 2015). In addition, it has been recognized that neurotrophic factors such as GDNF and growth factors such as TGF-B and BFGF are secreted by astrocytes, which supports their involvement in the induction and regulation of the BBB phenotype (Erdő et al., 2017).

On the other hand, the other fundamental cellular component of the BBB corresponds to pericytes (PCs) (Sorby-Adams et al., 2017), contractile cells embedded in the basement membrane that line 22-32% of capillary walls (Bagchi et al., 2019; Hall et al., 2014). In addition, the cytoplasm of PCs projects multiple cytoplasmic processes (Harrel et al., 2018), which contain actin, myosin and tropomyosin microfilaments, demonstrating the contractility capacity of these cells (Yang et al., 2017). Likewise, they interact with endothelial cells through holes in their shared basement membrane (Armulik et al., 2011) by means of 3 types of intercellular junctions: GAP junctions (connexin-43/30), adhesion plates similar to adherens junctions formed by integrins and peg-socket junctions, in which the cytoplasmic extensions of pericytes are inserted into the endothelial invaginations (Zhang et al., 2020). This interaction allows the achievement of the diverse functions of pericytes, as well as the control of BBB permeability, angiogenesis, regulation of cerebral blood flow, clearance of toxic metabolites, inflammatory processes, among other keys for the maintenance of cerebral homeostasis (Wilhelm et al., 2011; Winkler et al., 2011).

Basal Membrane

The basal membrane is a reticular structure that provides support to both endothelial and epithelial cells and is composed of extracellular matrix proteins, mainly type IV collagen, laminin, nidogen and perlecan (Thomsen et al., 2017). These proteins are involved in maintaining the integrity of tight junctions by participating in the expression of tight junction proteins (Erdő et al., 2017).

Type IV collagen is the predominant component of the extracellular matrix. These proteins consist of polypeptide chains that are organized into triple helices called protomers, which stabilize the basal membrane through interactions with other matrix proteins (Reed et al., 2019). On the other hand, laminins correspond to glycoproteins formed by a mixture of alpha beta and gamma chains, which are essential for the assembly of the basal membrane and the regulation of leukocyte infiltration; their absence is associated with disruptions in the BBB (Baeten and Akassoglou 2011).

Anatomically, two types of basal membrane are found in the CNS, the endothelial basal membrane, secreted by pericytes and endothelial cells, and the parenchymal basal membrane, secreted by astrocytes (Castro-Dias et al., 2019). These membranes are separated by pericytes, however, they share physiological roles such as providing cell anchoring, structural basis and signal transduction (Xu et al., 2018).

In addition, extracellular matrix proteins act as ligands and interact with two types of receptors: the dystroglycan and the integrin receptor (Obermeier et al., 2013). The latter activate growth factors and extracellular matrix ligands, favoring endothelial functions such as differentiation, migration, polarity and adhesion, so that integrin malfunction will be associated with BBB failures, including immaturity, Claudin-5 scarcity and deficient VE-cadherin signaling (Liebner et al., 2018; Sweeney et al., 2019).

Microglia

Microglia play a fundamental role in CNS immune responses because they are activated by brain injury and immunological stimuli. On the one hand, they can release proinflammatory cytokines such as IL-1β and TNF-α, which affect the integrity of tight junctions and adherens junctions, increasing the permeability of the BBB, while on the other hand, they participate in the release of vascular growth factor, phagocytosis of damaged neurons and activation of neurotrophic pathways in order to restore tissue damage (Keaney and Campbell 2015).

Transport System in the BBB

There are several mechanisms for the control of molecules and compounds that pass through the BBB:

- Passive diffusion: More than 98% of small molecules fail to cross the BBB, however, some low molecular weight fat-soluble molecules manage to cross it and enter the brain through the temporary formation of pores in the phospholipid bilayer (Kadry et al., 2020).
- Efflux pumps: ABC, or ATP-dependent, transporters function as efflux pumps from the endothelium into the blood limiting the entry

of xenobiotics, drugs, and other toxic compounds (Sweeney et al., 2019).

- Carrier-mediated transport (CMT): Genes of membrane transporter proteins called Solute Carrier (SLC) express CMT systems, which allow the entry of a large number of molecules into the BBB, such as amino acids, carbohydrates, hormones, fatty acids, vitamins, nucleotides, among others (Zhao et al., 2015).
- Transcytosis: Some types of molecules are transported into the CNS in vesicles, this type of transcellular transport is known as transcytosis, which can be receptor-mediated, where the ligand binds to receptors that allow its endocytosis, or absorption, where the charge of the molecules allows their interaction with binding sites on the plasma membrane, favoring their endocytosis, as is the case of albumin (Ayloo and Gu 2019).

Vasogenic Edema Due to Alteration of the Blood-Brain Barrier

The integrity of the BBB can be affected in the context of CNS injury due to different causes (trauma, inflammation, infection, tumors, ischemia, among others) (Dalby 2020). This lesion produces several molecular alterations in the NVU that lead to the creation of pores at the endothelial level, causing an increase in the permeability of the BBB with its consequent rupture (Stokum et al., 2016). One of the different mechanisms contributing to this is the increased expression of vascular endothelial growth factor (VEGF) (Halstead and Geocadin 2019), which is a glycoprotein capable of increasing microvascular permeability through decreased expression of tight junction proteins and uncoupling of tight junction proteins (Jha et al., 2019; Stokum et al., 2016). Likewise, increased matrix metalloproteinase (MMP) activity also plays an important role in this disruption by playing a significant role in extracellular matrix degradation and in inducing inflammatory cell recruitment and migration, thus disrupting endothelial integrity and leading to increased barrier permeability (Michinaga and Koyama 2015; Sorby-Adams et al., 2017). Similarly, the increased release of substance P during neurogenic inflammation also contributes to this process through its ability to intensify the infiltration of inflammatory cells to the site of brain injury and at the same time through its ability to aggravate the local neuroinflammatory response through the manufacture of proinflammatory cytokines (Sorby-Adams et al., 2017). These cytokines stimulate barrier disruption by different modalities, including those mentioned above, and others such as increased chemokine synthesis and expression of inflammatory cell adhesion molecules, which will consequently impair BBB integrity (Jha et al., 2019). On the other hand, pinocytic vesicles may also develop during brain injury and will be able to configure transendothelial channels through which the transport of water and solutes from one extracellular compartment to another will be allowed (Stokum et al., 2016).

In this sense, the disruption of the BBB will allow a direct connection between the vascular and interstitial compartments of the brain, where hydrostatic pressure gradients facilitate the passage and abnormal accumulation of fluid and plasma proteins from the intravascular space to the brain parenchyma, which corresponds to a pathological condition known as vasogenic edema (Michinaga and Koyama 2015; Stokum et al., 2016). In this type of edema, the white matter is more damaged than the gray matter, due to its various axonal tracts arranged in parallel, which have a greater capacity for distension and allow greater propagation of the exudate (Mahajan and Bhagat 2016). This accumulation results in an increase in brain volume (Mohanty et al., 2019) which, based on the Monro-Kellie doctrine, will try to be compensated for through the decrease of another of its constituent components (Mahajan and Bhagat 2016). However, if the compensatory mechanism fails, it will result in increased intracranial pressure (Mohanty et al., 2019) that can affect cerebral blood flow and cerebral perfusion pressure, presenting clinically with mild symptoms such as headache, to symptoms of cerebral herniation, ischemia, and even death (Jha et al., 2019; Mahajan and Bhagat 2016).

Diagnosis

Although CT does not allow a clear characterization of the affected area, it is the first-line study used for the diagnosis of vasogenic cerebral edema, which shows a hypodense lesion limited to the white matter, sometimes accompanied by calcified, hemorrhagic or necrotic foci (Ho et al., 2012). On the other hand, the heavy diffusion MRI technique is useful to differentiate vasogenic from cytotoxic edema, since the former has a high apparent diffusion coefficient, while the latter has a lower one; moreover, it is useful if a much more complete delineation of the extent of edema is sought, in which the edema is evidenced as a hyperintense lesion in a T2/FLAIR sequence (Esqueda-Liquidano et al., 2014).

Treatment

Untreated vasogenic edema leads to the development of serious complications that can threaten the patient's life (Mahajan and Bhagat 2016). Therefore, it is necessary to provide adequate medical management with the aim of maintaining ideal intracranial pressure levels, along with optimal blood flow to meet all the metabolic requirements of the brain (Jha et al., 2019).

Thus, the usual therapy used in vasogenic edema is based on a systemic approach that includes from general measures, such as ensuring an adequate head position and optimal oxygenation, hydration and blood pressure, to specific measures such as the administration of corticosteroids, diuretics, osmotics and, as a last resort, surgical management (Mohanty et al., 2019). However, interest has now emerged in identifying new, more targeted therapeutic targets due to the growing knowledge about the cellular mechanisms involved in edema formation (Bosma et al., 2018; Halstead and Geocadin 2019). Among these new therapeutic targets, which continue to be topics of research, are the following:

- *VEGF inhibitors:* Due to the contributing role of VEGF in the disruption of BBB and consequently in the formation of vasogenic edema, the use of VEGF inhibitors has been investigated in order to regulate the expression of tight junction proteins and consequently aiming to play a beneficial role in the context of vasogenic edema (Jha et al., 2019).
- *MMP inhibitors:* Some experimental studies in rodents have shown that early use (within 48 hours after injury) of MMP inhibitors can restore the integrity of the blood-brain barrier, so their administration in the context of vasogenic edema could be favorable (Mahajan and Bhagat 2016)
- *AQP-4:* Due to its function, several activators of this molecule have been studied to eliminate the abnormal fluid accumulated in the interstitial compartment of the brain in the context of vasogenic edema; however, further studies are still needed to obtain a clearer picture regarding its role in this clinical scenario (Mahajan and Bhagat 2016).
- *Selective endothelin B receptor (ETB-R) antagonists:* Stimulation of endothelin B receptors is responsible for activating resting astrocytes in the CNS (Mahajan and Bhagat 2016). These reactive astrocytes

manufacture factors such as VEGF and MMP that increase the permeability of the blood-brain barrier; because of this, the use of ETB-R antagonists with the consequent reduction of reactive astrocytes could be a timely therapeutic option in the context of vasogenic edema (Michinaga and Koyama 2015).

- *Peroxisome proliferator-activated receptor (PPAR) agonists:* The use of fenobrate as a PPAR agonist in the management of vasogenic edema has been investigated to reduce neurogenic inflammation (Halstead and Geocadin 2019). Studies have evidenced that this substance can stabilize BBB integrity by decreasing its permeability, however, further studies are considered necessary (Jha et al., 2019).

Conclusion

The BBB is an indispensable element for the maintenance of CNS integrity by blocking the entry of various neurotoxic substances from the peripheral circulation and by allowing the entry of energy and nutrients necessary for proper neuronal functioning and consequent brain homeostasis through the multiple and dynamic interactions between each of its components. Therefore, any type of dysfunction, whether at the mechanical or molecular level in the BBB, gives way to the development of several potentially serious clinical conditions, among which is the formation of vasogenic edema. Such edema represents a delicate pathological condition that must be managed in an adequate and timely manner in order to avoid the establishment of serious complications that threaten the patient's life.

References

Abdullahi, W., Tripathi, D. and Ronaldson, P. T. (2018). Blood-brain barrier dysfunction in ischemic stroke: targeting tight junctions and transporters for vascular protection. *Am J Physiol Cell Physiol,* 315: C343-C356.

Armulik, A., Genové, G. and Betsholtz, C. (2011). Pericytes: developmental, physiological, and pathological perspectives, problems, and promises. *Dev Cell,* 21: 193-215.

Ayloo, S. and Gu, C. (2019). Transcytosis at the blood-brain barrier. *Curr Opin Neurobiol,* 57:32-38.

Baeten, K. M. and Akassoglou, K. (2011). Extracellular matrix and matrix receptors in blood-brain barrier formation and stroke. *Dev Neurobiol,* 71: 1018-39.

Bagchi, S., Chhibber, T., Lahooti, B., Verma, A., Borse, V. and Jayant, R. D. (2019). In-vitro blood-brain barrier models for drug screening and permeation studies: an overview. *Drug Des Devel Ther,* 13: 3591-3605.

Bauer, H. C., Krizbai, I. A. and Bauer, H. (2014). Traweger A. "You Shall Not Pass" – tight junctions of the blood brain barrier. *Front Neurosci,* 8: 2392.

Beutel, O., Maraspini, R., Pombo-García, K., Martin-Lemaitre, C. and Honigmann, A. (2019). Phase Separation of Zonula Occludens Proteins Drives Formation of Tight Junctions. *Cell,* 179: 923-936.

Bosma, E. K., van Noorden, C. J. F., Schlingemann, R. O. and Klaassen, I. (2018). The role of plasmalemma vesicle-associated protein in pathological breakdown of blood-brain and blood-retinal barriers: potential novel therapeutic target for cerebral edema and diabetic macular edema. *Fluids Barriers CNS,* 15:24.

Castro-Dias, M., Mapunda, J. A., Vladymyrov, M. and Engelhardt, B. (2019). Structure and Junctional Complexes of Endothelial, Epithelial and Glial Brain Barriers. *Int J Mol Sci,* 20: 5372.

Costea, L., Mészáros, Á., Bauer, H., Bauer, H. C., Traweger, A., Wilhelm, I., Farkas, A. E., Krizbai, I. A. (2019). The Blood-Brain Barrier and Its Intercellular Junctions in Age-Related Brain Disorders. *Int J Mol Sci,* 20: 5472.

Dalby, T. (2020). Pathophysiology of Cerebral Edema - A Comprehensive Review. *J Neuroanaesthesiol Crit Care.*

Erdő, F., Denes, L. and de Lange, E. (2017). Age-associated physiological and pathological changes at the blood-brain barrier: A review. *J Cereb Blood Flow Metab,* 37: 4-24.

Esqueda-Liquidano, M. A., Gutiérrez-Cabrera, J. J., Cuéllar-Martínez, S., Vargas-Tentori, N., Ariñez-Barahona, E., Flores-Álvarez, E., Ruiz-Pérez, J., Esqueda-Liquidano, L. and Loo-Salomé, S. (2014). Brain edema I: pathophysiology, clinical manifestations, diagnosis and neurological monitoring. *Med Int Méx,* 30:584-590.

Garcia, M. A., Nelson, W. J. and Chavez, N. (2018). Cell-Cell Junctions Organize Structural and Signaling Networks. *Cold Spring Harb Perspect Biol,* 10.

Greene, C. and Campbell, M. (2016). Tight junction modulation of the blood brain barrier: CNS delivery of small molecules. *Tissue Barriers,* 4.

Greene, C., Hanley, N. and Campbell, M. (2019). Claudin-5: gatekeeper of neurological function. *Fluids Barriers CNS,* 16: 3.

Hall, C. N., Reynell, C., Gesslein, B., Hamilton, N. B., Mishra, A., Sutherland, B. A., O'Farrell, F. M., Buchan, A. M., Lauritzen, M. and Attwell, D. (2014). Capillary pericytes regulate cerebral blood flow in health and disease. *Nature,* 508: 55-60.

Halstead, M. R. and Geocadin, R. G. (2019). The Medical Management of Cerebral Edema: Past, Present, and Future Therapies. *Neurotherapeutics,* 16:1133-1148.

Harrell, C. R., Simovic-Markovic, B., Fellabaum, C., Arsenijevic, A., Djonov, V. and Volarevic, V. (2018). Molecular mechanisms underlying therapeutic potential of pericytes. *J Biomed Sci,* 25(1): 21.

Hatte, G., Prigent, C. and Tassan, J. P. (2018). Tight junctions negatively regulate mechanical forces applied to adherens junctions in vertebrate epithelial tissue. *J Cell Sci,* 131(3).

Ho, M. L., Rojas, R. and Eisenberg, R. L. (2012) Cerebral edema. *AJR Am J Roentgenol,* 199(3): W258-73.

Jha, R. M., Kochanek, P. M. and Simard, J. M. (2019). Pathophysiology and Treatment of Cerebral Edema in Traumatic Brain Injury. *Neuropharmacology,* 145(Pt B):230-246.

Kadry, H., Noorani, B. and Cucullo, L. (2020). A blood-brain barrier overview on structure, function, impairment, and biomarkers of integrity. *Fluids Barriers CNS,* 17: 69.

Keaney, J. and Campbell, M. (2015). The dynamic blood-brain barrier. *FEBS J,* 282: 4067-79.

Keep, R. F., Andjelkovic, A. V., Xiang, J., Stamatovic, S. M., Antonetti, D. A., Hua, Y. and Xi, G. (2018). Brain endothelial cell junctions after cerebral hemorrhage: Changes, mechanisms and therapeutic targets. *J Cereb Blood Flow Metab,* 38: 1255-1275.

Komarova, Y. A., Kruse, K., Mehta, D. and Malik, A. B. (2017). Protein Interactions at Endothelial Junctions and Signaling Mechanisms Regulating Endothelial Permeability. *Circ Res,* 120(1):179-206.

Liebner, S., Dijkhuizen, R. M., Reiss, Y., Plate, K. H., Agalliu, D. and Constantin, G. (2018). Functional morphology of the blood-brain barrier in health and disease. *Acta Neuropathol,* 135: 311-336.

Lochhead, J. J., Yang, J., Ronaldson, P. T. and Davis, T. P. (2020). Structure, Function, and Regulation of the Blood-Brain Barrier Tight Junction in Central Nervous System Disorders. *Front Physiol,* 11: 914.

Mahajan, S. and Bhagat, H. (2016). Cerebral oedema: Pathophysiological mechanisms and experimental therapies. *J Neuroanaesthesiol Crit Care,* 3:22-8.

Michinaga, S. and Koyama, Y. (2015). Pathogenesis of Brain Edema and Investigation into Anti-Edema Drugs. *Int J Mol Sci,* 16:9949-9975.

Mohanty, S., Swain, S. K. and Biswal, C. (2019). Brain Edema: Newer Concept of Treatment. *Ann Natl Acad Med Sci,* 55:189-192.

Obermeier, B., Daneman, R. and Ransohoff, R. M. (2013). Development, maintenance and disruption of the blood-brain barrier. *Nat Med,* 19(12):1584-96.

Reed, M. J., Damodarasamy, M. and Banks, W. A. (2019). The extracellular matrix of the blood-brain barrier: structural and functional roles in health, aging, and Alzheimer's disease. *Tissue Barriers,* 7(4): 1651157.

Sorby-Adams, A. J., Marcoionni, A. M., Dempsey, E. R., Woenig, J. A. and Turner, R. J. (2017). The Role of Neurogenic Inflammation in Blood-Brain Barrier Disruption and Development of Cerebral Oedema Following Acute Central Nervous System (CNS) Injury. *Int J Mol Sci,* 18:1788.

Stamatovic, S. M., Johnson, A. M., Keep, R. F. and Andjelkovic A. V. (2016). Junctional proteins of the blood-brain barrier: New insights into function and dysfunction. *Tissue Barriers,* 4(1): e1154641.

Stokum, J. A., Gerzanich, V. and Simard, J. M. (2016). Molecular pathophysiology of cerebral edema. *Journal of Cerebral Blood Flow & Metabolism,* 36(3).

Sun, J. D., Liu, Y., Yuan, Y. H., Li, J. and Chen, N. H. (2012). Gap junction dysfunction in the prefrontal cortex induces depressive-like behaviors in rats. *Neuropsychopharmacology,* 37(5):1305-20.

Sweeney, M. D., Zhao, Z., Montagne, A., Nelson, A. R. and Zlokovic, B. V. (2019). Blood-Brain Barrier: From Physiology to Disease and Back. *Physiol Rev,* 99(1): 21-78.

Thomsen, M. S., Birkelund, S., Burkhart, A., Stensballe, A. and Moos, T. (2017). Synthesis and deposition of basement membrane proteins by primary brain capillary endothelial cells in a murine model of the blood-brain barrier. *J Neurochem,* 140(5): 741-754.

Wilhelm, I., Fazakas, C. and Krizbai, I. A. (2011). In vitro models of the blood-brain barrier. *Acta Neurobiol Exp (Wars),* 71(1):113-28.

Winkler, E. A., Bell, R. D. and Zlokovic, B. V. (2011). Central nervous system pericytes in health and disease. *Nat Neurosci,* 14(11): 1398-1405.

Xu, L., Nirwane, A. and Yao, Y. (2018). Basement membrane and blood-brain barrier. *Stroke Vasc Neurol,* 4(2):78-82.

Yamazaki, Y. and Kanekiyo, T. (2017). Blood-Brain Barrier Dysfunction and the Pathogenesis of Alzheimer's Disease. *Int J Mol Sci,* 18(9): 1965.

Yang, S., Jin, H., Zhu, Y., Wan, Y., Opoku, E. N., Zhu, L. and Hu, B. (2017). Diverse Functions and Mechanisms of Pericytes in Ischemic Stroke. *Curr Neuropharmacol,* 15(6): 892-905.

Yuan, S., Liu, K. J. and Qi, Z. (2020). Occludin regulation of blood-brain barrier and potential therapeutic target in ischemic stroke. *Brain Circ.* 6(3): 152-162.

Zhang, Z. S., Zhou, H. N., He, S. S., Xue, M. Y., Li, T. and Liu, L. M. (2020). Research advances in pericyte function and their roles in diseases. *Chin J Traumatol,* 23(2): 89-95.

Zhao, Y., Xin, Y., He, Z. and Hu, W. (2018). Function of Connexins in the Interaction between Glial and Vascular Cells in the Central Nervous System and Related Neurological Diseases. *Neural Plast.* 2018: 6323901.

Zhao, Z., Nelson, A. R., Betsholtz, C. and Zlokovic, B. V. (2015). Establishment and Dysfunction of the Blood-Brain Barrier. *Cell,* 163(5): 1064-1078.

Chapter 3

Normal Pressure Hydrocephalus

Brajesh Kumar
Department of Neurosurgery, IGIMS, Patna

Abstract

Normal pressure hydrocephalus is term introduced by Hakim and Adams in 1963. The patient is usually in the seventh decade of life with gait disturbances (magnetic gait), dementia and urinary incontinence as a classical triad with an enlarged ventricular system and normal intracranial pressure. There are 2 types of NPH: (i) Idiopathic normal pressure hydrocephalus (iNPH) (ii) Secondary normal pressure hydrocephalus (sNPH) mostly due to meningitis, head injury, subarachnoid hemorrhage or encephalitis present in the younger population.

iNPH is a surgically treatable neurodegenerative disease with a favorable outcome in properly diagnosed and selected cases. Patents usually present this illness in the seventh decade of life and diagnosis is often difficult due to the presence of the ageing process, alzheimer's and Parkinson's disease. Neuro imaging (axial CT brain, MRI brain, 3D-phase contrast MRI, 3D-phase contrast cine MRI, pseudo continuous arterial spin labelling perfusion MRI, 3D volumetric study high-field 3D MRI) invasive tests for confirmation and predicting the response to success of CSF diversion procedures are- CSF removal test, CSF markers analysis (hsa-mir-4274, PTPRQ-protein tyrosine phosphatase receptor type Q, Tf-glycan isoform of transferrin,), computer aided intrathecal infusion test to measure resistance of CSF outflow. CSF diversion procedure is the only effective treatment of properly diagnosed and selected cases of iNPH. Types of CSF diversion procedure in iNPH - venticulo-peritoneal shunt (VP shunt); lumbo-peritoneal shunt (LP shunt); ventriculo-atrial shunt (VA shunt); ventriculo-epiplooic shunt;

In: Advances in Neurosurgery Research
Editors: Amit Agrawal, Pradeep Chouksey, Adesh Shrivastava et al.
ISBN: 978-1-68507-859-1

endoscopic 3rd ventriculostomy (ETV). When an elderly patient in 7th decade of life presents with relevant signs and symptoms which matches with the noninvasive and invasive diagnostic procedure, a diagnosis of iNPH can be considered. These patients can also have other diseases considering their old age like Parkinsonism, amyloid disease, vascular and white matter diseases. The CSF diversion procedure may not have the desired response considering the presence of other neurodegenerative diseases.

Keywords: normal pressure hydrocephalus, gait disturbance, dementia, urinary incontinence, shunt surgery

Introduction

Normal Pressure Hydrocephalus (NPH) is usually present in the 6th or 7th decade of life. Common presenting complaints are; difficulty in walking (magnetic gait), increased forgetfulness and difficulty in holding urine which was described by Hakim and Adams as a triad in 1965 [1]. A small number of patients present with the full triad and the most common clinical presentation is gait difficulty with other symptoms in varying severity. As the name suggests there is a presence of ventriculomegaly along with the normal range of CSF pressure on lumbar puncture in NPH. Alzheimer's dementia, Parkinson's disease, multi-infarct dementia, cervical and lumbar stenosis are other differential diagnosis of NPH. NPH has been divided into *idiopathic* (iNPH) and *secondary* (sNPH) (post meningitis, post head injury or post subarachnoid haemorrhage, after posterior fossa surgery, Alzheimer's disease etc.) subtypes. We will focus our discussion on iNPH which is surgically treatable, if diagnosed properly.

Aetiology

Many hypotheses have been given to explain the normal range of CSF pressure with increasing ventricular dilatation. There is *decreased* CSF resorption at levels of arachnoid granulations and brain parenchyma probably due to leptomeningeal fibrosis and *increased vascular resistance*. The decrease in CSF resorption increases the pressure difference between ventricle and subarachnoid space which causes ventricular dilatation [2]. Ventricular dilatation more than sulcal enlargement differentiates it from cortical atrophy

[3]. There is decreased blood supply in the area between perforators of the middle cerebral artery and the medullary branches from the pial arteries. These ischemic changes decrease the elasticity of periventricular tissue and causes ventricular enlargement. CSF seeps into periventricular parenchyma causing a decrease in the flow of interstitial fluid which causes accumulation of *vasoactive metabolite* leading to local autoregulation failure. This causes a high incidence of periventricular white matter hyperintensities in theses ischemic areas.

Diagnostic Criteria [4]

The definitive diagnosis of iNPH can be made when there is improvement of symptoms after shunt surgery. They are also called shunt responders. Those patients *likely* having NPH who are having 2 of the below features:

1. More than one symptom of clinical triad: gait disturbance, cognitive impairment, and urinary incontinence, which cannot be completely explained by other neurological or non-neurological disease or having any other previous disease which may cause ventricular dilatation (subarachnoid haemorrhage, meningitis, head injury, congenital/ developmental hydrocephalus, and aqueductal stenosis).
2. CSF pressure of 200 mm of H_2O or less and normal CSF content and improvement in the symptoms after CSF drainage.
3. MRI feature of narrowing of the sulci and subarachnoid space over the high-convexity/midline surface (DESH) with short and unstable gait as if feet glued to earth (magnetic gait)

Clinical Signs

The triad of gait disturbance, dementia and urinary incontinence is present in only one third of patients in age group more than 60 years of age.

Gait Disturbance

This is most frequent symptom in patients with NPH. Characteristics of gait are:

- Wide based gait
- Short and shuffling steps
- Difficulty in initiating step
- Unsteadiness in turning

They walk like feet are glued to the floor, also called magnetic or wobbly gait. This gait differentiates NPH from dementia. Gait in patients suffering from dementia is normal. In NPH there is difficulty in standing upright without assistance with forward leaning and motor incoordination. The wider sway and imbalance increase on eye closure. The ventricular dilation causes the compression of corticospinal tract passing through the corona radiata. Involvement of the pyramidal tract due to subcortical white matter damage causing extensor plantar response. Dopaminergic nigrostriatal pathway impairment and decreased input to reticular formation in the tegmentum contribute to gait difficulty [5, 6]. Parkinson's disease is another important differential diagnosis of the disease in which there is resting tremor, cogwheel rigidity and improves with levodopa administration. Cerebellar disease can also mimic NPH having a predominantly cerebellar gait ataxia, cerebellar speech, gaze evoked nystagmus and appendicular dysmetria. Patients of NPH presenting with gait disturbance exhibit better response to CSF shunting.

Dementia

Patients mainly have memory impairment with decreased attention, inertia and slowness in thought. Patients become withdrawn and apathetic. As the disease progresses, memory deficit may be associated with motor slowness and gait apraxia. Dementia is unlikely to recover even after shunting. Cortical dementia is characteristically associated with aphasia-apraxia-agnosia syndrome w*hich differentiates it from NPH.*

Urinary Incontinence

Disturbance in bladder control can present as an increase in urinary frequency, urgency and incontinence. This is not specific for NPH. Bladder symptoms, if present, may not improve or resolve with CSF diversion [7]. The problem of urinary function may be due to the involvement of sacral fibres of corticospinal tract or dementia.

D/D

- *Neurodegenerative diseases* e.g., Alzheimer's disease, Parkinson's disease, amyotrophic lateral sclerosis (ALS) and multisystem atrophy
- *Diseases causing vascular dementia* - Cerebrovascular disease, multi-infarct dementia, vertebrobasilar insufficiency
- *Disorders presenting with hydrocephalus* - Aqueductal stenosis, arrested hydrocephalus, non- communicating hydrocephalus
- *CNS Infections* - CNS tuberculosis, HIV
- *Urological disorder with urinary incontinence-* Urinary tract infection, benign prostatic hyperplasia, prostate carcinoma, cystitis and other causes of neurogenic bladder.
- *Other Causes* - Vitamin B12 deficiency, traumatic brain injury, chiari malformation, spinal stenosis and spinal cord tumors.

Diagnosis

NPH is mainly a clinical diagnosis and should always be considered in elderly males with symptoms suggestive of NPH. With advancement in the imaging techniques, various imaging modalities have been added to strengthen the clinical diagnosis. Considering the age of presentation of disease, many other diseases overlap and make the diagnosis difficult mainly in borderline cases. Both clinical and imaging evidence can help in the diagnosis of NPH with accuracy and can help in choosing the treatment protocol for the disease.

Clinical Tests

CSF Tap Test

In this test, a large volume 40-50 ml CSF [8, 9] is drained which creates a short acting physiological effect of shunt. The opening pressure of CSF should be in the range of 5-18 mm of Hg (70-245 mm of water). The patient should be examined in detail before and after the lumbar puncture (LP), so that the response to CSF removal can be documented and quantified. A preoperative video of the gait should be made before and after the removal of CSF, which shows immediate improvement after the adequate removal of CSF.

Revaluation of patient's gait (step length, step height, time to travel, difficulty in turning and walking pattern) should be done between 2-4 hours of CSF removal. This CSF removal has the specificity of (60-100%) and sensitivity of (50-80%). This test can be repeated after a week to reconfirm the response, or some may respond in a second test who have not responded in the 1st test. Though LP in lateral recumbent position gives intracranial pressure (ICP) or CSF pressure as a definition of NPH, it must be between 5-18 mm of Hg (68 and 244.8 mm of H_2O, nearly 70-250 mm H_20 [13] measurement of ICP is not mandatory and not always possible for the diagnosis of NPH. In a normal person, the CSF opening pressure is in the range of 122 ± 34mm H_2O (8.8 ± 0.9 mm Hg). In patients with iNPH, the CSF average opening pressure is 11±3.3 mm Hg (150 ± 45 mm H_2O) which can vary between 4.4 mm Hg and 17.6 mm hg (60-240 mm H_2O). The diagnosis of iNPH is unlikely if the pressure is not present in this range. CSF opening pressure in iNPH is slightly higher than normal but remains within the normal range. There may be transient high pressure CSF waves (B wave) found in continuous intraventricular pressure monitoring but they are not sustained.

Continuous Intracranial Pressure Monitoring

Continuous ICP recording over 24 hours having normal or slightly elevated ICP and increased frequency of B wave occupying more than 50% of monitoring period is indicative of low compliance to shunt. It has been proposed that amplitude and duration rather than frequency of B or A waves are important [10]. Controlled continuous lumbar drainage is not routinely done due to a high complication rate e.g., severe back pain due to nerve root irritation and infection further increasing the hospitalization cost [11].

Other Tests

- Slow vasogenic ICP waves [12]
- CSF markers:
  - Expression of has-miR-4274 [13]
  - Glycan isoforms of transferrin (Tf) [14]
- Computer aided intrathecal infusion test showing resistance to CSF outflow [15, 16]

Neuroimaging

MRI plays important role in the diagnosis of iNPH and if image findings match the clinical tests, only then can a decision be made regarding the CSF diversion procedures for the definitive treatment. A CT brain scan is the first radiological investigation usually done.

Radiological Diagnosis

Axial CT of the brain [17] - The CT findings of NPH for diagnosis:

- Enlargement of the lateral and third ventricle,
- Enlargement of the temporal horn,
- Prominent basilar cistern,
- Enlarged suprasellar cistern and the
- Non-visualization of the high cerebral convexity sulci.

A temporal horn enlargement is more specific for the diagnosis of NPH. Primary cortical atrophy may cause ex-evacuo dilatation of the ventricle. Patients with cortical atrophy and symptoms of NPH respond to shunting. The mean value of silver index (ratio between the areas of Sylvian fissure (SF) and the subarachnoid space (SS) at the vertex) in possible iNPH was 11.52+/-!.68 compared to 1+/-0.98 in the control group.

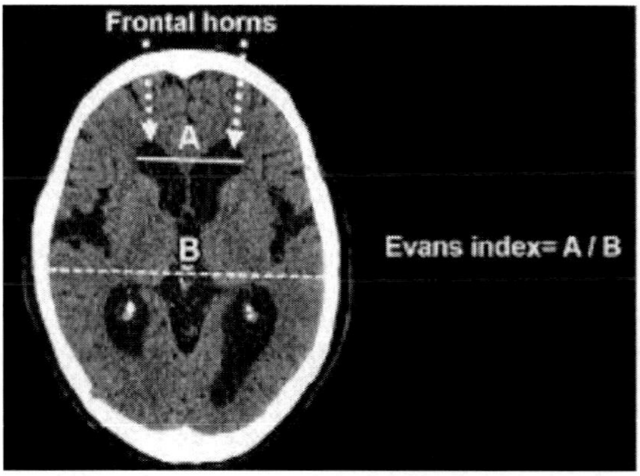

Figure 1. CT scan showing measurement of Evan's Index.

- *Evan's Index (EA) & Callosal Angles (CA)* - EA [18] are markers of ventricular volume: EI>0.3 indicate pathological VF (17) cut-off value is different in males/females in various age groups:

  - 65-69 yrs- 0.34/0.32
  - 70-74 years-0.36/0.33
  - 75-79 years- 0.37/0.34
  - 80-84 years- 0.37/0.36

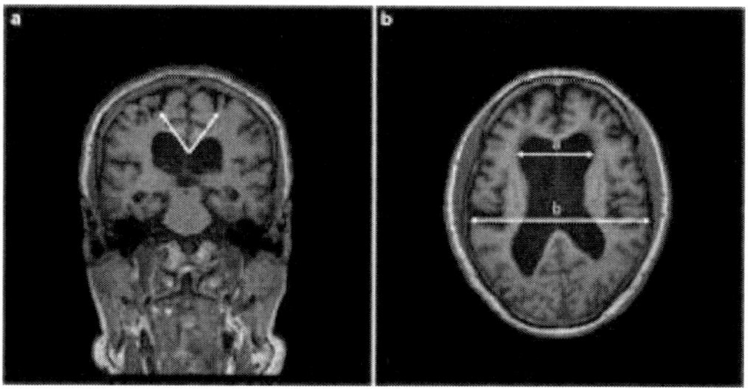

Figure 2. MRI showing (a) measurement of callosal angle and (b) Evan's Index

- *Callosal angle* is measured at the level of midpoint of the corpus callosum in mid-sagittal plane oriented parallel to the floor of 4th ventricle (Figure 2A). Cut off for CA is 105.4 and there is an increase in surgical response with decrease in callosal angle [19].
- *MR Phase- contrast –cine* [20] is done for the quantitive assessment of the flow of CSF in the aqueduct. There is increase in the velocity of fluid motion when larger volume moves through decreasing cross-sectional area. This produces a signal void (jet sign) in the region of cerebral aqueduct. The CSF peak velocity (V peak), minute flow volume (min V) and flow volume of systole and diastole significantly increase in iNPH as compared to normal control. The degree of rise in the diastolic phase more than systolic phase in iNPH resulting in reversal of net flow direction, likely causes ventriculomegaly in iNPH patients. Although aqueductal flow void may be seen in a normal person, its extension to the adjacent third and fourth ventricle is more marked in the iNPH group than in the normal person.
- *MRI Elastography* [21] - Analyse the parenchymal viscoelastic properties with clinical symptoms and compare with normal controls.

There is increased stiffness in the cerebrum (region of interest-ROI) and decreased stiffness in periventricular ROI.

- *T2W MRI* [20] – There is altered cerebral compliance and autoregulation leading to periventricular ischemia seen as hyperintensity in the periventricular region. Hyperdynamic CSF motion is seen as flow void within the ventricular system on T2W MR scans [22]
- *Glymphatic MRI* [23] - There is delayed clearance of godobutrol at sylvian fissure presenting as delayed enhancement in that region in patients of NPH.
- *3D Phase Contrast MRI* [24] - This measures hyperdynamic CSF motion between iNPH and normal control. The CSF pressure gradient in the aqueduct was found to be significantly different in patients of iNPH and control.
- *High field 3D MRI* [25] - The study of subarachnoid space- INPH has ventricular enlargement (VE) with large subarachnoid space at basal cisterns (BC) and sylvian fissure (SF) but diminished at convexity while in the secondary NPH there is VE with diminished subarachnoid space at BC, SF as well as convexity due to decreased CSF drainage from subarachnoid space.
- *CT cisternography* - There is a persistence of ventricular reflux for more than 24 hours with slow cortical uptake, this help discriminating NPH from cerebral atrophy.
- *CT Perfusion* [26] - A significant reduction in cerebral blood flow in the periventricular white matter.
- *CT Volumetric assessment of intracranial CSF distribution* [27] - In comparison to the subarachnoid spaces and basal cisterns the CSF volume in the ventricular system was found greater in NPH patients, when compared with the patients with brain atrophy.

Treatment Modality

When the patient shows slowly progressive clinical signs of NPH with an enlarged ventricular system without intracranial organic lesion and improvement of clinical signs by CSF removal by LP, then NPH is strongly suspected and shunt surgery should be considered.

Shunt may not always arrest the progression of iNPH. The neurological decline after shunt placement may be due to progression of co-morbid conditions. Shunt surgery is already established as the only durable and effective treatment of NPH. Even a temporary improvement after shunt placement for 1-3 year brings a significant difference to the quality of life. The placement of a ventriculo -peritoneal (VP) shunt is a current standard of treatment.

How a shunt improves the symptomatology of patients- it diverts the excess amount of CSF which leads to modulation of pulse pressure, interstitial edema decreases, leading to improvement in perfusion and decrease in ischemia. This is probably the reason endoscopic 3rd ventriculostomy has also been found effective in these cases [28].

Types of CSF diversion procedure in NPH are [29]:

- VP shunt
- Lumbo-Peritoneal (LP) Shunt
- Ventriculo Atrial (VA) Shunt
- Ventriculo-epiploic (VE) Shunt
- Endoscopic Third Ventriculostomy (ETV)

VP shunt with programmable valve is the most common and recommended procedure with the least complication and revision rates [13]. The programmable shunt allows for the correction of over drainage externally which is the most common complication of nonprogrammable shunt placement. Non programmable shunts are placed most commonly considering their low cost. Medium pressure shunts are the most commonly used shunt in the treatment of NPH. These pressure valves have an antisiphon device to prevent gravity dependent overdrainge in the upright position but in case of iNPH, CSF pressure is in normal range which make these antisiphon device ineffective. Efficacy and safety rates of LP shunts for patient with INPH with programmable valves are comparable to those of VP shunts [30, 31], however shunt revisions were more common in LP shunt treated patient [19]. A modification of VP shunt by putting the peritoneal end of the catheter between the epiploic layer of the greater omentum showed a favourable outcome without any significant complication [32]. Patients who have multiple intraabdominal operations or history of peritonitis may have decreased absorptive capacity of the peritoneal cavity; VA shunts may be preferred in these cases. Systemic review done by Tudor et al. found that there was no difference in the outcome in ETV and standard VP shunt without programmable valve [33].

Outcome and Prognosis

About 40% iNPH patients improved after shunt surgery. All the symptoms in NPH may improve after the shunt surgery but cognitive improvement is not commonly anticipated. In the first 6–12-month regular follow up is needed to look for any complications and symptoms related to overdrainge.

Complication from CSF Diversion Procedure iNPH

Subdural Hygroma/Hematoma

This is the most common complication due to shunt overdrainge. There is high risk when low pressure valve shunts are used which cause over drainage of CSF in patients with gross cerebral atrophy. In the case of a programmable valve, pressure should be increased externally and in the presence of a fixed valve, there is the need for the replacement with a programmable valve, and the addition of an anti-siphon device or revision with a high pressure valve.

Complications Related to Shunt

Shunt malfunction, shunt Infection, shunt obstruction, shunt migration and shunt disconnection are common complications. Hung et al. found that 36% in VA and 42.5% in VP shunted patients experienced shunt complications [34]. They also found VA shunted patient were less likely to experience shunt blockage and shunt revision in comparison to VP shunted patient.

Intracerebral Haemorrhage

Surface, deep and intraventricular can happen during shunt introduction or with patients on anticoagulants or with a coagulation disorder. An immediate CT scan should be done if any new cognitive deficit appears postoperatively.

Seizure and CSF Infection

Adequate precautions should be taken and should be managed as per hospital policy of using antiepileptics and antibiotics.

Conclusion

NPH is one of the most common causes of treatable gait disturbance, urinary incontinence and dementia. The lumbar tap test is a useful diagnostic and therapeutic procedure. It is important to advise having a CT or MRI in patients of old age having these symptoms. If diagnosed properly, surgery can be very rewarding and enhance the quality of life in such elderly patients. Whenever there is no improvement, even with proper selection of cases and exclusion of shunt malfunction, other comorbid conditions of the patient should be considered and a revaluation of the disease should be done.

References

[1] Hakim S, Adams RD. (1965). The special clinical problem of symptomatic hydrocephalus with normal CSF pressure. *J Neurol Sci*, 2 :307-327.

[2] Conner ES, Foley L, Black PM. (1984). Experimental normal pressure hydrocephalus is accompanied by increased transmantle pressure. *J Neurosurg,* 61:322-7.

[3] Katano H, Karasawa K, Sugiyama N, Yamashita N, Ohkura A, Kamiya K. (2003). Clinical evaluation of shunt implantations using Sophy programmable pressure valves: comparison with Codman-Hakim programmable valves. *J Clin Neurosci*, 10: 557-61.

[4] Madoka Nakajima, Shigeki Yamada, Masakazu Miyajima . (2021). Guidelines for Management of Idiopathic Normal Pressure Hydrocephalus (Third Edition): Endorsed by the Japanese Society of Normal Pressure Hydrocephalus. *Neurol Med Chir*, 61(2):63-97.

[5] Stolze H, Kuhtz-Buschbeck JP, Drucke H, Johnk K, Diercks C, Palmie S, Mehdorn HM, Illert M, Deuschl G. (2000). Gait analysis in idiopathic normal pressure hydrocephalus- which parameters responds to the CSF Tap test? *Clin Neurophysiol*, 111:1678-86.

[6] Vanneste JA. (2003). Diagnosis and management of normal pressure hydrocephalus. *J Neurol,* 247:5-14.

[7] Ahlberg J, Norlen L, Blomstrand C, Wikkelso C. (1998). Outcome of shunt operation on urinary incontinence in normal pressure hydrocephalus predicted by lumbar puncture. *J Neurol Neurosurg Psychiatry*, 273:117-26.

[8] INPH GUIDELINE STUDY GROUP. (2005). Guidelines for the diagnosis and management of idiopathic normal pressure hydrocephalus. *Neurosurgery,* 57(3): 1-52.

[9] Huchche AM, Bharucha NE, Patil ND. (2017). Practical Neurosurgery: Analysis of Clinical Cases-A patient with Dementia. *Thieme,* Chapter 6.

[10] Vanneste JA. (2003). Diagnosis and management of normal pressure hydrocephalus. *J Neurol,* 247:5-14.

[11] Chen IH, Huang CI, Liu HC, Chen KK. (1994). Effectiveness of shunting in patients with normal pressure hydrocephalus predicted by temporary, controlled resistance, continuous lumbar drainage: a pilot study. *J Neurol Neurosurg Psychiatry*, 57:1430-2.

[12] Spiegelberg A, Krause M, Meixensberger J, Seifert B, Kurtcuoglu V. (2018). Significant association of slow vasogenic ICP waves with normal pressure hydrocephalus diagnosis. *Acta Neurochir Suppl*, 126: 243-246.

[13] Jurjevic I, Miajima M, Ogino I, Akiba C, Nakajima M, Kondo A. (2017). Decreased expression of has-miR-4274 in cerebrospinal fluid of normal pressure hydrocephalus mimic with Parkinsonian syndrome. *J Alzheimers Dis*, 56: 317-25.

[14] Murakami Y, Matsumoto Y, Hoshi K, Ito H, Fuwa TJ, Yamaguchi Y. (2018). Rapid increase of 'brain type' transferrin in cerebrospinal fluid after shunt surgery for idiopathic normal pressure hydrocephalus: A prognosis marker for cognitive recovery. *J Biochem,* 164:205-213.

[15] Nabbanja E, Czosnyka M, Keong NC, Garnett M, Pickard JD, Lalou DA. (2018) Is there a link between ICP -derived infusion test parameters and outcome after shunting in normal pressure hydrocephalus? *Acta Neurochir Suppl*, 126:229-232.

[16] Meier U, Bartels P. (2002). The importance of the intrathecal infusion test in the diagnosis of normal pressure hydrocephalus. *J Clin Neurosci*, 9: 260-7.

[17] Benedetto N, Gambacciani C, Aquila F, Di Carlo DT, Morganti R, Perrini P. (2017). A new quantitative method to access disproportionately enlarged subarachnoid space (DESH) in patients with possible idiopathic normal pressure hydrocephalus: The Silver index. *Cin Neurol Neurosurg*, 158:27-32.

[18] Brix MK, Westman E, Simmons A, Ringstad GA, Eide PK, Wagnet-Larsen K (2017). The Evans' Index revisited: new cut-off levels for use in radiological assessment of ventricular enlargement in the elderly. *Eur J Radiol*, 95:28-32.

[19] Grahnke K, Jusue-TorresI, Szujewski C, Joyce C, Schneck M, Prabhu VC (2018). The quest for predicting sustained shunt response in normal pressure hydrocephalus: An analysis of the callosal angle's utility. *World Neurosurg*, 115: e712-722.

[20] Yin LK, Zheng JJ, Zhao L, Hao XZ, Zhang XX, Tian JQ. (2017). Reversed aqueductal cerebrospinal net flow in idiopathic normal pressure hydrocephalus. *Acta Neurol Scand*, 136: 434-439.

[21] Perry A, Graffeo CS, Fattahi N, ElSheikh MM, Cray N, Arani A, Ehman RL, Glaser KJ, Manduca A, Meyer FB, Huston J. (2017). Clinical correlation of abnormal finding on magnetic resonance elastography in idiopathic normal pressure hydrocephalus. *World Neurosurg*, 99:695-700.

[22] Dixon GR, Friedman JA, Luetmer PH, Quast LM, McClelland RL, Peterson RC, Maher CO, Ebersold MJ. (2002). Use of cerebrospinal fluid flow rates measured by

phase contrast MR to predict outcome of ventriculoperitoneal shunting for idiopathic normal pressure hydrocephalus. *Mayo Clin Proc*, 77:509-14.

[23] Ringstad G, Vatnehol SA, Eide PK. (2017). Glymphatic MRI in idiopathic normal pressure hydrocephalus. *Brain,* 140: 2691-705.

[24] Takizawa K, Matsumae M, Hayashi N, Hirayama A, Yatsushiro S, Kuroda K. (2017). Hyper dynamic CSF motion profiles found in idiopathic normal pressure hydrocephalus and alzheimer's disease assessed by fluid mechanics derived from magnetic resonance images. *Fluid barriers CNS*, 14:29.

[25] Yamada S, Ishikawa M, Iwamuro Y, Yamamoto K. (2016). Choroidal fissure acts as an overflow device in cerebrospinal fluid drainage: Morphological comparison between idiopathic and secondary normal pressure hydrocephalus. *Sci Rep,* 6:39070.

[26] Ziegelitz D, Arvidsson J, Hellstrom P, Tullberg M, Wikkelso C, Starck G. (2016). Pre-and post-operative cerebral blood flow changes in patients with idiopathic normal pressure hydrocephalus measured by computed tomography (CT) perfusion. *J Cereb Blood Flow Metab*, 36:1755-66.

[27] Czerwosz L, Szczepek E, Nowinski K, Sokolowska B, Jurkiewicz J, Czernicki Z, Koszewski W. (2018). Discriminant analysis of intracranial volumetric variables in patients with normal pressure hydrocephalus and brain atrophy. *Adv Exp Med Biol,* 1039:83-94.

[28] Gammal TE, Allen Mb Jr, Brooks BS. MR evaluation of hydrocephalus. (1987). *AJR Am J Roentfenol,* 149:807-13.

[29] Liew BS, Takagi K, Kato Y, Duvuru S, Thanapal S, Mangaleswaran B. (2019). Current updates on idiopathic normal pressure hydrocephalus. *Asian J Neurosurg,* 14:648-656.

[30] Miyajima M, Kazui H, Mori E, Ishkawa M. (2016). On behalf of the SINPHONI-2 Invesigators. One year outcome in patients with idiopathic normal pressure hydrocephalus: Comparison of lumboperitoneal shunt to ventriculoperitoneal shunt. *Neurosurg,* 125: 1483-92.

[31] Bayer MA, Tekiner A, Celik H, Yilmaz A, Menekse G, Yildirim T, Algoz F, Guvenc Y, Erdem Y. (2018). Efficacy of lumboperitoneal shunting in patients with normal pressure hydrocephalus. *Turk Neurosurg*, 28:62-66.

[32] Grigorean VT, Sandu AM, Popescu M, Florian IS, Lupascu CD, Ursulescu CL. (2017). Our initial experience with Ventriculo-epiploic shunt in treatment of hydrocephalus in two centers. *Neurol Neurochir Pol*, 51: 290-298.

[33] Tudor KI, Tudor M, McCleery J, Car J. (2015). Endoscopic third ventriculostomy (ETV) for idiopathic normal pressure hydrocephalus (iNPH). *Cochrane Database Syst Rev*, (7): CD010033.

[34] Hung AL, Vivas-Buitrago T, Adam A, Lu J, Robison J, Elder BD, Goodwin CR, Tores IJ, Rigamonti D. (2017). Ventriculoatrial versus ventriculoperitoneal shunt complications in idiopathic normal pressure hydrocephalus. *Clin Neurol Neuro Surg*, 157:1-6.

Chapter 4

Neuromonitoring in the Brain and Spinal Cord

Arjun Shankar Dasgupta and Sandip Chatterjee*

Park Clinic, Kolkata,India

Abstract

Intraoperative neurophysiological monitoring (IONM) is a tool that we use to assess the integrity of our central and peripheral nervous system during the operation. It helps us to know about any iatrogenic injury to the neural tissue and most importantly we can prevent or rectify the same and have an objective data that can predict our operative outcome. We can also achieve the maximum safe resection of tumours or correction of deformity. This tool can well be used in both cranial and spinal surgeries. It can be used to localise eloquent areas in brain by cortical and subcortical mapping; can monitor most of the cranial nerves by triggered electromyography (EMG), brainstem auditory evoked potential (BAER); can monitor spinal cord motor and sensory pathways by means of motor evoked potentials (MEP) and somatosensory evoked potential (SSEP) respectively. Thus, it has become an inevitable tool in brain surgery in and around eloquent areas, epilepsy surgery, surgery for spinal cord tumors and spinal deformity and lot more. In this chapter we shall try to give an overview of IONM, its physiological basis, anaesthetic consideration and different modalities used in contemporary neurosurgical practices.

* Corresponding Author's Email: sandipchat@gmail.com.

In: Advances in Neurosurgery Research
Editors: Amit Agrawal, Pradeep Chouksey, Adesh Shrivastava et al.
ISBN: 978-1-68507-859-1

Introduction

The basis of intraoperative neurophysiological monitoring relies on the fact that one can get a response at the effector organs by stimulating the central nervous system and the signal can go from periphery also by an afferent pathway to create electrical changes in brain. Intra operative neuromonitoring has replaced the neurological examination in an anaesthetized patient [1]. Any loss of integrity in the circuit will cause interruption of signal transmission and this interruption or decrement in the level of signal intensity (like amplitude of waves or latency after stimulation) can be recorded and reproduced. Thus, use of this neurophysiological monitoring can be helpful for brain and spine surgery not only to predict the outcome but also can detect intra operatively any injury so that early intervention can be planned because post operative neuro-deficit not only increases the post operative morbidity and mortality but also it inflates the cost of treatment [2]. Ankle clonus test [3] and Stagnara wake up test [4] were used before to assess the functional status of the spinal cord in patients undergoing surgery. These tests could predict only the gross injury to the motor tract and required emergence from anesthesia so it was very difficult to use them repeatedly. Hence there was need for some modalities which could monitor the functional status of the brain and spinal cord effectively and continuously without waking the patient up periodically during the surgical procedure. In this chapter we shall be discussing in brief about the basic modalities of intra operative neurophysiological monitoring and its usefulness, the anesthetic consideration and the challenges associated with it.

IONM data are either obtained quasi continuously [sensory and motor evoked potentials (SSEP and MEP), electroencephalography (EEG), and free-run electromyography (fEMG)] or at specific time points such as for functional-anatomic localization (direct nerve and cortical stimulation).

History

Wilder Penfield (1891-1976) in his publication with Edwin Boldrey in the journal Brain summarized his work on the motor and sensory system's organization in the cerebral cortex of humans with the help of intra-operative electrical stimulation. This brilliant experiment laid the foundation for the field of intraoperative neurophysiological monitoring [5]. By the late 1970s somatosensory evoked potential (SSEP) became a routine need for intraoperative assessment of functional integrity of somatosensory system in spinal surgery [6]. The first surgeon to mention the need for developing this technology was Dr. Jacquelin Perry, working at Rancho Los Amigos Hospital. With the advent of noninvasive trans cranial electrical stimulation, motor responses were first reported in 1980 by Merton and Morton [7]. These authors succeeded in recording evoked muscle action potentials after stimulating the human brain motor cortex transcranially. The key to their success was high-voltage stimulation with a 0.1 μF condenser charged to ~2,000 V delivered through electroencephalogram electrodes, although this did not work in the operating theatre. Then in 1987 Levy first described the use of trans cranial electrical motor evoked potentials (TcMEP) in an anaesthetized individual, marking the beginning of the modern era of intra-operative neurophysiological assessment of motor function [8]. Nakagawa et al., [*] carried out an animal experimental study and found that CMAP (muscle MEP), used for multimodal spinal cord monitoring, provided the most sensitive method of monitoring possible ischemic and compressive insults to the spinal cord during surgical procedures.

In India, intraoperative neuromonitoring was started in CMC Vellore in the late eighties, but was mainly used as a research tool. Its widespread acceptance in neurosurgery occurred after its start in spinal deformity surgery by orthopaedic spinal colleagues in the early part of this century.

Anaesthesia in IONM

The main challenge in obtaining a response during IONM in an anesthetized patient is to minimize the effects of different drugs. The basic requirement is to use a short acting muscle relaxant at the time of intubation and then to maintain the patient on total intra venous anesthesia. Though the halogenated compounds have very minimal effect in somatosensory evoked potential but they can definitely decrease the amplitude of the same and for motor evoked potential the patient should be completely free from the effects of muscle relaxants. At our institution we use total intravenous anesthesia (TIVA) with Propofol infusion at a dose of 100-150 microgram/kg/hr and Fentanyl infusion at 1-2 microgram/kg/hr after small dose of short acting muscle relaxant for endotracheal intubation [9]. Intra operative monitoring of bi spectral index (BIS) and train of four (TOF) count helps to determine the depth of anaesthesia and weaning from muscle relaxant respectively. For any motor evoked potential a TOF count of more than 80 is desirable.

Modalities of IONM used in neurosurgery can be classified broadly into 2 groups. One where continuous monitoring of spontaneous electrical activities are monitored and another is evoked potentials. Raw Electromyography (EMG), electro encephalography or electrocorticography are monitored as spontaneous electrical activities of CNS and motor evoked potential (muscle MEP), Somatosensory evoked potential (SSEP), Triggered EMG, brainstem auditory evoked potential (BERA) etc., belong to the second category. Which modalities are to be used during a neurosurgical procedure depends on the discretion of surgeon and neurophysiologists, and proper planning as a team before the surgery is essential for smooth conduction of IONM and to achieve the best possible outcome.

Technical Consideration

A dedicated team of personnel is desired for proper conduction of IONM. The scalp electrodes are attached according to 10-20 system of EEG recording and the muscles of interests are monitored for motor evoked potential. (Figure 1). It is to be noted that to get a desired baseline for muscle MEPs the muscle of interest should at least have grade 3 preferably grade 4/5 power [10]. The checklist for the technicians are to see and minimize noise artifact, proper placement of electrodes in muscle for stimulating electrode not in subcutaneous tissue, to minimize the intensity of simulation and to maintain collaboration with anaesthesia team. Proper positioning and use bite blocks can prevent untoward incidents. We prefer to use transparent drapes during the procedures as then the muscle twitching can be easily observed.

Analysis of electrophysiological signals is based on 3 properties of the recorded signals: (1) the amplitude, or height of the response, referenced to some baseline or between the highest and lowest recorded points; (2) the latency, or time of the response from the start of the stimulation; and (3) the wave shape (determined by the frequency or spectral content of the activity).

Motor Evoked Potential

Motor evoked potential is obtained from the effector organs on stimulation over the motor cortex. It can be obtained directly from spinal cord as direct wave (D wave) or from the muscles as muscle MEPs. The physiology behind the generation of MEP is explained below.

In a normal awake patient, electrical stimulus to cortex or sub cortical white matter with a single electrical pulse produces a number of responses that can be recorded by thoracic epidural electrode. First recorded wave is called D-wave and subsequent waves, generated due to synaptic activity are called I-waves. Hence, I wave can be strongly suppressed with general anesthesia. The anterior horn cell (AHC) which is the beginning of final common pathway for motor responses respond optimally to a multiple sequential time locked stimulus i.e., train of stimuli [1, 11]. Trans cranial motor evoked potential in an anesthetized person is a bit complex due to lack of synaptic activity (Figure 1). So, there will be lack of I wave and the AHC senses a single D wave and there is lack of firing resulting in no muscle response. In addition, there is a reduction in spontaneous activity in the inter-neurons of the spinal cord during General Anesthesia reducing overall level of excitation reaching the AHCs. The solution lies in giving trains of stimuli. As the depression of intrinsic activity of spinal cord is maximum with halogenated anesthetics and nitrous oxide, they are generally avoided during intra operative monitoring of MEP [12]. The use of total intravenous anesthesia with Propofol is preferred while monitoring muscle MEP as it suppresses the intrinsic response to a lesser degree than inhalational anesthetic agents. A good understanding of neural anatomy, impact of physiology and anesthetic medications can allow effective intra operative monitoring and good team decision making when changes in recording occurs [13]. Since the D-wave is a purely nerve action potential and does not involve synaptic activity, it is relatively insensitive to the effects of muscle relaxants [1, 14].

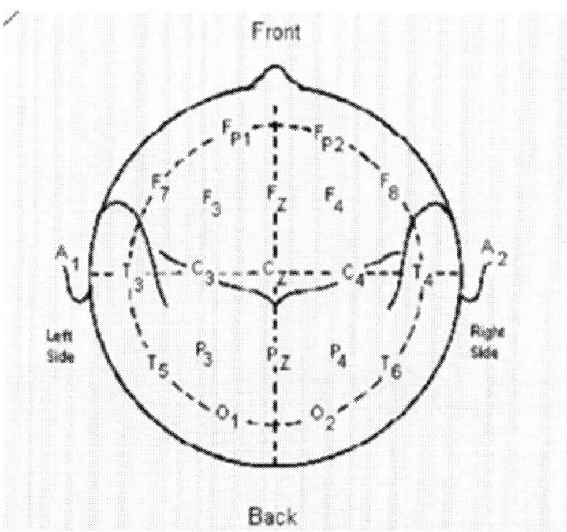

Figure 1. The 10-20 system of electrodes on the scalp.

The preoperative muscle power if less than MRC grade 3/5, the baseline m MEPs are not satisfactory most of the time. The muscle MEP monitoring has a high sensitivity in most series but is often criticized to have low specificity. Sensitivity and specificity of m MEP in predicting post operative neurological status is shown in table 1.

Table 1. Different studies showing sensitivity and specificity of m MEP in predicting post operative outcome. (m MEP- myogenic motor evoked potential)

Study	Year	Diagnosis	Criteria for significant fall in m MEP	Sensitivity	Specificity
Krammer et al., [15]	2009	Spinal tumor	50% fall in amplitude	83%	86%
Hyun and Rhim [16]	2009	Intramedullary spinal SOL	50% fall in amplitude	100%	25%
Forster et al., [17]	2012	Spinal tumor	Presence or absence	95%	98.9%
Choi et al., [18]	2014	Intra medullary spinal SOL	75% fall in amplitude	94%	94%

Direct Wave

Direct wave is actually a motor evoked potential recorded directly from spinal cord with stimulation over motor cortex. It helps in real time assessment of pyramidal tract and is more sensitive than muscle motor evoked potentials to assess its integrity. The stimulating electrodes are same as muscle motor evoked potential that is corkscrew electrodes placed at C3-C4 over scalp or it can also be placed epidurally or subdurally proximal to the lesion at spinal cord for direct cord to cord stimulation. The recording electrode can be placed epidurally or subdurally distal to the lesion. Placing subdurally blindly has its risk of damaging any vascular structure. In our institution we routinely place the electrode epidurally (Figure 2). The wave forms can be obtained repeatedly and there is no need to discontinue the procedure. Drop in amplitude by more than 50% is taken as significant.

D-wave recording is used mainly for intramedullary spinal cord tumor and is regarded as the gold standard for it [14]. D wave has a very high negative predictive value and many a time we can find the muscle MEPs are significantly reduced in amplitude with preserved D wave, and this indicates almost all the time that post operative deficit if any is going to be transient and the surgeon can safely perform the surgery as long as the D waves are preserved (Figure 3) [11, 14].

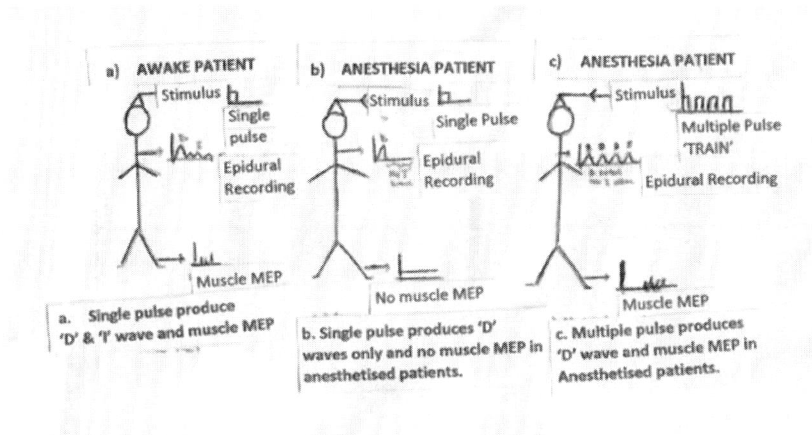

Figure 2. Effect of transcranial stimulus at different levels of motor path way.

Only disadvantage of this modality of monitoring is it cannot be used for lesions below D10 spinal level as it is difficult to place the catheter below that and obtain satisfactory waveform from the pyramidal tract.

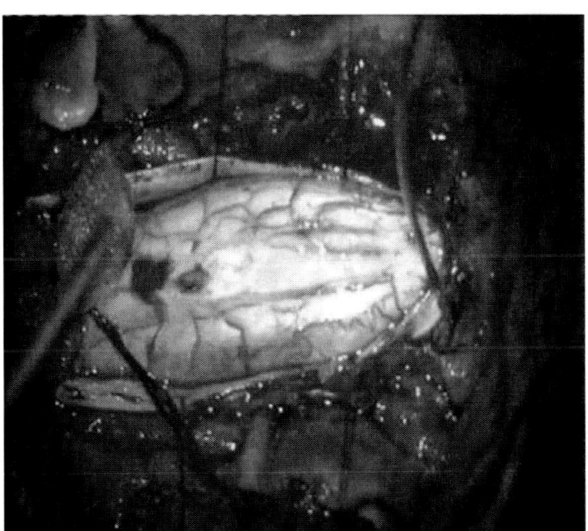

Figure 3. Epidurally placed D wave electrode.

Somatosensory Evoked Potential

SSEP is recorded from the peripheral nerve, spinal cord or sensory cortex following stimulation of peripheral nerves. It shows the integrity of sensory pathway more precisely the dorsal column. It is monitored continuously and the averaging is done after few fixed number of stimuli and the latency and the amplitude is monitored. Both of these parameters are well influenced by halogenated anesthetic agents and nitrous oxide and so we need to be cautious about this [19]. The SSEPs are mainly recorded by surface electrodes from median nerve for lesions above C8 and from posterior tibial nerve for lesions below it. Prolongation of latency of more than 10% and drop in amplitude of more than 50% is taken as significant [20]. It is very useful as minute ischemic insults that can occur with surgical manipulation can show change in SSEP which can be restored by rectifying the insult rendered.

SSEP monitoring is now indispensable for correction of spinal deformity as it can guide us as to precisely the amount of distraction we can do safely without inflicting any ischemia to the cord. SSEP is now widely used during spinal vascular malformation surgery, for surgery of aortic aneurysms where cord ischemia has to be monitored closely. In cranial surgery also we use SSEP monitoring in phase reversal technique to locate the central sulcus, during carotid endarterectomy and also surgery for aneurysms and other vascular lesions. Like D wave the SSEP also has a very high negative predictive value of 99.9%.

SSEP monitoring is not very effective in intramedullary spinal cord lesions as we tend to lose it if the myelotomy is not done exactly at physiological midline [21].

Triggered Electromyography

It is a modality of IONM used mostly in lesions around cauda equina, peripheral nerves and during procedures such as Dorsal rhizotomy. We can use this modality to identify the filum terminale before detethering of spinal cord as the filum is regarded as relatively electrophysiologically inert [22]. Around 2 mAmp current is used to stimulate the structure in question and bipolar electrodes are most often used to prevent antidromic spread of current. The principle of triggered EMG is also used in brain surgeries to surgically map the motor cortex. In many centers placement of pedicle screws are sometimes done with triggered EMG monitoring to avoid medial or inferior cortical breach [23].

IONM in Cranial Surgeries

The main use of IONM in cranial procedure are – 1) in lesions in and around the motor cortex or other eloquent cortex to achieve maximal safe resection. 2) in lesions with direct proximity to the cranial nerves where it is mandatory to preserve its function. 3) in epilepsy surgery, to know the extent of resection and completeness of the procedure. Along with functional MRI and Diffusion tensor imaging, IONM is an added adjunct that has made neurosurgery safer like never before.

Phase Reversal Technique and Motor Cortex Mapping

Phase reversal technique is a procedure where we use Somatosensory evoked potential to be recorded by a strip or grid electrode placed anteroposteriorly over the bare cortex and see the phase reversal of the SSEP which is the guide to locate the central sulcus (Figure 4). The stimulation is made over the contralateral median or posterior tibial nerve most often to detect the central sulcus. Then after locating the sulcus, direct cortical stimulation is used anteriorly to evoke responses same as triggered EMG and to precisely map the motor cortex [24, 25]. The stimulation is often delivered by bipolar stimulating electrode and generally 0.5-2 m Amp stimulation is used. It is our practice to then label the hand, face and leg areas before beginning any resection around the motor cortex. The stimulation can also be done subcortically to locate eloquent areas and to save the same. We at our institution routinely use a stimulating electrode which goes through the suction, the so-called suction stimulator during resection of lesions in close proximity to the motor cortex. Generally it is a dictum that if response is obtained by 1m Amp stimulation the corresponding area is at most within 1 cm from our surgical site, and thus we can achieve maximum safe resection.

Use of this technique is now invaluable during surgery of lesions in and around motor cortex.

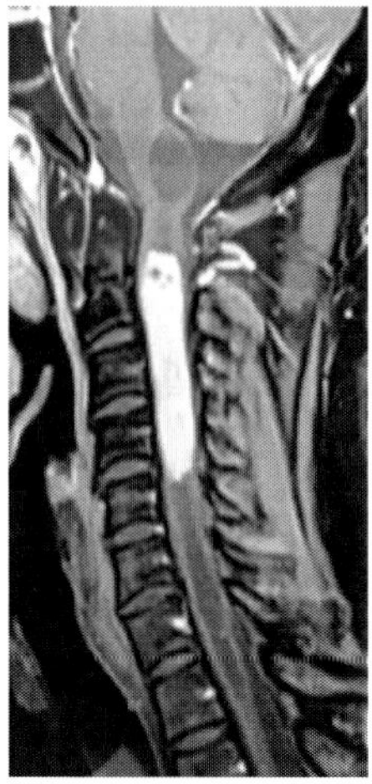

(A)

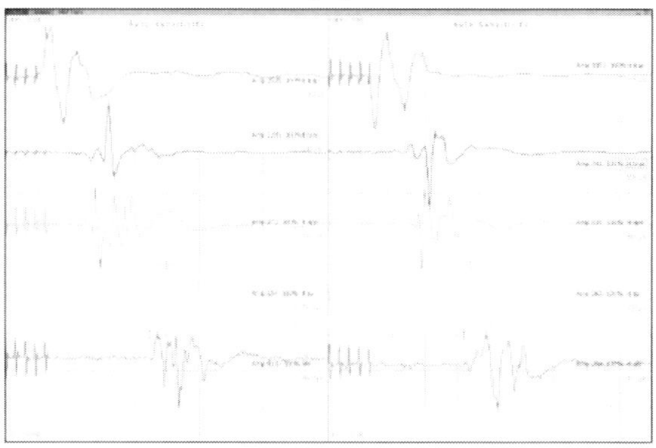

(B)

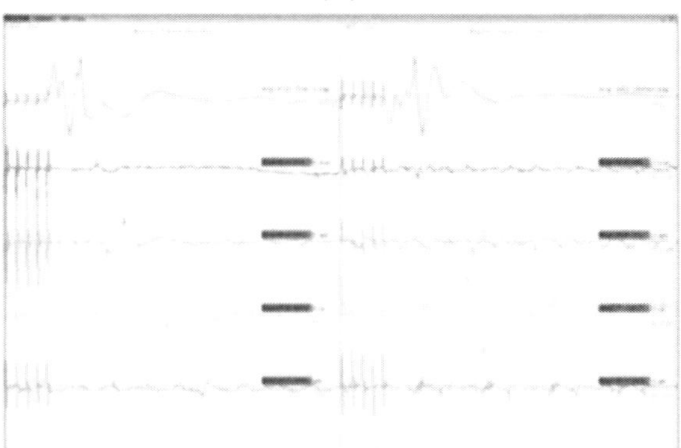

(C)

Figure 4. (Continued).

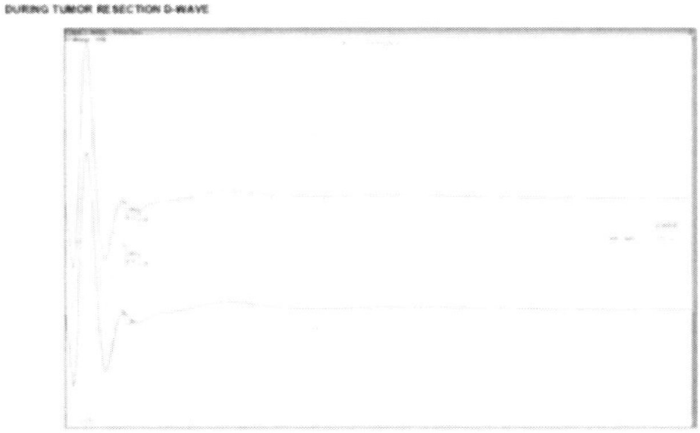

(D)

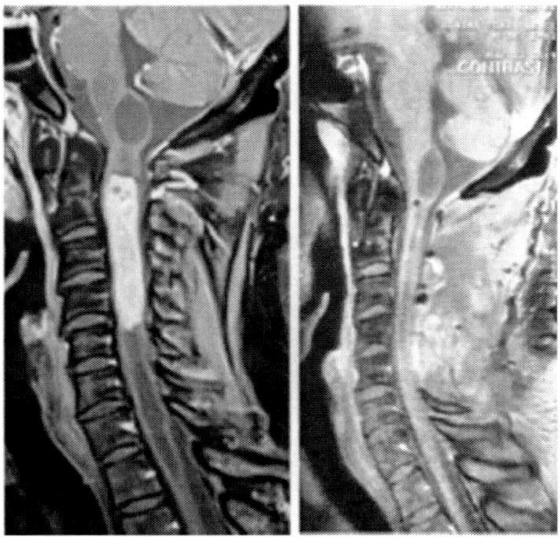

(E)

Figure 4. (A-E): showing role of D wave in intramedullary spinal tumor. (A) cervical intramedullary spinal cord tumor with syringomyelia. (B) satisfactory baseline m MEP. (C) significant fall in m MEP during tumor dissection. (D) preserved D wave. (E) complete excision of tumor possible without any permanent neurodeficit.

Electrocorticography

Electrocorticography is now routinely used for epilepsy surgeries specially for resection technique. The grid electrode is placed in the area of interest and the resection is continued till we achieve electrically stable recordings in electrocorticography. It helps in complete removal of epileptogenic zone [26].

Monitoring of Cranial Nerves

Can be done by muscle motor evoked potential for 5th, 7th, 10th, 11th and 12th cranial nerves. The same needle electrodes used for monitoring limb muscles can be used here. At our institution we routinely use Massetor for 5th, orbicularis oris for 7th, trapizeus for 11th and tongue muscles for 12th cranial nerves. Specially designed endotracheal tubes can be used for 10th nerve monitoring that can obtain response from laryngeal muscles. Many institutions use invasive techniques to obtain responses from extraocular muscles to monitor 3rd, 4th and 6th cranial nerves. Intra operative brainstem auditory evoked response and even visual evoked response can be obtained to monitor 8th and 2nd nerves respectively. Intra operatively triggered EMG can help us to localize 7th cranial nerve during acoustic neuroma surgery [27].

We can use cranial nerve monitoring in surgeries for cerebellopontine angle lesions [27], brain stem lesions, lesions around jugular foramen, petroclival lesions and lesions in close proximity to cavernous sinus [27, 28].

Limitations and Adverse Effects

Although intra operative neuromonitoring has made a neurosurgeon's life safer, it has its limitations. Judicious use of muscle relaxants and inhalational anaesthetic agents is an essential prerequisite for neuromonitoring. The waveforms can be influenced by operating room noise, use of diathermy, blood pressure, temperature etc. The procedure itself warrants presence of specialized person in the theatre and can cause overcrowding.

Adverse effects are also documented. Seizure is a possibility with trans cranial stimulation or direct motor cortex stimulation. Tongue bite is another potential hazard which can be prevented by use of bite blocks or Guedel's airway [11]. Dislodgement of needle electrodes can cause serious problem which we have also encountered. The main limitation about the use of this adjunct is its cost. In developing countries we have to use it judiciously to cut down the overall expenditure.

There is no doubt that IONM has positive effects in identifying neurological deficits, but it has the disadvantage of increasing surgical time and costs. Anesthesia needs to be modified, and there are medicolegal ramifications if a neurological event occurs. Additionally, IONM may not identify or avoid further neurological injury once neural tissue damage has occurred.

Future Directions

The science of IONM is continuously evolving. Now from mapping of motor cortex, we are moving towards brainstem mapping and spinal cord mapping by collision technique [11]. With spinal phase reversal we can detect the physiological midline and do a myelotomy safely, and we can do dorsal column mapping. IONM combined with neuronavigation, imunofluoroscence and DTI techniques are being done now more commonly to achieve maximum safe resection [25] in tumours. The basis of neural prosthesis is also related to neuromonitoring techniques and we are now a part of never-ending technological revolution.

Conclusion

Intraoperative neuromonitoring is now an inevitable tool for neurosurgical procedures. Judicial use of IONM can justify the extra cost it carries. It needs teamwork inside the theatre to achieve its maximum potential. It helps patients to have a better post operative outcome and definitely helps neurosurgeons during surgeries by reducing chances of adverse events and also helps to avoid and fight future litigations.

References

[1] Stecker Mark M; A review of intra operative monitoring for spinal surgery; *Surg. Neurol. Int.* 2012; 3 (supp l3): S174-S187.

[2] Szelenyi A, Langer D, Kothbauer K, De Camargo A B, Flamm E S, Deletis V. Monitoring of muscle motor evoked potentials during cerebral aneurysm Hoppenfeld S, Gross A, Andrews C, Lonner B. The ankle clonus test for assessment of the integrity of the spinal cord during operations for scoliosis. *J. Bone Joint Surg. Am.* (1997) 79:208–12.

[3] Hoppenfeld S, Gross A, Andrews C, Lonner B. The ankle clonus test for assessment of the integrity of the spinal cord during operations for scoliosis. *J. Bone Joint Surg. Am.* (1997) 79:208–12.

[4] Vauzelle C, Stagnara P, Jouvinroux P. Functional monitoring of spinal cord activity during spinal surgery. *Clin. Orthop. Relat, Res.,* (1973) 93:173–8.

[5] Penfield W, Boldrey E; Somatic motor and sensory representation in the cerebral cortex of man as studied by electrical stimulus; *Brain*; 1937; vol 60: 339-443.

[6] Engler G L, Spelholz N I, Bernhard W N, Danziger F, Merkin H, Wolff T; Somatosensory evoked potentials during Harrington instrumentation for scoliosis; *J. Bone joint surg*.; 1978; vol 60: 528-532.
[7] Merton P A, Morton H B; Stimulation of the cerebral cortex in the intact human subject; *Nature*; 1980; 285 (5762): 227.
[8] Levy W J Jr; Clinical experience with motor and cerebellar evoked potential monitoring; *Neurosurgery*; 1987; 20(1): 169-182.
[9] Kothbauer K F; Intraoperative neurophysiological monitoring in spinal cord surgery; *European neurological review*; 2008; 3(1): 56-58.
[10] Rajshekhar V, Velayutham P, Joseph M, Babu K S; Factors predicting the feasibility of monitoring lower limb muscles motor evoked potentials in patients undergoing excision of spinal cord tumors; *J. Neurosurg. Spine*. 2011 Jun; 14(6) :746-53.
[11] Deletis V, Sala F; Intraoperative neurophysiological monitoring of the spinal cord during spinal cord and spine surgery: a review focus on the corticospinal tracts; *Clin. Neurophysiol*. Feb 2008; vol 119(2):248-64. E pub. 28 Nov, 2007.
[12] Sloan T. Anesthesia and motor evoked potential monitoring; In: Deletis V, Stils J Editors; *Neurophysiology in Neurosurgery*. San Diego, California. Academic Press; 2002 pp. :452-74.
[13] Jameson L C, Sloan T B; Monitoring of the brain and spinal cord; *Anaesthesiol. Clin.;* Dec 2006; Vol 24(4):777-91.
[14] Costa P, Peretta P, Faccani G; Relevance of intraoperative D wave in spine and spinal cord *surgeries; Eur. Spine. J.*; 2013; vol22:840-848.
[15] Krammer M J, Wolf S, Schul D B, Gerstner W, Lumenta C B: significance of intraoperative motor function monitoring using transcranial electrical motor evoked potential (MEP) in patients with spinal and cranial lesions near the motor pathway. *Br. J. Neurosurg*. 2009 (23) : 48-55.
[16] Hyun S J, Rhim S C; Combined motor and somato sensory evoked potential monitoring for intramedullary spinal cord tumor surgery: correlation of clinical and neurophysiological data in 17 consequtive procedures. *Br. J. Neurosurg*. 2009 (23): 393-400.
[17] Forster M T, Marquardt G, Seifert V, Szelenyi A: Spinal cord tumor surgery – importance of continuous intraoperative neurophysiological monitoring after tumor resection. *Spine* (Phila Pa 1976) 2012; 37 : E1001-08.
[18] Choi I, Hyun S J, Kang J K, Rhim S C: combined muscle motor and somato sensory evoked potentials for intra medullary spinal cord tumor surgery. *Yonsei. Med. J.* 2014 (55):1063-1071.
[19] Peterson DO, Drummond JC, Todd MM. Effects of halothane, enflurane, isoflurane, and nitrous oxide on somatosensory evoked potentials in humans. *Anesthesiology*. 1986 Jul;65(1):35-40.
[20] Kundnani V K, Zhu L, Tak H, Won H; Multimodal intraoperative neuromonitoring in corrective surgery for adolescent idiopathic scoliosis: evaluation of 354 consecutive cases; *Indian J. Orthop*. 2010; 44: 66-72.
[21] Park J H, Hyun S J. Intraoperative neurophysiological monitoring in spinal surgery. *World J. Clin. Cases*. 2015;3(9):765-773.

[22] Quiñones-Hinojosa A, Gadkary C.A, Gulati M, von Koch C.S, Lyon R, Weinstein PR, Yingling CD. Neurophysiological monitoring for safe surgical tethered cord syndrome release in adults. *Surg. Neurol.* 2004 Aug;62(2):127-33.
[23] Mikula A L, Williams S K, Anderson P A. The use of intraoperative triggered electromyography to detect misplaced pedicle screws: a systematic review and meta-analysis. *J. Neurosurg. Spine.* 2016 Apr;24(4):624-38.
[24] Simon M V, Sheth S A, Eckhardt C A, Kilbride R D, Braver D, Williams Z, Curry W, Cahill D, Eskandar E N. Phase reversal technique decreases cortical stimulation time during motor mapping. *J. Clin. Neurosci.* 2014 Jun;21(6):1011-7.
[25] Romstöck J, Fahlbusch R, Ganslandt O, et al. Localisation of the sensorimotor cortex during surgery for brain tumours: feasibility and waveform patterns of somatosensory evoked potentials; *Journal of Neurology, Neurosurgery & Psychiatry* 2002;72:221-229.
[26] Kuruvilla A, Flink R. Intraoperative electrocorticography in epilepsy surgery: useful or not? *Seizure.* 2003 Dec;12(8):577-84.
[27] Yingling C D, Gardi J N. Intraoperative monitoring of facial and cochlear nerves during acoustic neuroma surgery. *Otolaryngol. Clin. North Am.* 1992 Apr;25(2): 413-48.
[28] Kartush J M, Larouere M J, Graham M D, Bouchard K R, Audet BV. Intraoperative cranial nerve monitoring during posterior skull base surgery. *Skull Base Surg.* 1991;1(2):85-92.

Chapter 5

Traumatic Brain Injury and Point of Care Ultrasound in Emergency Departments

Tej Prakash Sinha[*], MS and Ayush Srivastava, MD

Department of Medicine (Trauma Centre), Emergency Medicine,
All India Institute of Medical Sciences, New Delhi, Inda

Abstract

Point of care ultrasonography (POCUS) has become an indispensable tool for patient evaluation and management in the Emergency and Intensive care unit. It is an easy to deploy, non-invasive, and repeatable diagnostic tool that can be utilized by the treating physician to augment physical examination and decision making. Patients with traumatic brain injury are often detected with conditions that might have adverse effect on outcome, if not attended to promptly. Stabilization of airway, breathing and circulation takes precedence in such patients and POCUS can assist in management of airway, as well as help in early detection of Pneumothorax, Hemothorax and Intraperitoneal bleed. As a part of Disability assessment, POCUS can help in assessment of pupillary size and reflex especially in patients with severe periorbital edema due to trauma. Ultrasonographic measurement of optic nerve sheath diameter (ONSD) has been found to correlate well with the intracranial pressure and can be repeated as per convenience and need. Similarly, in presence of an optimal acoustic window, such as an open fontanelle in neonates and defects in patients with decompressive craniotomy, excellent sonographic views of the brain parenchyma and related structures can be obtained. As such, point of care ultrasonography can be utilized in management of all aspects of emergency care in a patient with Traumatic brain injury.

[*] Corresponding Author's Email: drsinha123@gmail.com.

In: Advances in Neurosurgery Research
Editors: Amit Agrawal, Pradeep Chouksey, Adesh Shrivastava et al.
ISBN: 978-1-68507-859-1

Introduction

The concept of seeing things through sound waves comes from nature. Bats use ultrasound to create an image of their surroundings in the pitch-dark caves so as to navigate through it. The same concept was applied to submarines in the First World War that later found its way into medical diagnostics. The pioneer of diagnostic ultrasound was Karl Thoedore Dussik, an Austrian Neurologist and Psychiatrist at university of Vienna, who in the year 1942 used ultrasound beams for the purpose of diagnosing brain tumors. Ultrasound was incorporated into medical diagnostic system by the year 1965. The ultrasound machine later found its way to the bedside of the patient by the year 1980 and since then has become an indispensable part of patient evaluation and care in Emergency department and ICUs. Point of care Ultrasonography (POCUS) is an easy to deploy, non-invasive, non-radiating and repeatable diagnostic tool that can be used as an adjunct to clinical and physical examination of a patient.

Knobology

Ultrasonography requires a probe or transducer that emits sound waves of high frequency through a patient's body. The core of the transducer consists of piezoelectric material that converts electric energy into a mechanical pulse of sound that is then directed towards the body. The sound wave crosses the skin and traverses through the internal anatomy propagating through different tissues. A part of the sound energy is reflected at the surface between tissues of different densities, the proportion of which depends upon the difference in acoustic impedance of the two tissues. The reflected echo returns to the transducer, where it is converted to an electric signal and then processed to form the ultrasound image displayed on the screen.

The image obtained is a grayscale image, where the tissues and organs are usually represented as dots of variable brightness, the brightness depending on the amplitude of the reflected echo.

The tissues or medium with a higher acoustic impedance appear white, like the bone cortex, calcified gallstones and air. As these structures strongly reflect sound waves, there is a signal void behind these structures, leading to an imaging artifact, known as Acoustic Shadowing.

Homogenous fluids (blood, urine, effusions) transmit sound waves without producing echoes and appear black.

Organs like the liver are partway between the above two and appear gray.

The present-day ultrasonography machines use transducers that may either be linear array, or phased array.

- Linear Probe: Also known as the linear sequential array, is designed for superficial imaging. It utilizes high frequencies (5-13 MHz) that are useful in obtaining high-resolution images of superficial structures. They produce a rectangular field of view with uniform beam density throughout.
- Curvilinear Probe: Also called the convex probe. It is basically a linear array system but the crystals are arranged along a curved surface, thereby resulting in a wider field of view. The curvilinear probe uses low-frequency sound waves for deeper penetration and is best suited for abdominal and pelvic examination.

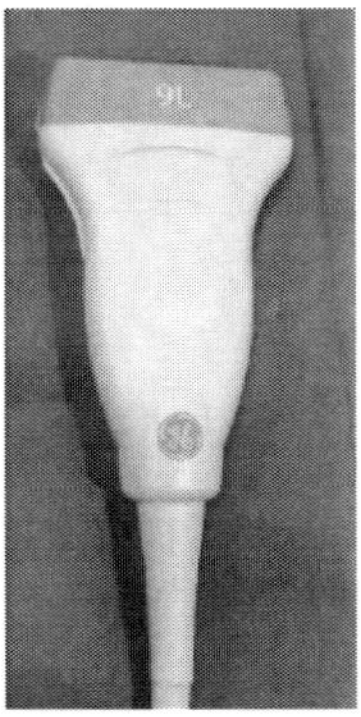

Figure 1. Linear probe.

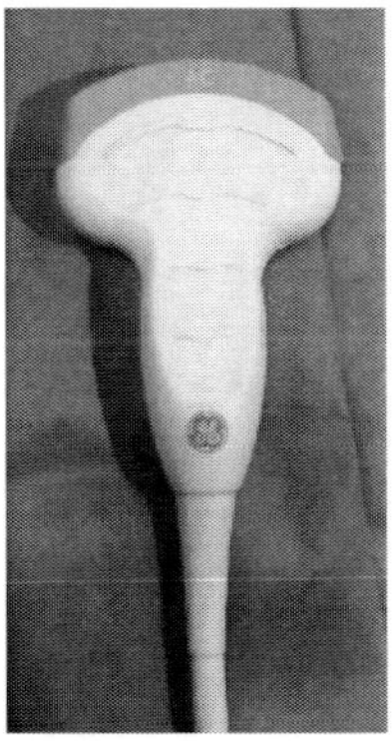

Figure 2. Curvilinear probe.

- Phased Array Probe: Phased array probes usually have a smaller footprint, but produce an electronically steerable and focused beam which helps obtain a wider field of image despite the smaller footprint. The probe is best suitable for areas with a limited acoustic window, such as the rib cage. It can also be used for Trans fontanelle ultrasonography of infant brain.

Orientation

Correct orientation of the probe is always important to obtain reliable images. While obtaining a longitudinal image, make sure the probe marker points towards the head of the patient. Similarly, while obtaining a transverse image, the marker should point towards the right side of the body.

Depth

While performing the ultrasound, the Depth should be so adjusted, that the area of interest lies at the center of the screen.

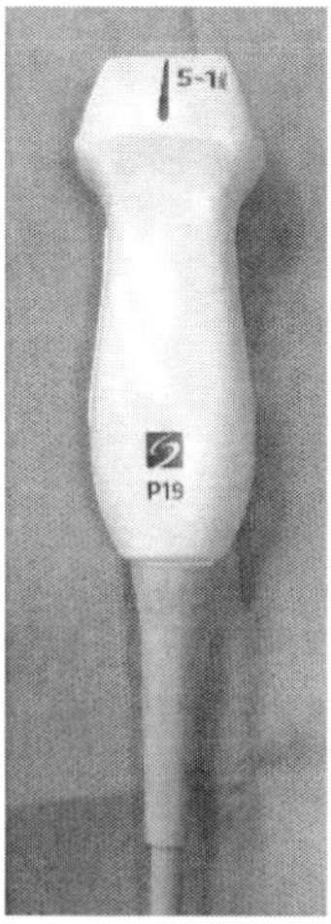

Figure 3. Phased array probe.

Gain

Gain controls the brightness of the image. It can be used for appropriate amplification of the organ of interest. Gain should be used in such a way that the image is neither too bright nor too dark and is uniform in distribution.

Ultrasound in Trauma Emergency

Airway Management: ET Tube Confirmation

Head injury patients with a low GCS (Glagow Coma Scale) often require their airways to be secured by means of endotracheal intubation and mechanical ventilation. Though, in a chaotic emergency department, the intubating conditions may not always be favorable and may result in accidental esophageal intubation. Early detection of any such complications is critical as it may have devastating consequences for the concerned patient. There are multiple methods available to confirm the position of endotracheal tube (ETT), although directly visualizing the passage of the tube in between the vocal cords is the best method. Other clinical assessments include the 5-point auscultation, observation for tube condensation or symmetric chest wall expansion.

The 2015 American Heart Association/Advanced Cardiovascular Life Support guidelines recommend employing quantitative capnography as the criterion standard to confirm ETT placement [1]. Capnographs measure the carbon dioxide in expired air escaping the ETT, the absence of which is suggestive of ETT misplacement. However, capnography has its own limitations including a wait for 4-5 breaths until the appearance of the capnograph waveform. False negative results in patients with cardiac arrest, and false positive results in patients with a hypopharygeal tube placement are not uncommon. Also, quantitative capnograph is not available in many emergency departments.

The use of ultrasound has thus been gaining popularity as it is available bedside, is easy to perform and is non-invasive. It provides a real-time visualization of the ET tube passing through the vocal cords. In case of inadvertent esophageal intubation, one can visualize air-filled esophagus adjacent to the trachea, referred to as the “Double Track Sign.” Necessary steps to correct this can be taken immediately while using ultrasound as compared to waiting for traditional methods of confirming tube placement. A recent meta-analysis demonstrated the excellent performance of ultrasonography in confirmation of ETT placement with an overall sensitivity of 98% and specificity of 95% [2].

Technique

- Tracheal ultrasound can be performed in real-time during the process of intubation, but is not necessary for intubation.
- The examination is conducted using a high-frequency linear probe.
- The probe is initially placed transversely approximately 1 inch above the sternal notch to identify the trachea.
- The trachea appears as a curvilinear structure with posterior shadowing.
- The probe is then moved laterally towards the left sterno-cleidomastoid muscle. Here the esophagus can be visualized just lateral to the trachea, as an oval structure with a hyperechoic wall and hypoechoic center.
- Endotracheal tube in the esophagus will appear as a hyperechoic curvilinear structure with posterior shadowing, situated posterolateral to the trachea.

Cervical Spine Assessment

Head Injury is associated with a cervical spine injury in about 5-10% of cases [3]. Performing airway maneuvers in such patients may aggravate a preexisting undiagnosed injury. Airway management with cervical spine immobilization takes utmost priority during primary survey of the trauma patients. Cervical spine immobilization involves the application of a hard-cervical collar early in the management of patients with significant head injury. In such cases, CT is the screening tool most commonly used to rule out any cervical spine injury because of the high negative predictive value [4]. Ultrasonography in such cases may be used to detect certain cervical spine injuries early in the process, though its use as a screening tool is still uncertain. Vishnu et al. [5] in a study on patients with known cervical spine injuries, demonstrated that POCUS could to identify vertebral body fractures and listhesis between C4 and C7 in 92-100% of the patients. Though there are many limitations as well.

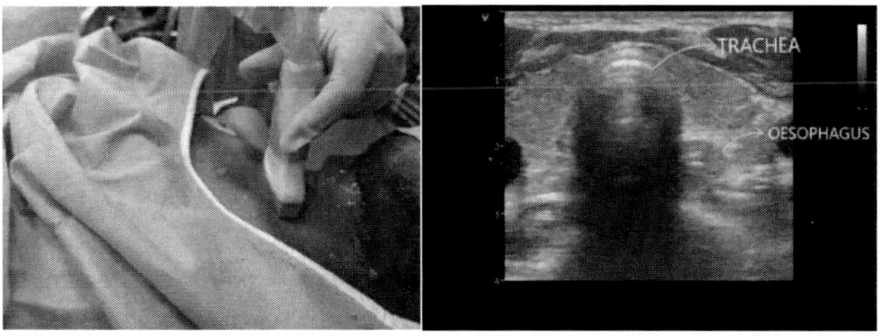

Figure 4. Airway Ultrasound. Left: Liner array probed placed centrally just above the suprasternal Notch. Right: Ultrasound Image showing the trachea and the esophagus.

The major disadvantages of POCUS in evaluating for cervical spine injuries include:

- Availability of only anterior approach for examination as the posterior approach is not feasible in an acutely injured patient.
- Difficulty in the visualization of injuries of the posterior column, transverse process fractures, pedicle fractures and injuries of C1 and C2 [5].

Technique for Cervical Spine examination Using POCUS from anterior approach.

- The ultrasonographic assessment of the cervical spine usually requires the presence of two persons with one person maintaining the in-line stabilization of the spine while the ultrasound is performed by the other person. The anterior part of the cervical collar is first removed before starting the procedure.
- A curvilinear or adult linear probe may be used for the examination. The linear probe provides better image quality, whereas the curvilinear probe is better in terms of visualization of the extent and alignment of vertebrae.
- The probe is initially placed over the neck anteriorly in the midline and maneuvered to identify the thyroid cartilage first.
- Once identified, the probe is then slid down to identify the cricoid cartilage.
- Once the cricoid cartilage is identified, the probe is then moved laterally to visualize the vertebrae, which is identified as a

hyperechoic line with posterior shadowing. The cricoid usually corresponds to the 6th cervical vertebrae

- At this point, the probe is rotated 90° to lie in the longitudinal axis, with the probe marker pointing cranially. The probe is initially fanned to first identify the internal jugular vein and the carotid artery and then moved medially to visualize the cervical spine.

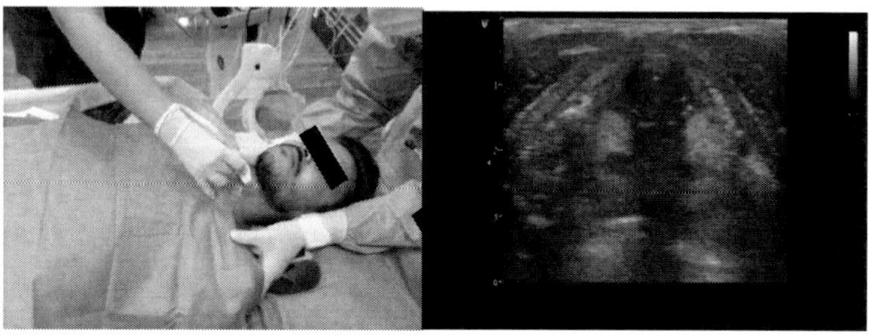

Figure 5. Left: Linear probe positioned transversely at the level of thyroid cartilage. Right: Ultrasonographic image of mid transverse view of the thyroid.

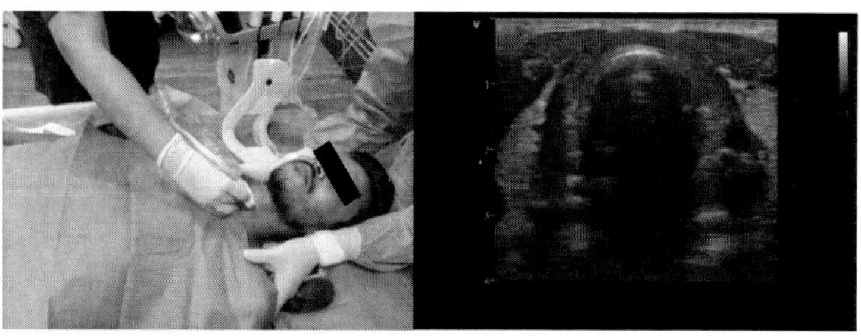

Figure 6. Left: Linear Probe positioned transversely at the level of cricoid cartilage. Right: Ultrasonographic image of the cricoid cartilage.

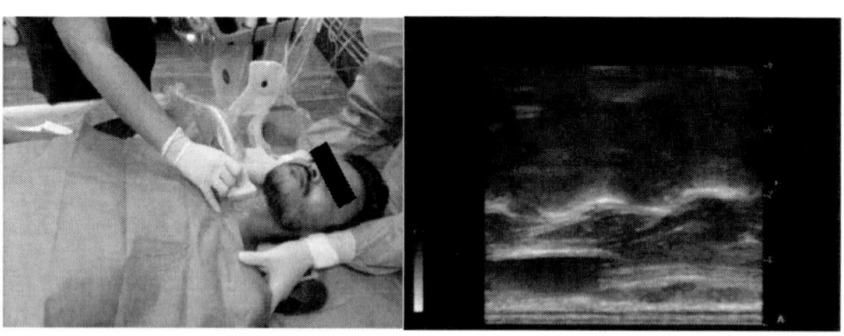

Figure 7. Left: Transducer rotated longitudinally at the level of cricoid. Right: Ultrasonographic image of vertebral bodies corresponding to cricoid cartilage (C5, C6, C7).

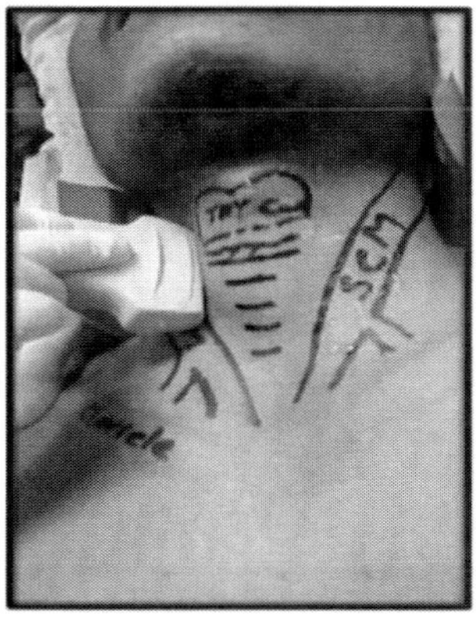

Figure 8. Anatomical landmark for placing the probe probe anteriorly in order to view the cervical spine.

Breathing and Circulation

An important aspect of managing a neurotrauma patient in the emergency department is prevention of secondary insult that may result from conditions such as hypoxia and hypotension. A single episode of hypotension and hypoxia in patients with neurotrauma can increase mortality by up to 150% [6]. Hence, early management of secondary insults can result in reduced morbidity and mortality. These conditions are addressed as a part of the primary survey while evaluating a patient.

Focused Assessment by Sonography in Trauma (FAST) is an adjunct to the primary survey. The sole purpose of the investigation is to look for fluid in 4 areas (hepatorenal, splenorenal, pelvic and pericardial spaces). The investigation answers the question of the presence of fluid in a binary fashion of yes or no, without going into details of the injury. Presence of fluid in any of the above-mentioned spaces is assumed to be blood in the context of trauma, until proven otherwise. E-FAST or the extended version of FAST examination includes assessment for the presence of hemothorax by scanning bilateral hemi thoraces, and also mandates the scanning of bilateral anterior chest wall in order to rule out pneumothorax. E- FAST is now the standard of care in trauma patients as it is a quick, bedside examination that can be performed within minutes of a patient arriving in the Emergency Department. It is also repeatable and can be performed by the clinician (non-radiologist) himself with results comparable to the radiologist [7].

Disability

Ultrasonographic evaluation of the brain has been considered unsuitable in the past because of the presence of the thick bony covering-the skull. Though with the unceasing improvements in sonographic technology, it is now possible to acquire better images of the intracranial anatomy. This is usually done by using low frequency sound waves through a Transtemporal approach in B-Mode [8-10]. The 'Temporal Window' represents the region where the temporal bone is thin enough to allow the passage of the low-frequency ultrasound waves and is located just above the zygomatic arch. Aaslid et al. [11] were the first to describe the 'Temporal Window' in their research work 'Noninvasive Transcranial Doppler Ultrasound recording of flow velocity in basal cerebral arteries.' In 1993, Becker and Boghdan [12] utilized the same window to precisely describe the sonoanatomy of the cerebrum. This led to TCS being extensively studied for various other purposes. However, the temporal window may still be inadequate in about 5-18% of patients [13], with even higher rates of failure being noticed in patients of Asian Ethnicity [14]. One important component of Transcranial Ultrasound that has gained much traction in recent times is the Transcranial Ultrasound Doppler. More will be discussed in the chapter separately.

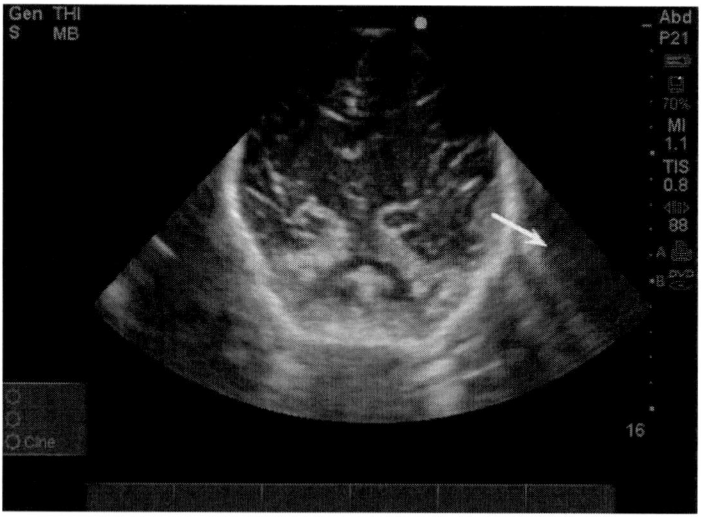

Figure 9. (Continued).

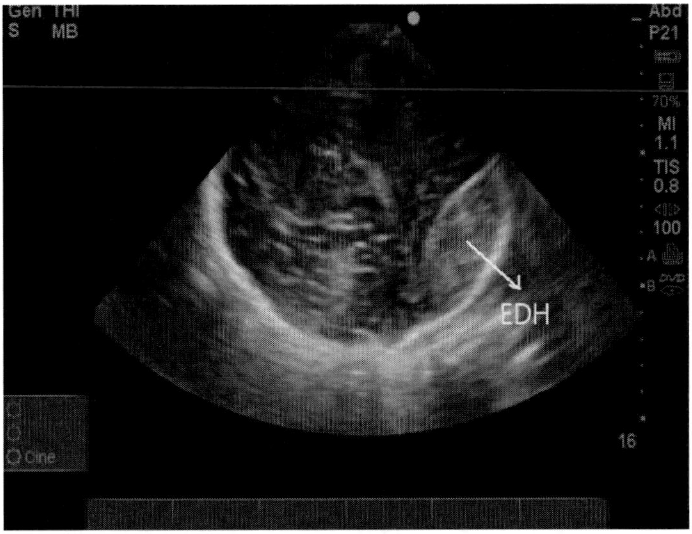

Figure 9. Infant transfontanelle ultrasound: Ultrasound image through anterior fontanelle of a 6-month-old Infant with a history of fall, depicting a right bi-convex hyperechoic lesion (EDH).

Examination in Presence of Acoustic Window

In presence of an optimal acoustic window, such as an open fontanelle in neonates and defects in patients with decompressive craniotomy, excellent sonographic views of the brain parenchyma and related structures can be obtained. Operative neurosurgical patients commonly seek follow-up care in the emergency department for a myriad of symptoms ranging from fever to altered sensorium. These patients usually undergo computed tomography for the diagnosis of any adverse pathology, but ultrasonography now provides an exciting alternative for evaluation and diagnosis.

In patients with *Decompressive Craniotomy*, low-frequency curvilinear probe can be used to obtain images in B-Mode.

- The Probe is placed on an axis parallel to the orbitomeatal line. The initial aim is to identify the butterfly-shaped mesencephalic brainstem with the surrounding echogenic basal cistern.
- Fanning the probe by 10° results the probe to lie in the transverse plane of the diencephalic brainstem. This plane can be used to

measure the dimensions of the third ventricle and frontal horn of the contralateral lateral ventricle.

- In surgical decompressed patients a multiplanar freehand approach may be adopted, but standardized approach are more helpful for comparison and, follow-up sonographic findings.

Raised Intracranial Pressure (Optic Nerve Sheath Diameter)

Cranium is an enclosed space with a fixed volume. Neurotrauma usually leads to change in volume of one or more constituents of the cranium leading to an increase in intracranial pressure. This can lead to secondary brain Injury either by direct compressive damage to the tissues or by causing vascular compromise. Raised ICP may also lead to brain parenchyma herniation and brain death. Prompt reduction of ICP can improve cerebral blood flow, cerebral perfusion pressure (CPP) and brain metabolism. Hence ICP measurement and monitoring assumes important role in the management of patient with head trauma.

The gold standard for ICP measurement is ventriculostomy and intraparenchymal microtransducers, which are invasive procedures. They have the distinct advantage of providing accurate values and continuous monitoring but are associated with risks such as infection and hemorrhage [15, 16] and are not always feasible in the emergency department.

Non-invasive methods for evaluation of ICP are being sought [17], of which optic nerve sheath diameter (ONSD) measurement has gained significant traction. Point of care ultrasonography brings with it several advantages which include the convenience of being performed at the bedside, is radiation-free and repeatable.

The eye is a superficial organ consisting of fluid-filled compartments making it an ideal structure for ultrasound imaging. The optic nerve is the connecting link between the eye and the CNS. It is surrounded by the cerebrospinal fluid and is sheathed by all three layers (dura, pia and arachnoid). Any rise in the intracranial pressure is transmitted through the subarachnoid space to the retrobulbar aspect of the optic nerve sheath. Therefore, the measurement of ONSD can be used as a surrogate marker for intracranial pressure.

Technique

- ONSD is measured with the patient lying supine with up to 20° head elevation.
- The eye of the patient needs to remain shut throughout the process, this can be achieved by applying a Tegaderm or any other barrier. Application of Tegaderm also facilitates the liberal use of gel. This may help in obtaining better resolution with minimal pressure application. Take care to avoid air trapping under the Tegaderm while applying.
- The probe is initially placed on the superior-lateral margin of the eyelid. Be sensitive while transferring pressure over the orbit.
- Fan the probe slowly in the medial direction, scanning through the globe to obtain the image of the optic nerve, which is visualized as an oblique hypoechoic tract posterior to the globe.
- ONSD is measured 3 mm behind the optic disc. Two measurements are usually noted, one in the sagittal plane and the other in the transverse plane. The average of the two is taken as the value of ONSD
- The procedure is performed in both eyes.

An increased ONSD strongly correlates with an elevated ICP. A range of ONSD (4.8 mm to 5.9 mm) measurements are used to correlate with adult ICP > 20 mmHG. In a recent meta-analysis, the cut-off value of 5.0 mm showed a pooled sensitivity of 92-97% and specificity of 86%. It is suggested that in case the value of ONSD lies between 5-6 mm, it is better to take into account the pre-test probability of the patient having a high ICP.

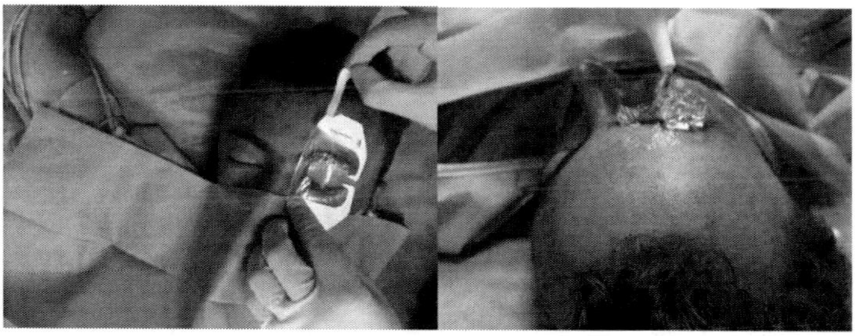

Figure 10. Left: Application of Tegaderm over the closed eyelid. Right: Liberal use of ultrasound gel over the Tegaderm.

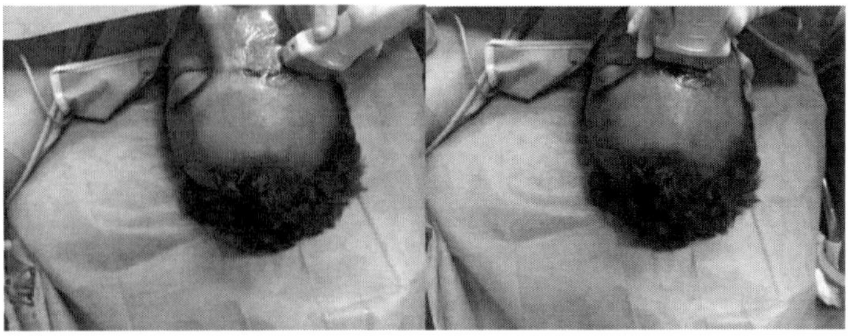

Figure 11. Left: The linear probe was initially placed over the lateral margin of superior eyelid. Right: The probe is then moved medially and directed caudally.

Pupillary Examination

Pupillary Assessment is an important aspect of disability assessment in patients with neurotrauma. The size, equality and reactivity of pupils can provide answers to vital clinical questions. The assessment though may be difficult in certain sets of patients with periorbital swelling which may accompany the trauma. Ultrasound can be used in these patients to assess the size and reactivity.

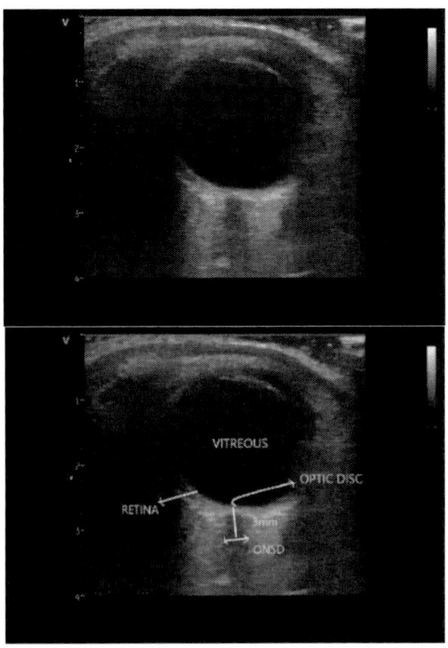

Figure 12. Ultrasound Image of the eyeball with optic nerve posteriorly.

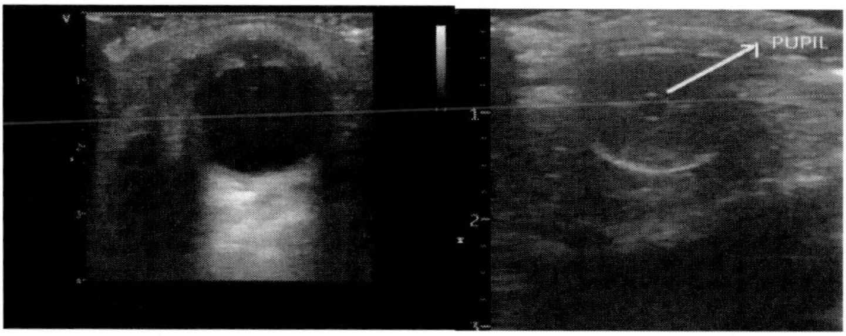

Figure 13. Left: Ultrasound image of the eyeball with pupil anteriorly, Right: coronal view of the globe at the level of the iris.

The reactivity can be assessed by applying the principle of consensual light reflex. The ultrasound is moved over the affected eye after applying a barrier and ultrasound gel buffer. The iris is located and an image is captured to measure the size. Now the light is shown in the opposite eye and reactivity is checked in the affected as well as in the normal eye.

The examination is carried out with the patient lying in a supine position, and the examiner at the head end position.

Pupils are visualized by applying the probe flatly over the lower eyelid, and the pupillary diameter is measured in a frozen still image of the pupil.

Conclusion

Lack of adequate acoustic window has prevented clinicians from using ultrasound as a diagnostic tool in patients with TBI. But with recent advances and novel developments, it is now more frequently integrated in the examination of TBI patients. Basic knowledge of ultrasonography can also help clinicians in early detection of other life-threatening conditions that might be associated with Trauma. With the inherent advantages of ultrasonography (Portable, cost- effective, repeatable, non-invasive, etc.), it will certainly have an important role in the management of patient with TBI in future.

References

[1] Link MS, Berkow LC, Kudenchuk PJ, et al. Adult advanced cardiovascular life support: 2015 American Heart Association guidelines update for cardiopulmonary

resuscitation and emergency cardiovascular care. *Circulation* 2015; 132 (supply 2): S444-S464.

[2] Sahu AK, Bhoi S, Aggarwal P, et al. Endotracheal tube placement confirmation by ultrasonography: A systematic review and meta-analysis of more than 2500 patients. *J. Emerg. Med.* 2020.

[3] Demetriades D, Charalambides K, Chahwan S, Hanpeter D, Alo K, Velmahos G, et al. Nonskeletal cervical spine injuries: epidemiology and diagnostic pitfalls. *J. Trauma Inj. Infect. Crit. Care.* 2000; 48(4): 724-7.

[4] Holmes JF, Akkinepalli R. Computed Tomography versus plain radiography to screen for cervical spine injury: A meta-analysis. *J. Trauma* 2005; 58(5): 902-5.

[5] Vishnu VK, Bhoi S, Aggarwal P. Diagnostic Utility of Point of care ultrasound in identifying cervical spine injury in emergency settings. *Australasian Society for Ultrasound in Medicine*. 2021.

[6] Marmarou A, Lu J, Butcher I, et al. Prognostic value of the Glasgow Coma Scale and pupil reactivity in traumatic brain injury assessed pre-hospital and on enrollment: an IMPACT analysis. *J. Neurotrauma* 24: 270,2007.

[7] Bhoi S, Sinha TP, Ramchandani R, Kurrey L, Galwankar S. To determine the accuracy of focused assessment with sonography for trauma done by nonradiologists and its comparative analysis with radiologists in emergency department of a level 1 trauma center of India. *J. Emerg. Trauma Shock.* 2013 Jan. 6(1):42-6.

[8] Gerriets T, Stolz E, Konig S, et al. Sonographic Monitoring of midline shift in space occupying stroke: An early outcome predictor. *Stroke*, 2001:32:442-447.

[9] Behnke S, Becker G: Sonographic Imaging of Brain Parenchyma. *Eur. J. Ultrasound* 2002: 16:73-80.

[10] Dohrmann GJ, Rubin JM: Neurotraumatology: Ultrasonographic evaluation of the central nervous system. *Neurol. Res.* 1997: 19: 317-322.

[11] Aaslid R, Markwalder TM, Nornes H. Noninvasive Transcranial Doppler Ultrasound recording of flow velocity in basal cerebral arteries. *J. Neurosurg.* 1982; 57: 769-774.

[12] Becker G, Winkler J, Hofmann E et al. Differentiation between ischemic and hemorrhagic stroke by transcranial color-coded real-time sonography. *J. Neuroimaging* 1993, 3(1): 41-7.

[13] Wijnhound AD, franckena M, van der Lught A, koudstaal PJ, Dippel ED. Inadequate acoustical temporal bone window in patients with a transient ischemic attack or minor stroke: role of skull thickness and bone density. *Ultrasound Med. Biol.* 2008; 34: 923-929.

[14] Yoshimura S, Koga M, Toyoda K, Mukai T, Hyun BH, Naganuma M, Nagatsuka K, Minematsu K. Frontal bone window improves the ability of transcranial color-coded sonography to visualize the anterior cerebral artery of Asian patients with stroke. *AJNR Am. J. Neuroradiol.* 2009; 30: 1268-1269.

[15] Holloway KL, Barnes T, Choi S et al. (1996) Ventriculostomy infections: The effect of monitoring duration and catheter exchange in 584 patients. *J. Neurosurg.* 85:419-424. https://doi.org/10.3171/jns.1996.85.3.0419.

[16] Hoefnagel D, Dammers R, Ter Laak-Poort MP, Avezaat CJJ (2008) Risk Fators for Infections related to external ventricular drainage. *Acta Neurochir.* 150:209-214. https://doi.org/10.1007/s00701-007-1458-9.

[17] Robba, Bacigaluppi S, Cardim D, Donnely J, Bertuccio A, Czosnyka M (2016) Non-invasive assessment of intracranial pressure. *Acta Neurochir.* 150:209-214. https://doi.org/10.1111/ane.1257.

Chapter 6

Functional MRI: A Simplified Approach

Niharika Prasad*, MD, FRCR

Consultant Radiologist, Image Core Lab, Bangalore, India

Abstract

F-MRI has gained increased popularity in recent times in functional connectivity analysis of healthy subjects as well as patients suffering from neurological and psychiatric diseases. Task based approach was formerly used; however, resting state f-MRI does not require a stimulus/task. Both are based on the measurement of metabolic activity using BOLD (blood oxygen level-dependent) contrast imaging. This chapter highlights the various methods of data analysis and newer developments in this field of neuroimaging. The following discussion on the pearls & pitfalls of f-MRI, advantages, and limitations, will benefit radiologists as well as non-experts. It illustrates applications such as pre-surgical planning, follow-up imaging and mapping eloquent areas of brain in patients with epilepsy.

Introduction

There are two important concepts in the field of neuroimaging - '*localization*' and '*connectivity.*' These two relate to physiological processes in the brain, both at the neuronal level, as well as at the macroscopic level. The purpose of localization is to assign specific functions to different regions of the brain. The concept of connectivity implies the way of communication between different areas of the brain [1].

---

* Corresponding Author's Email: vats.niharika248@gmail.com.

In: Advances in Neurosurgery Research
Editors: Amit Agrawal, Pradeep Chouksey, Adesh Shrivastava et al.
ISBN: 978-1-68507-859-1

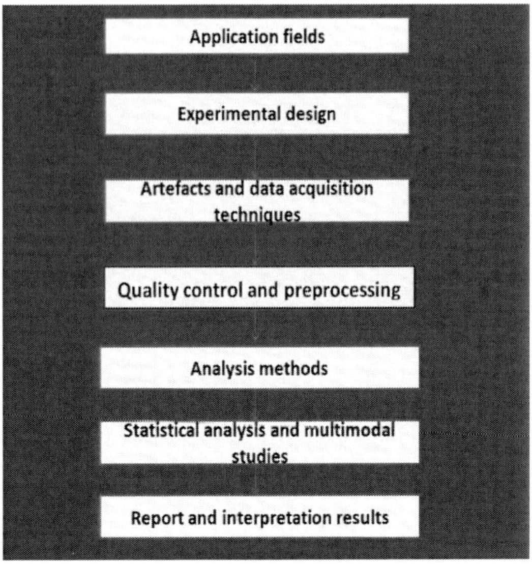

Figure 1. A typical fMRI workflow chart.

The use of fMRI is both in the study of healthy and diseased individuals. It requires a broad knowledge of structural and functional anatomy of the brain, various MRI acquisition techniques, analysis methods and MRI artifacts [2].

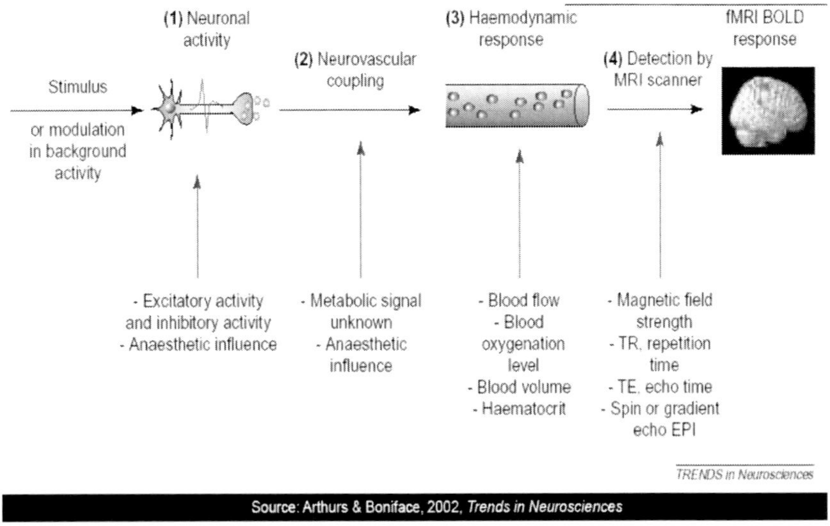

Figure 2. Blood oxygen level-dependent (BOLD) contrast imaging.

Blood Oxygen Level-Dependent (BOLD) Contrast Imaging

There is an increase in neuronal activity causes both higher energy consumption and increased blood flow. This results in a change in the relative levels of oxyhemoglobin and deoxyhemoglobin that can be detected by MRI on the basis of their differential magnetic susceptibilities. The amount of the BOLD signal, indirectly, gives a measure of the neuronal activity. This is represented as a statistical map which is a representation of regional activity [3].

The change in the BOLD signal is the cornerstone of functional MR imaging.

Types

Task-Based fMRI

In this approach stimuli are presented to the subject as a function of time. There are three main types of experimental designs:

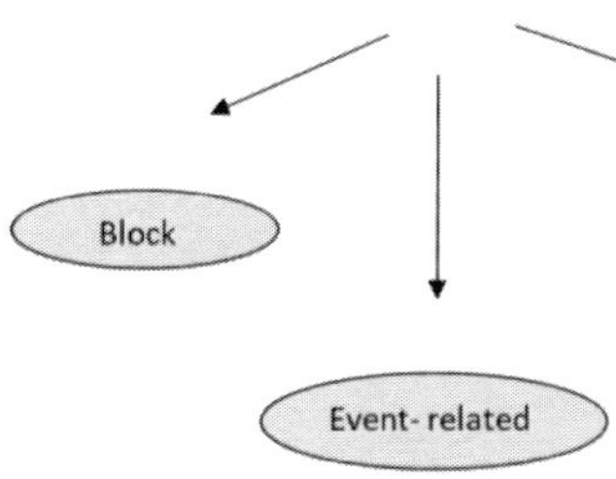

Figure 3a. Designs of task-based f-MRI.

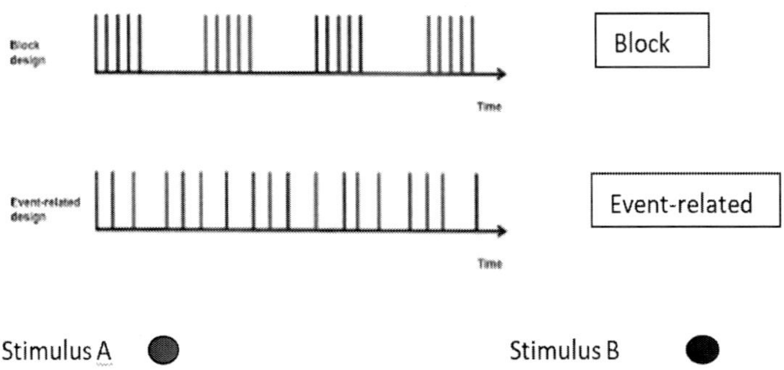

Figure 3b. Designs of task-based f-MRI.

Case Example

History: Six-year old child with refractory epilepsy. A known case of Dysembryoplastic neuroepithelial tumor (DNET) of the left temporal lobe.

Resting State fMRI

The Human Brain Is Constantly Working, Even While Relaxing or Daydreaming.

In contrast to task-based design, resting-state fMRI does not require the subject to perform a specific task. A resting state network is a set of regions in the brain that show similarities in their BOLD changes obtained during rest. The most well-known among these is the ***Default Mode Network*** (DMN) which contains regions in the brain that show reduced activity when the brain is performing a task as compared with when it is at rest. Such areas have been identified with the use of fMRI and PET (positron emission tomography) [2]. The major areas of this network include:

- Posterior cingulate cortex
- Precuneus
- Medial prefrontal cortex
- Inferior parietal lobule
- Lateral temporal cortex

The dorsal attention network (DAN) is a task-positive network, consisting of regions that are activated during various types of goal-directed response [1].

The most traditional acquisition includes instructing the subject to keep the eyes closed and neither falling off to sleep, nor thinking of anything in particular.

The default mode is more active in creative people!

Regular yoga leads to increased gray matter volume in the insula and hippocampus, increased activation of prefrontal cortical regions, and functional connectivity changes mainly within the default mode network! [10]

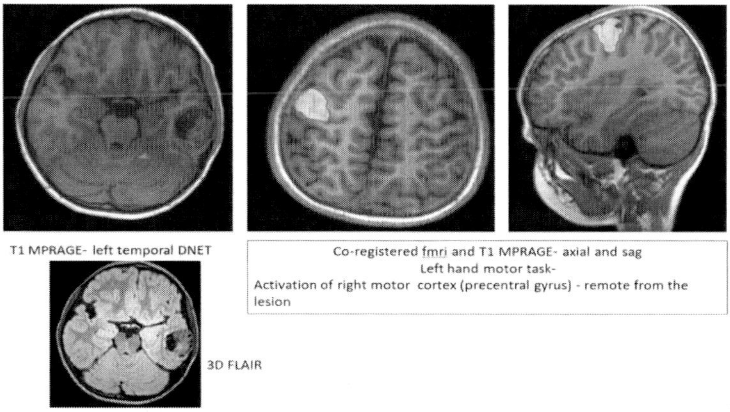

(A)

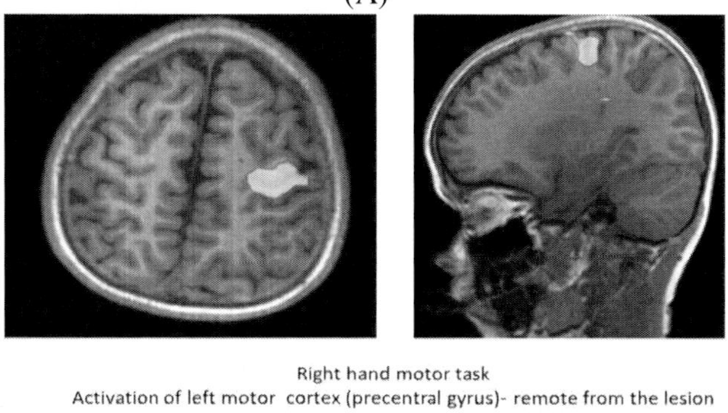

(B)

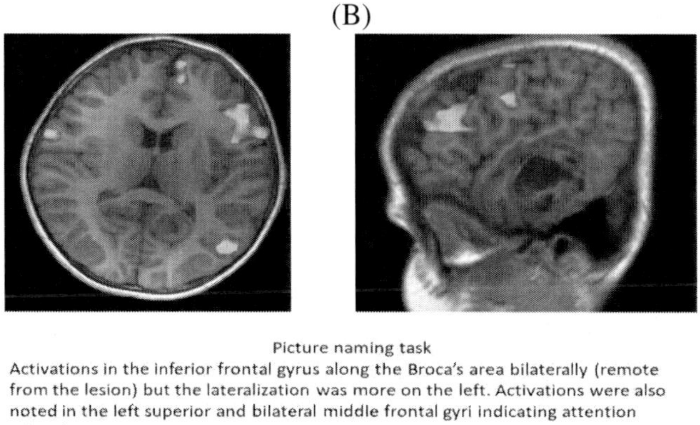

(C)

Source: Department of Neuroimaging and Interventional Radiology (NIIR), NIMHANS.

Figure 4. All the details are there with individual images.

The American College of Radiology recommends that a MRI scanner of 1.5 Tesla or higher field strength be used. A high performance head coil aids in achieving a higher signal-to-noise ratio (SNR). A gradient echo or echo planar pulse sequence is used [4].

Analytics Methods

Seed-Based Analysis

Most commonly, Echo planar imaging (EPI) sequence is used, parameters which need adjustment include - *repetition time, voxel size and coverage.* One has to achieve a balance between temporal and spatial resolution.

Another important factor is noise correction.

- The user chooses a single or multi-voxel ROI
- The objective is to obtain an entire brain connectivity map that shows the correlation of each voxel with the ROI.
- The voxel wise correction is performed followed by Fischer's r-to-Z transformation.
- Bias may be possible as the network depends on seed size and location

Independent Component Analysis

- Automatic/semi automatic data driven method [3, 6]
- It segregates the whole brain resting state BOLD data into a mixture that reflects neuronal signal and structured noise [1].
- At the end, the data is separated from the noise using regression analysis.
- Dual regression is usually used along with this method.

The factors which play a role in the final analysis/interpretation include:

1. Psychology of the subject
2. Physiology of the BOLD signal
3. Methodology used for the analysis

Clinical Applications

- Pre-surgical planning
- Assessment of eloquent cortex in relation to a tumor or mass
- Therapeutic follow up
- Planning epilepsy surgery
- Radiation treatment planning
- Studying psychiatric diseases
- Study of neurodegenerative conditions

Challenges and Limitations

- Controlling motion artifacts especially in pediatric patients
- Task based approach depends on individual's age and ability to perform the task
- Neuroplasticity in pediatric population
- Reorganization of domains after brain injury can lead to atypical dominance patterns [5]
- Complex neurophysiology necessitates good knowledge of anatomy and neuroscientific techniques
- Requirement of expensive and complex hardware and software tools [4].

New Headways

- A *hybrid of EEG and fMRI* has been developed for further research related to neurodegenerative and psychiatric diseases. It is used to correlate the electrical brain activity with hemodynamic mutation [7, 8].
- This method combines the advantages of high spatial resolution of MRI with that of high temporal resolution of EEG.
- A combined approach incorporating an MR-compatible EEG system in the hybrid MR-PET scanner has been proposed.
- fMRI *'neurofeedback'* is a type of biofeedback in which real-time online fMRI signals are used to self-regulate brain function. Newer

medications of this such as decoded neurofeedback (DecNef) and functional connectivity-based neurofeedback (FCNef) help to study the relation between brain functions and behaviour. Connectivity-based neurofeedback has enabled modification of the connectivity of a targeted network [8].
- *'Connectome'* is a relatively new concept in epilepsy imaging where network analyses have the capacity to explain cognitive deficits extending beyond the seizure focus and to identify relevant reorganization patterns in patients [1, 9].

Conclusion

Blood oxygen level-dependent functional magnetic resonance imaging has multiple clinical applications. Although it has a few limitations, it has the benefit of being a non-invasive method. It has grown from just a research tool to having an emerging role in surgical planning and has found several new applications in the present era.

Acknowledgment

I thank Dr. Richa Singh Chauhan, Final year DM SR from National Institute of Mental Health and Neurosciences (NIMHANS), Bangalore for her valuable contribution of patient images.

References

[1] Bijsterbosch J, Smith SM, Beckmann CF. (2017). *An introduction to resting state fMRI functional connectivity*. Oxford University Press.

[2] Soares JM, Magalhães R, Moreira PS, Sousa A, Ganz E, Sampaio A, Alves V, Marques P, Sousa N. (2016). A hitchhiker's guide to functional magnetic resonance imaging. *Frontiers in Neuroscience*. 10:515.

[3] Lv H, Wang Z, Tong E, Williams LM, Zaharchuk G, Zeineh M, Goldstein-Piekarski AN, Ball TM, Liao C, Wintermark M. (2018). Resting-state functional MRI: everything that nonexperts have always wanted to know. *American Journal of Neuroradiology*. 39(8):1390-9.

[4] American College of Radiology. (2014). *ACR-ASNR-SPR practice parameter for the performance of functional magnetic resonance imaging (fMRI) of the brain*. Amended.

[5] Jones JY, Selvaraj B, Ho ML. (2020). Pediatric Functional Neuroimaging: Practical Tips and Pearls. *American Journal of Roentgenology*. 214(5):995-1007.

[6] Poldrack RA, Mumford JA, Nichols TE. (2011). *Handbook of functional MRI data analysis*. Cambridge University Press.

[7] Mele G, Cavaliere C, Alfano V, Orsini M, Salvatore M, Aiello M. (2019). Simultaneous EEG-fMRI for functional neurological assessment. *Frontiers in Neurology*. 10:848.

[8] Watanabe T, Sasaki Y, Shibata K, Kawato M. (2017). Advances in fMRI real-time neurofeedback. *Trends in Cognitive Sciences*. 21(12):997-1010.

[9] Schmidbauer V, Bonelli S. (2020) Recent developments in cognitive fMRI for temporal lobe epilepsy. *Zeitschrift für Epileptologie*. 33(1):30-6.

[10] van Aalst J, Ceccarini J, Demyttenaere K, Sunaert S, Van Laere K. (2020). What has neuroimaging taught us on the neurobiology of yoga? a review. *Frontiers in Integrative Neuroscience*. 8;14:34.

Chapter 7

Non-Invasive ICP Monitoring

Sandra Marcela Mass-Ramírez, Carmen Sofía Sierra-Ochoa and Ivan David Lozada-Martínez*

Grupo Prometheus y Biomedicina Aplicada a las Ciencias Clínicas, School of Medicine, Universidad de Cartagena, Cartagena, Colombia and
Colombian Clinical Research Group in Neurocritical Care, Latin American Council of Neurocritical Care, Cartagena, Colombia

Abstract

Monitoring is a key tool in the context of acute brain pathology, which is used to effectively measure intracranial pressure and thus provide a timely diagnosis on occasions when it is elevated. There is a great variety of monitoring methods that have been implemented for a long time, being the invasive methods the "gold standard" techniques in the medical field, such as external ventricular drainage and intraparenchymal monitoring, but these carry great risks for the patient with the possibility of even worsening his clinical condition. For this reason, new techniques have been implemented, which carry a lower risk of complications and their results are comparable to those obtained with invasive methods. These are known as non-invasive measures and will be the subject of study in this chapter.

* Corresponding Author's Email: ilozadam@unicartagena.edu.co.

In: Advances in Neurosurgery Research
Editors: Amit Agrawal, Pradeep Chouksey, Adesh Shrivastava et al.
ISBN: 978-1-68507-859-1

Introduction

Monitoring constitutes a therapeutic guide in acute neurological processes with risk of intracranial hypertension. This clinical parameter was introduced as a novel modality in clinical practice by Guillaume and Janny in 1951 [1], but it was not until 1960 that its use was systematized and established as a protocol in the neurointensive care area [2]. For the next three decades, intracranial pressure monitoring was considered for research purposes only until 1995, when the Brain Trauma Foundation published guides for healthcare personnel and recommendations, which have been modified over time.

Hospital visits for acute brain pathology that can lead to elevated intracranial pressure (ICP), being the main trigger of death and disability in these patients, are increasingly frequent. Therefore, ICP assessment is an indispensable measure in the neurocritical care unit [3]. Traditionally, invasive ICP monitoring has been used because it is considered the gold standard for its measurement; however, it exposes the patient to certain risks such as bleeding and infection, making it not useful in all clinical events [3].

With the advance of technology, new monitoring measures have been implemented that involve fewer complications for the patient and are less invasive, such as near infrared spectroscopy, optical nerve sheet diameter or transcranial Doppler ultrasound, whose main objective is to evaluate cerebrovascular dynamics through cerebral blood flow velocity [4]. In this chapter, the noninvasive methods for measuring intracranial pressure will be discussed in a global manner, establishing their usefulness and importance in the timely diagnosis of the patient.

Essentials of Intracranial Pressure

The mean intracranial pressure should be kept in the range of 7-15 mmHg for adults, 3-7 mmHg in children and between 1.5-6 mmHg in term newborns [5]. Clinical practice guidelines recommend maintaining a ICP of <20-25 mmHg in the neurocritical care unit for acute brain pathology, including traumatic brain injury (TBI) [5], therefore, ICP reduction therapy is initiated when values exceed this range [6].

Intracranial hypertension (ICH) is a neurological status caused by elevated pressures within the skull, and has a major impact on patient mortality and morbidity [7, 8]. The increase in ICP can occur as a consequence of TBI, which is the most frequent cause, as well as due to other neurological entities that occupy a space as an expansive process, such as stroke, hemorrhage, intracranial infection, hydrocephalus, hematomas, primary brain tumors, among others [5]; these are closely related to brain masses, intracranial edema, stasis of cerebrospinal fluid (CSF) flow or obstruction of venous flow [9]. In turn, the consequence of high ICP is a decrease in cerebral perfusion pressure (CPP), resulting in secondary parenchymal lesions such as ischemia or cerebral herniation, leading to a greater likelihood of disability and increased mortality [5, 10]. This secondary brain injury is considered to be any physiological condition that may occur in minutes, hours or days after the primary lesion and results in a major injury to the nervous system [11].

Pathophysiological Aspects of Intracranial Hypertension

The intracranial cavity contains three main components: blood flow formed by a network of arteries and veins, parenchymal tissue and CSF. Its mean volume is about 1500 mL, composed of 88% brain matter, 7.5% blood and 4.5% CSF [12, 13]. It can be said that these components are part of a closed system, since they are contained within the skull, which constitutes a bony structure without expansion capacity [5]; therefore, any variation in the volume of these elements results in a modification of ICP (directly proportional relation) [5]. This volume - pressure relationship is based on the Monroe - Kellie theory

$$Vc + Vs + Vlcr = K$$

where, Vc is the brain volume, Vs is the circulating blood volume and Vlcr is the CSF volumen.

Initially, the imbalance and volume increase of some component of this system can be attenuated by variations (decrease) in the volume of the other constituents, which are usually the movement of CSF and cerebral venous blood; thus, if one intracranial element increases it must be accompanied by a compensatory decrease in the volume of another constituent, or the pressure will raise [5, 12, 13]. However, when these mechanisms are exhausted, ICP starts to rapidly increase [5]. Accordingly, cerebral blood flow and the proper equilibrium between CSF production and absorption or drainage are the most important components that contribute to the maintenance of ICP, since cerebral volume is constant under normal conditions [5, 14].

This ratio gives a compensatory reserve denominated spatial compensation, which varies from 60 to 80 ml in the young and from 100 to 140 ml in the old people, as a result of cerebral atrophy [15]. Thus, at first, the increase in pressure is very limited because there is a compensatory reserve sufficient to adjust the additional volume, but once the reserve is overcome, there is a fast elevation of pressure [15].

As mentioned above, when ICP rises, CPP decreases. The latter is estimated by subtracting ICP from mean arterial pressure (MAP) [15]. MAP is defined as the sum of diastolic pressure added to one third of the difference between systolic and diastolic pressure.

Cerebral autoregulation is the process within which cerebral blood flow is modified to maintain adequate cerebral perfusion, maintaining a constant flow of blood to the brain by dilation or contraction of arterioles; it is only effective when MAP is between 50 and 150 mmHg [7, 15]. When the MAP is high, hyperemia and cerebral edema are generated, while if it is under the borderline, there is deficient blood flow and brain ischemia, which favors the formation of edema, which is associated with a poor prognosis for the patient [15]. In this sense, any injury to the brain can induce an imbalance in brain autoregulation and the flow will depend exclusively on CPP, so that the brain becomes sensitive to even minimal changes in CPP [15]. An elevated ICP may be associated with a reduction in CPP and, therefore, with focal or global ischemic damage at the level of brain tissue.

Clinical Picture of Intracranial Hypertension

The clinical manifestations of intracranial hypertension are nonspecific, however, it may be suspected if a patient manifests clinical signs and symptoms such as: headache, often described as palpitations or bursts that are exacerbated by exertional activity such as coughing; nausea and projectile vomiting, which are not relieved by medication; and altered level of consciousness [7, 11, 16, 17, 18]. Visual symptoms may vary from hazy vision, double eyesight due to cranial nerve disorders to photophobia [7, 16, 17, 18]. Papilledema is a reliable sign, but may appear days after the increase in ICP and does not occur in all patients [11, 12].

The increased ICP may also cause displacement of the brain substance, which can lead to structural injury to the brain and herniation across the tentorial hiatus or foramen magnum. This event would result in a Cushing's triad, consisting of severe hypertension, bradycardia (caused by pressure in the brainstem), and irregular breathing, which if not treated promptly, can lead to respiratory depression and death [11, 13].

Intracranial Pressure Monitoring

Early identification, monitoring, and treatment of elevated IH in neurocritical care settings is essential for better short- and long-term neurological outcomes [5]. In fact, ICP monitoring has been shown to improve prognosis in certain pathologies such as TBI, cerebrovascular infections like meningitis and brain tumors [19].

The Brain Trauma Foundation has stated that ICP should be monitored in every patient with TBI in whom hematoma, contusion, bruising, herniation or compression of the basal cisterns are evident on brain computed tomography [20, 21]. The guidelines further suggest that ICP monitoring should be conducted in such patients at risk for elevated ICP, in patients with Glasgow scale <8 and in patients in whom critical management is warranted, and in those patients who have two or even more of the following criteria: age more than 40 years, unilateral or bilateral motor posturing, and systolic blood pressure less than 90 mm Hg [17, 21]. Similarly, late onset or complete absence of signs and symptoms may delay the timing of treatment initiation, so early ICP monitoring is recommended in patients considered to be at high risk for IH [20].

The correct measurement of ICP and its interpretation by trained personnel at the right time represents a key strategy for the diagnosis and establishment of an adequate treatment in the neurology area [19]. In clinical practice, different invasive and non-invasive ICP monitorization tools are available to determine the optimal ICP [11]. The choice of device is dictated by the patient's clinical picture, the expected function of the device, the physician's preference and skills, and institutional policies, and ideally this choice should be made on the basis of the best current evidence. ICP monitors are also categorized according to final location in the brain and according to their function (diagnostic or therapeutic) [22]. The most commonly used methods of monitorization in clinical acute situations are fluid-based systems, implantable transducers, and Doppler ultrasound [14, 22].

Brief Approach to the Most Commonly Used Invasive Methods

Invasive ICP measurement is performed by means of specific catheters inserted in the intraventricular, intraparenchymal, epidural, subdural or subarachnoid space. The ideal ICP monitoring device should be accurate, reproducible, inexpensive and have minimal complications [11]. Currently, the "gold standard" method used for monitoring is the intraventricular catheter, because it is the most reliable method and measures global ICP, assuming there is no CSF flow restriction [11, 18, 23].

- *External ventricular drainage (EVD):* This method consists of introducing a hollow catheter into one of the lateral ventricles. This catheter is attached through a tube to a pressure transmitter, which gives a computerized signal that can be saved or viewed virtually electronically in mm Hg or centimeters of water (cm H_2O) [18, 23]. This technique offers diagnostic and therapeutic answers as it provides information regarding the patient's ICP and at the same time allows CSF drainage, thus reducing the ICP in case it is increased [14, 18].
  The fact that this measurement is currently considered the "gold standard" does not necessarily mean that it is the most accurate assessment technique, but it is the most widely used technique with which to monitor a clinical parameter, in this case ICP values [8]. It should be noted that external ventricular drainage is not suitable for monitoring ICP over a prolonged period of time because the longer the patient remains with the catheter, the greater the risk of intracranial infection [14].
- *Intraparenchymal monitoring:* In this method, the brain parenchyma is the location chosen for ICP monitoring. These devices are used when the patient does not require CSF drainage or when insertion of the catheter in the ventricle is not an option, as in the presence of ventricular compression caused by cerebral edema. Their benefits include reduced techniques difficulties in device insertion and, in theory, a reduced risk of infection and hemorrhage. But the use of these devices may be limited due to the impossibility of recalibrating them once the device is in place and the high cost of these devices compared to the EVD [18, 22, 24].

Non-Invasive Methods for ICP Monitoring

New measures have now been introduced that allow ICP monitoring from outside the skull, which are known as noninvasive [19]. These methods are intended to make ICP measurement easier and to avoid complications such as bleeding and infection [25]. To evaluate the precision of a noninvasive technique, the Association for the Advancement of Medical Instrumentation declared that, when ICP is between 0 and 20 mmHg, a difference of 2 mmHg is acceptable compared to an invasive method; however, when ICP is between 20 and 100 mmHg, the discrepancy may not exceed 10% [26].

Table 1. Comparison between invasive and non-invasive methods for PCI monitoring

	Advantages	Disadvantages
Invasive ICP Monitoring	More accurate and reliable methods for ICP measurement. Diagnostic and therapeutic utility (EVD). Numerous scientific trials have supported the application of these methods in institutions.	Costly methods so not all patients can have access to them. Risk of bleeding and infection. Requires hospitalization in ICU for at least 24 - 48 hours after the procedure. Needs to be performed by an expert neurosurgeon. Requires properly equipped facilities for its implementation. Contraindications: concurrent use of anticoagulants, bleeding disorders, scalp infection and brain abscess.
Non-Invasive ICP Monitoring (nICP).	Helps to decide which patient deserves invasive PCI monitoring There is no risk of complications as in invasive methods . Provides continuous long-term ICP measurements without the need to insert a new instrument every measurement. Has more affordable methods. It may be done at the patient's bedside.	There is not enough evidence to establish them as a standard procedure in the institutions. Trained personnel are needed to perform and interpret them

New techniques proposed include computed tomography, transcranial doppler ultrasound, magnetic resonance imaging, near infrared spectroscopy, among others. The eye, as an extent of the central nervous system, has been utilized as a monitoring device for ICP by examining the optic nerve. These noninvasive methods study the 3D structure of the skull, brain, ventricles, optic nerve or cerebral blood flow function, which are related to ICP [18].

Radiological Techniques

Brain Computed Tomography

It has been mentioned that clinicians may base on qualities that can suggest ICP pathology, demonstrable by computed tomography (CT), which quickly evaluates for the detection of particular finds or markers that improve the diagnostic of ICH [11]. This may include mass effect, displacement of the midline, absence or compression of the basal cisterns, cerebral hemorrhage, enlargement of the ventricles, cerebral edema, or the loss of distinction of gray and white matter [11, 25]. It is important to mention that all these markers are only studied in the background of TBI and its use in other environments is debatable. Moreover, CT is not a very sensitive tool and its predictive value remains unclear, as it can remain normal even with elevated ICP [25]. Therefore, a normal cerebral CT scan on hospital admission does not eliminate the potential risk of premature IH or the risk of possible high ICP [20]. Overall, CT-based approaches showed high specificity but decreased sensitivity for predicting IH, so there is a strong possibility of false negatives [20]. Therefore, magnetic resonance imaging (MRI) could be more accurate than CT, however, it has limitations such as low availability and time constraints for imaging [20].

Magnetic Resonance Imaging

MRI is a non-invasive technique for measuring ICP based on parameters such as flow velocity, intracranial elastance (derived as the exponential relationship between intracranial volume and pressure) and optic nerve sheath diameter (ONSD) [18].

MRI has also been used in the examination of indirect signs indicative of elevated ICP. Among these imaging findings are empty sella turcica or flattened pituitary gland, dilatation and tortuosity of the optic nerve sheaths, transverse sinus stenosis, effacement of the subarachnoid space, and flattened of the posterior globes [27, 28].

This technique has been successfully applied in the evaluation of ICP in patients with cerebral arteriovenous malformations and as a diagnostic aid in determining prognosis in patients with symptomatic hydrocephalus. It should be noted that the use of MRI in the assessment of ICP was effectively used in the correlation of headaches caused by acute mountain sickness and changes in ICP [20].

MRI is also utilized to quantify the volume of subarachnoid fluid surrounding the optic nerve, which can be observed more precisely, allowing accurate calculation of the diameter of the sheath. In patients presenting with papilledema it is possible to observe the dilated subarachnoid space, the compressed optic nerve and the distended optic nerve sheath, all through MRI [17].

Despite its advantages and wide use in various fields of medicine, this technique is not suitable for constant monitoring and repetitive evaluation of ICP; moreover, the use of this technique demands a conscientious screening of significant imaging sections and the correct selection of relevant blood vessels, which requires highly trained personnel [20]. Among the disadvantages of this method we find that its cost is very high, that it is not an equipment that can be easily transported and the relatively long period of time it requires, including sedation in young children [18].

Transcranial Doppler Ultrasound

Transcranial Doppler (TCD) is an effective, noninvasive method that can detect improper cerebral blood flow and evaluate cerebral autoregulation [11]; it can determine red blood cell flow velocity in real time and can estimate ICP [26]. Similarly, it can also indicate which patients need invasive brain monitoring, causing them not to undergo the latter method in the first instance.

TCD has the ability to determine blood flow velocity (VF) through the main intracranial vessels, of which the most frequent is the middle cerebral artery (MCA) [11, 29]. Thus, the changes reflected in VF are the result of increased external pressure in the cerebral vessels when ICP increases [11]; detection of decreased VF suggests impaired cerebral blood flow and an indirect increase in ICP [11]. MCA is used for insonation and different indices, such as the Pourcelot resistance index and the Gosling pulsatility index, have been explored for correlation with ICP [25, 29].

In addition to mean VF, the pulsatility index (PI) has been correlated with ICP. PI is referred to as the difference between systolic and diastolic flow velocity divided by mean flow velocity [26]. It has been found that changes in PI in the MCA are associated with changes in ICP, when the latter is between 5 and 40 mmHg [11]. One of the advantages of the PI is that the ratio is obtained from the difference between the systolic and diastolic velocities, so it is not affected by the angle of insonation [25].

Among the limitations of TCD are that it is susceptible to intra- and inter-observer variability, so the veracity of the technique depends on the experience of the observer. In addition, in 10-15% of patients, the characteristics of the skull restrict the transmission of ultrasound waves, which complicates the interpretation of TCD [11, 14]. On the other hand, several studies have been conducted to investigate the reliability and safety of this method in relation to ICP [30, 31].

Transcranial Time-of-Flight

Transcranial time-of-flight (TOF) for noninvasive measurement of volume and ICP was first proposed in 1995 by Ragauskas et al. [32]; later the option of incorporating an acoustic trajectory through the head was considered [25]. The technique is based on the measurement of the acoustic properties of intracranial components, such as ultrasound velocity and frequency-dependent attenuation along an acoustic path [25]. Thus, a change in the content of the intracranial components within this trajectory has an impact on the overall acoustic characteristics of the intracranial environment and on the monitored parameters of the ultrasonic signal [20].

Optic Nerve Sheath Diameter

The optic nerve is an important component of the central nervous system. When the optic nerve leaves the intracranial space behind to go into the orbit, it is surrounded by the dural sheath, indicating that the subarachnoid space surrounding the optic nerve is closely linked to the intracranial subarachnoid space. This confirms the close relationship between ophthalmology and brain pathologies; thus, when ICP elevation occurs, it can be transmitted through the CSF into the subarachnoid space and leads to dilatation of the optic nerve sheath, more specifically the anterior and retrobulbar segment [14, 20, 33]. This increase in ICP pressure directly and linearly increases optic nerve sheath strain; this increase in pressure also causes axoplasmic transport stasis which is related to papilledema [17].

One modality implemented in recent years as a method of evaluating ICP has been ophthalmic ultrasound with a frequency between 5 and 10.5 MHz to assess the ONSD [17]. The use of ocular ultrasonography in the measurement of ONSD has become a useful method in the detection of elevated ICP. Among the advantages of this technique are that it is a noninvasive method, it is portable, it can be performed at the patient's bedside in a short period of time, the evaluation can be repeated if necessary, and there is no radiation risk for the patient [33]. To perform this method, the physician sits at the head of the patient's bed, who should be in a supine position with the head and trunk of the body elevated 20-30° so that there is no pressure on the eye. The patient should be held in this position for at least one minute before obtaining data. Before placing the transducer, a gel cover should be applied to the closed upper eyelid. When the transducer is placed, it should be positioned on the temporal side of the eye. The patient is asked to look forward with closed eyes in order to reduce eye movement and thus achieve a more precise observation of the anatomical structures of interest for the study (optic nerve and crystalline lens) [34]. An ONSD of 5.8 mm as a cutoff value provides high specificity and sensitivity for establishing a diagnosis of elevated ICP. A clinical picture of increased ICP is unlikely when the ONSD is less than 5.0 mm [35].

The use of this technique is not recommended in patients with facial trauma or pathologies that may alter the ONSD, such as Graves' disease and sarcoidosis [14].

CT and MRI are useful tools to detect elevated ICP in a non-invasive way, but in cases of ONSD measurement they are not highly recommended due to their high cost, requirement of patient transport that is not always possible and the longer time spent in the study compared to ultrasonography. Because of this, ONSD ultrasound represents the best option due to its affordable cost, its ease of use at the patient's bedside, especially in those patients who are not in an intensive care unit and require real-time monitoring of ICP [35, 36].

Pupillometry

Quantitative pupillometers, which have the ability to measure subtle changes in pupil constriction in response to a light stimulus, are used to perform this method. Studies by Meeker et al. [37] and Du et al. [38] established that pupillometers are more specific than manual scoring and have the ability to measure subtle pupillary constrictions that would go unnoticed with manual examination.

In healthy subjects, the light reflex usually causes a 34-36% reduction in pupil size. Taylor et al. [39] demonstrated that in patients with head injuries the pupil constriction after stimulation is approximately 20%. They were also able to demonstrate that a decrease in pupil size of less than 10% is related to an ICP of more than 20 mmHg [17, 39].

Although this method has yielded good results in the detection of increased ICP in patients with severe TBI, it has several limitations. One of the main limitations is the anatomical variability between individuals, which makes it difficult to implement universal guidelines in institutions; in addition, optic disc swelling in cases of elevated ICP occurs late, so this technique is not recommended in acute situations [20].

Tympanic Membrane Displacement

The tympanic membrane displacement (TMD) method for ICP monitoring takes advantage of the communication of CSF and perilymph through the cochlear duct, where the increase in ICP is able to displace the tympanic membrane to its initial position, since this is transmitted directly to the stapes base [11]; in this way, if the displacement is inward it indicates a high ICP and if it is outward it indicates normal or low ICP [11].

Its technique is based on the proximity between the stapes and the oval membrane, where the pressure of the liquid in the cochlea affects the position of the membrane and the stapes and its movement, due to the fact that the stapes rests on the oval window which is covered by a flexible membrane [15, 25]. TMD can be estimated indirectly in response to auditory stimulation by means of the stapedial reflex that causes a movement of the tympanic membrane, which correlates with ICP [15, 25].

Although the current evidence indicates that it is a good screening method that can be useful in the assessment and follow-up of patients with elevated ICP, this technique lacks precision, does not allow establishing specific ICP values, and is an unreliable method for its quantitative assessment [25]. It has been shown that the mean of TMD and invasively measured ICP precludes the clinical use of this technique as an absolute figure [20]. Shimbles et al. [40], tested the technique in 148 patients with benign intracranial hypertension or hydrocephalus and in 77 healthy controls; as a result, the technique was successfully applied in 70% of the healthy controls, but only in 40% of the patients, which was attributed to the perilymphatic duct being less traversable with age, particularly after the age of 40 years.

Among its limitations are those derived from the technique itself (failed tympanometry), as well as other anatomical factors such as the integrity of the ossicles, the existence of masses in the middle ear or the permeability of the Eustachian tube and the cochlear duct [20].

Near Infrared Spectroscopy

Transcranial near infrared spectroscopy (NIRS) is a non-invasive technique used for monitoring regional cerebral oxygen saturation (rSO2) [17]. This technique, as its name indicates, uses light in the near infrared spectrum, and is based on the principle that light (wavelength 700-950 nm) passing through biological tissues is absorbed by the blood depending on its oxygenation state. The attenuation of the light allows calculation of the oxygen status in the tissue volume reached by the light [41]. Thus, NIRS makes it possible to detect changes in brain tissue oxygenation, volume and cerebral blood flow by recording given changes in oxygenated and deoxygenated hemoglobin concentration [42]. Currently, almost all NIRS cerebral oximeters consist of a light source and sensor combination that is designated to the patient's head and connected to a monitor that outputs regional saturation values calculated from algorithms unique to each particular oximeter [18].

The ability of cerebrovascular smooth muscle to react to transmural pressure fluctuations is called "cerebrovascular pressure reactivity" (PRx). Thus, when cerebral vessels are reactive, any change in blood pressure will produce an inverse change in cerebral blood volume, which directly influences ICP [43]. A positive PRx indicates passive pressure which is associated with death in adults with a clinical picture of traumatic brain injury. Conversely, a negative PRx indicates reactivity to pressure which is associated with survival in adult patients with traumatic brain injury [44].

This method has proven to be very effective for long-term patient monitoring especially in the area of neurovascular pathologies [20]. A limitation of NIRS is that it only allows monitoring of brain reactivity with the use of sensors located specifically in the frontal region of the brain [17].

Visual Evoked Potentials

Measurement of visual evoked potentials (VEP) accurately reflects electrical disturbances in the visual pathway [26]. Increased ICP interferes with the physiological function of the visual pathway and can therefore be detected as a disturbance of VEPs [17]. VEPs are the electrical signals generated by the occipital lobe in response to visual stimuli. VEP waveforms have many components, such as the number of positive or negative waves, latency, and their shape. VEP peaks are labeled as P or N, indicating whether the deflection is positive or negative, with a numerical subindex that indicates the mean latency of the peak after the stimulus. VEPs give a picture of the state of the visual system from the optic nerve to the primary visual cortex [18].

ICP is calculated from the latency of the second negative wave (N2) of the VEP or the latency of the third positive wave (P3) of the VEP [20]. A study by York et al. [45, 46], in children with hydrocephalus and young adults with closed head trauma, evidenced a close linear association between increased VEP N2 wave latency and ICP elevations.

Currently, VEPs are used in the treatment of optic nerve pathologies and the monitoring of brain activity in the performance of certain surgeries [18]. This method is not recommended in patients with frontal hematomas, retinal lesions or optic nerve pathologies [26]. VEPs are not yet fully developed and have several limitations such as the requirement for neurophysiological expertise; in addition, VEPs are significantly affected by anesthesia, and since the purpose of the study is to measure brain electrical activity, their use would be limited in sedated and intubated patients [18, 26].

Electroencephalogram

Since elevated ICP alters cerebral perfusion, neuronal activity and brain metabolism may also be affected. It has been shown that there are changes in the electroencephalogram (EEG) of patients with increased ICP, demonstrating that the entropy and bispectral index values correlate with CPP [20]. Chen et al. [47] evaluated a novel technique based on EEG power spectrum analysis as a noninvasive method for ICP monitoring. The authors performed EEG power spectrum analysis and an intracranial pressure index was calculated; results from 62 patients showed a relatively strong correlation between the pressure index and ICP.

EEG patterns linked to elevated ICP involve focal slowing of underlying rhythms or global EEG suppression progressing to burst suppression or flat EEG [11]. Similarly, it can detect cerebral ischemia, as it can show changes in neuronal function prior to structural damage ([11].

Continuous monitoring of ICP from EEG is theoretically possible, which can be recorded for 8-12 hours before the conductive gel in the electrodes dries out and the electrodes need to be replaced [25]; however, it is not an immediately available technique and therefore may not be suitable in an emergency setting [20].

Future Directions

As noted above, numerous noninvasive methods of ICP have been pursued for their reduced complication rate and their potential predictive value in the diagnosis of elevated ICP. Methods such as ONSD measurement and transcranial Doppler ultrasound, have been widely studied and therefore recommended for application in certain clinical circumstances where highly favorable results have been evidenced; however, there are many non-invasive monitoring methods, such as those categorized in the ophthalmic and otic group, which have not aroused sufficient interest but have the potential to be effective in clinical practice, so further studies on their implementation in the neurocritical care area are suggested.

Recently, Kostick et al. [48], described a non-invasive technique of ICP monitoring known as "Brain stethoscope," which consists of the modification of a conventional stethoscope, where the dome is replaced by a magnetic reluctance pressure sensor; the latter allowed the measurement of the pulsations of the tympanic membrane, which is directly related to the ICP. The cerebral stethoscope was found to be useful in detecting alterations in ICP from the pulsatile waveform of the tympanic membrane in healthy individuals. Further studies in patients with pathologically elevated ICP are needed before this technique can be implemented in clinical practice.

Conclusion

Intracranial hypertension is a pathological entity that leads to many pathological scenarios of poor prognosis for the patient. For this reason, its diagnosis and timely treatment should be the main objective in intensive care units. For years, intracranial pressure monitoring has been a very valuable tool, but nowadays, with the advent of technology, new methods have been developed that provide an effective diagnostic result and safeguard the integrity of the patient, so they could become a reliable alternative to replace invasive monitoring methods. For this reason, the scientific community should take an interest in this subject to provide evidence-based support and thus implement them in a systematized manner in hospital institutions.

References

[1] Guillaume, J., & Janny, P. (1951). Continuous intracranial manometry; importance of the method and first results. *Revue neurologique,* 84(2), 131–142.

[2] Lundberg, N. (1960). Continuous recording and control of ventricular fluid pressure in neurosurgical practice. *Acta psychiatrica Scandinavica. Supplementum,* 36(149), 1–193.

[3] Robba, C., Pozzebon, S., Moro, B., Vincent, J. L., Creteur, J., & Taccone, F. S. (2020). Multimodal non-invasive assessment of intracranial hypertension: an observational study. *Critical care* (London, England), 24(1), 379.

[4] Roldán, M., Abay, T. Y., & Kyriacou, P. A. (2020). Non-Invasive Techniques for Multimodal Monitoring in Traumatic Brain Injury: Systematic Review and Meta-Analysis. *Journal of neurotrauma,* 37(23), 2445–2453.

[5] Canac, N., Jalaleddini, K., Thorpe, S. G., Thibeault, C. M., & Hamilton, R. B. (2020). Review: pathophysiology of intracranial hypertension and noninvasive intracranial pressure monitoring. *Fluids and barriers of the CNS,* 17(1), 40.

[6] Munakomi, S., & M Das, J. (2021). *Intracranial Pressure Monitoring*. In StatPearls. StatPearls Publishing.

[7] Pinto, V. L., Tadi, P., & Adeyinka, A. (2021). *Increased Intracranial Pressure*. In StatPearls. StatPearls Publishing.

[8] March K. (2005). Intracranial pressure monitoring: why monitor? *AACN clinical issues*, 16(4), 456–475.

[9] Holbrook, J., & Saindane, A. M. (2017). Imaging of Intracranial Pressure Disorders. *Neurosurgery,* 80(3), 341–354.

[10] Marehbian, J., Muehlschlegel, S., Edlow, B. L., Hinson, H. E., & Hwang, D. Y. (2017). Medical Management of the Severe Traumatic Brain Injury Patient. *Neurocritical care,* 27(3), 430–446.

[11] Schizodimos, T., Soulountsi, V., Iasonidou, C., & Kapravelos, N. (2020). An overview of management of intracranial hypertension in the intensive care unit. *Journal of anesthesia,* 34(5), 741–757.

[12] Wolfe, T. J., & Torbey, M. T. (2009). Management of intracranial pressure. *Current neurology and neuroscience reports,* 9(6), 477–485.

[13] Smith M. (2008). Monitoring intracranial pressure in traumatic brain injury. *Anesthesia and analgesia,* 106(1), 240–248.

[14] Harary, M., Dolmans, R., & Gormley, W. B. (2018). Intracranial Pressure Monitoring-Review and Avenues for Development. *Sensors* (Basel, Switzerland), 18(2), 465.

[15] Raboel, P. H., Bartek, J., Jr, Andresen, M., Bellander, B. M., & Romner, B. (2012). Intracranial Pressure Monitoring: Invasive versus Non-Invasive Methods-A Review. *Critical care research and practice,* 2012, 950393.

[16] Robba, C., Cardim, D., Tajsic, T., Pietersen, J., Bulman, M., Rasulo, F., Bertuetti, R., Donnelly, J., Xiuyun, L., Czosnyka, Z., Cabeleira, M., Smielewski, P., Matta, B., Bertuccio, A., & Czosnyka, M. (2018). Non-invasive Intracranial Pressure Assessment in Brain Injured Patients Using Ultrasound-Based Methods. *Acta neurochirurgica. Supplement,* 126, 69–73.

[17] Rosenberg, J. B., Shiloh, A. L., Savel, R. H., & Eisen, L. A. (2011). Non-invasive methods of estimating intracranial pressure. *Neurocritical care,* 15(3), 599–608.

[18] Xu, W., Gerety, P., Aleman, T., Swanson, J., & Taylor, J. (2016). Noninvasive methods of detecting increased intracranial pressure. *Child's nervous system: ChNS: official journal of the International Society for Pediatric Neurosurgery,* 32(8), 1371–1386.

[19] Ganslandt, O., Mourtzoukos, S., Stadlbauer, A., Sommer, B., & Rammensee, R. (2018). Evaluation of a novel noninvasive ICP monitoring device in patients undergoing invasive ICP monitoring: preliminary results. *Journal of neurosurgery,* 128(6), 1653–1660.

[20] Robba, C., Bacigaluppi, S., Cardim, D., Donnelly, J., Bertuccio, A., & Czosnyka, M. (2016). Non-invasive assessment of intracranial pressure. *Acta neurologica Scandinavica,* 134(1), 4–21.

[21] Munakomi, S., & M Das, J. (2021). *Intracranial Pressure Monitoring.* In StatPearls. StatPearls Publishing.

[22] Heck C. (2016). *Invasive Neuromonitoring. Critical care nursing clinics of North America*, 28(1), 77–86.

[23] Olson, D. M., Batjer, H. H., Abdulkadir, K., & Hall, C. E. (2014). Measuring and monitoring ICP in Neurocritical Care: results from a national practice survey. *Neurocritical care,* 20(1), 15–20.

[24] Valadka A. B. (2015). Are External Ventricular Drains Better than Parenchymal Intracranial Pressure Monitors in Trauma Patients? *World neurosurgery,* 84(2), 211–213.

[25] Nag, D. S., Sahu, S., Swain, A., & Kant, S. (2019). Intracranial pressure monitoring: Gold standard and recent innovations. *World journal of clinical cases,* 7(13), 1535–1553.

[26] Zhang, X., Medow, J. E., Iskandar, B. J., Wang, F., Shokoueinejad, M., Koueik, J., & Webster, J. G. (2017). Invasive and noninvasive means of measuring intracranial pressure: a review. *Physiological measurement,* 38(8), R143–R182.

[27] Patterson, D. F., Ho, M. L., Leavitt, J. A., Smischney, N. J., Hocker, S. E., Wijdicks, E. F., Hodge, D. O., & Chen, J. J. (2018). Comparison of Ocular Ultrasonography and Magnetic Resonance Imaging for Detection of Increased Intracranial Pressure. *Frontiers in neurology,* 9, 278.

[28] Wong, H., Sanghera, K., Neufeld, A., Maxner, C., & Shankar, J. (2020). Clinico-radiological correlation of magnetic resonance imaging findings in patients with idiopathic intracranial hypertension. *Neuroradiology,* 62(1), 49–53.

[29] Khan, M. N., Shallwani, H., Khan, M. U., & Shamim, M. S. (2017). Noninvasive monitoring intracranial pressure - A review of available modalities. *Surgical neurology international,* 8, 51.

[30] Robba, C., Donnelly, J., Bertuetti, R., Cardim, D., Sekhon, M. S., Aries, M., Smielewski, P., Richards, H., & Czosnyka, M. (2015). Doppler Non-invasive Monitoring of ICP in an Animal Model of Acute Intracranial Hypertension. *Neurocritical care,* 23(3), 419–426.

[31] Cardim, D., Robba, C., Bohdanowicz, M., Donnelly, J., Cabella, B., Liu, X., Cabeleira, M., Smielewski, P., Schmidt, B., & Czosnyka, M. (2016). Non-invasive Monitoring of Intracranial Pressure Using Transcranial Doppler Ultrasonography: Is It Possible? *Neurocritical care,* 25(3), 473–491.

[32] Ragauskas A, Daubaris G. (1995); *A method and apparatus for non- invasively deriving and indicating of dynamic characteristics of the human and animal intracranial media.* Patent 5388583.

[33] Shirodkar, C. G., Rao, S. M., Mutkule, D. P., Harde, Y. R., Venkategowda, P. M., & Mahesh, M. U. (2014). Optic nerve sheath diameter as a marker for evaluation and prognostication of intracranial pressure in Indian patients: An observational study. *Indian journal of critical care medicine: peer-reviewed, official publication of Indian Society of Critical Care Medicine,* 18(11), 728–734.

[34] Lochner, P., Czosnyka, M., Naldi, A., Lyros, E., Pelosi, P., Mathur, S., Fassbender, K., & Robba, C. (2019). Optic nerve sheath diameter: present and future perspectives for neurologists and critical care physicians. *Neurological sciences: official journal of the Italian Neurological Society and of the Italian Society of Clinical Neurophysiology,* 40(12), 2447–2457.

[35] Munawar, K., Khan, M. T., Hussain, S. W., Qadeer, A., Shad, Z. S., Bano, S., & Abdullah, A. (2019). Optic Nerve Sheath Diameter Correlation with Elevated Intracranial Pressure Determined via Ultrasound. *Cureus,* 11(2), e4145.

[36] Chen, L. M., Wang, L. J., Hu, Y., Jiang, X. H., Wang, Y. Z., & Xing, Y. Q. (2019). Ultrasonic measurement of optic nerve sheath diameter: a non-invasive surrogate approach for dynamic, real-time evaluation of intracranial pressure. *The British journal of ophthalmology,* 103(4), 437–441.

[37] Meeker, M., Du, R., Bacchetti, P., Privitera, C. M., Larson, M. D., Holland, M. C., & Manley, G. (2005). Pupil examination: validity and clinical utility of an automated pupillometer. *The Journal of neuroscience nursing: journal of the American Association of Neuroscience Nurses,* 37(1), 34–40.

[38] Du, R., Meeker, M., Bacchetti, P., Larson, M. D., Holland, M. C., & Manley, G. T. (2005). Evaluation of the portable infrared pupillometer. *Neurosurgery,* 57(1), 198–203.

[39] Taylor, W. R., Chen, J. W., Meltzer, H., Gennarelli, T. A., Kelbch, C., Knowlton, S., Richardson, J., Lutch, M. J., Farin, A., Hults, K. N., & Marshall, L. F. (2003). Quantitative pupillometry, a new technology: normative data and preliminary observations in patients with acute head injury. Technical note. *Journal of neurosurgery,* 98(1), 205–213.

[40] Shimbles S., Dodd C., Banister K., Mendelow A.D., and Chambers I.R. (2005) "Clinical comparison of tympanic membrane displacement with invasive intracranial pressure measurements," *Physiological Measurement;* 26 (6), pp. 1085–1092.

[41] Oddo, M., Bösel, J., & Participants in the International Multidisciplinary Consensus Conference on Multimodality Monitoring (2014). Monitoring of brain and systemic oxygenation in neurocritical care patients. *Neurocritical care,* 21 Suppl 2, S103–S120.

[42] Weerakkody, R. A., Czosnyka, M., Zweifel, C., Castellani, G., Smielewski, P., Keong, N., Haubrich, C., Pickard, J., & Czosnyka, Z. (2010). Slow vasogenic fluctuations of intracranial pressure and cerebral near infrared spectroscopy--an observational study. *Acta neurochirurgica,* 152(10), 1763–1769.

[43] Zweifel, C., Castellani, G., Czosnyka, M., Helmy, A., Manktelow, A., Carrera, E., Brady, K. M., Hutchinson, P. J., Menon, D. K., Pickard, J. D., & Smielewski, P. (2010). Noninvasive monitoring of cerebrovascular reactivity with near infrared spectroscopy in head-injured patients. *Journal of neurotrauma,* 27(11), 1951–1958.

[44] Lee, J. K., Kibler, K. K., Benni, P. B., Easley, R. B., Czosnyka, M., Smielewski, P., Koehler, R. C., Shaffner, D. H., & Brady, K. M. (2009). Cerebrovascular reactivity measured by near-infrared spectroscopy. *Stroke,* 40(5), 1820–1826.

[45] York, D. H., Pulliam, M. W., Rosenfeld, J. G., & Watts, C. (1981). Relationship between visual evoked potentials and intracranial pressure. *Journal of neurosurgery,* 55(6), 909–916.

[46] York, D., Legan, M., Benner, S., & Watts, C. (1984). Further studies with a noninvasive method of intracranial pressure estimation. *Neurosurgery,* 14(4), 456–461.

[47] Chen H, Wang J, Mao S, Dong W, Yang H. (2012). A new method of intracranial pressure monitoring by EEG power spectrum analysis. *Can J Neurol Sci;* 39 (4):483–7.

[48] Kostick, N., Manwaring, K., Dhar, R., Sandler, R., & Mansy, H. (2021). The "Brain Stethoscope": A Non-Invasive Method for Detecting Elevated Intracranial Pressure. *Cureus,* 13(3), e13865.

Chapter 8

Neurosurgical Management of Stroke

Randy Reina-Rivero[1], Ivan David Lozada-Martínez[2] and Maria Paz Bolaño-Romero[2]
[1]School of Medicine, Universidad de Cartagena, Cartagena, Colombia
[2]Colombian Clinical Research Group in Neurocritical Care,
Latin American Council of Neurocritical Care, Cartagena, Colombia

Abstract

Cerebro-cardiovascular diseases are the leading cause of death worldwide. Each year, more people die from cerebrovascular diseases than from any other cause. Specifically, they represent 31% of all deaths registered worldwide. Of these deaths, 6.7 million are stroke-related. The gold standard for treating ischemic stroke is pharmacological thrombolysis, leaving endovascular therapy for specific cases. In case of hemorrhagic stroke, the classic treatment is the evacuation of the hematoma by neurosurgical intervention, considering other types of coadjuvant interventions that will depend on the type and location of bleeding. Considering that medicine is advancing rapidly and accurately, different therapies have been proposed, and classical therapies are constantly reevaluated to ensure efficacy and safety. The present chapter aims to present basic and clinical concepts on the neurosurgical management of stroke, both ischemic and hemorrhagic components.

Introduction

Stroke is defined as an abrupt onset of a neurologic deficit that is attributable to a focal vascular cause [1]. This disease constitutes the second most common

In: Advances in Neurosurgery Research
Editors: Amit Agrawal, Pradeep Chouksey, Adesh Shrivastava et al.
ISBN: 978-1-68507-859-1

cause of morbidity and mortality worldwide, with more than 15 million people affected every year and a lifetime risk for adults of approximately 24.9% [2, 3]. The global burden of stroke has been increasing, and prevention of stroke may require other strategies, in order to improve understanding of the risks among younger persons [3]. However, while stroke has grown in incidence worldwide, it is declining among the high-income countries and rising among low-income and middle-income countries [1]. In the United States, the incidence of stroke has declined steadily since 1958, and currently is the fifth leading cause of death. Despite this progress, stroke remains the most common disabling disease in the US [1, 4]. Conversely, the increase of stroke incidence in the low-income and middle-income countries can be explained due to differences in stroke prevention strategies owing to disparity in access to health care, health technologies, and relative rates of risk factors for stroke [3].

There are two main types of strokes: ischemic and hemorrhagic. Ischemic stroke is the most common type (accounts for 85% of all acute strokes), and is caused by interruption of blood flow to a certain area of the brain [4]. On the other hand, hemorrhagic strokes represent 15% of all acute strokes and are caused by bursting of a blood vessel (acute hemorrhage) [4]. The principal goal of therapy in the acute phase of ischemic stroke is reperfusion of salvageable brain tissue, chiefly the penumbra. With advancements in medical and surgical treatment, reperfusion can be accomplished via thrombolysis, namely in the form of intravenous thrombolytic therapy or mechanical thrombectomy in eligible patients [5].

Endovascular Treatment

As mentioned earlier, stroke is a major cause of death worldwide. However, due to the use of reperfusion therapies, the outcome of many patients with acute ischemic stroke (AIS) have changed, preventing death and incapacity [6]. Intravenous (IV) recombinant tissue plasminogen activator (rtPA) is safe and effective in reducing disability in patients with AIS, but some limitations (such as the narrow therapeutic time window and poor effect in the recanalization of large vessels) prevent its more widespread use. Recently, endovascular therapy has been proven a safe and effective therapy for patients with large vessel occlusion who do not respond to or are ineligible for IV thrombolysis [6].

Mechanical Thrombectomy Devices

Mechanical thrombectomy is an interventional procedure that uses endovascular devices to remove a thrombus or blood clot from occluded blood vessels. Mechanical thrombectomy is performed under image guidance and implement diverse catheter-based therapies, such as stent-retrieval, direct aspiration, or a mixture of both [7].

The Merci® Retrieval System (First Generation Device)

The Merci® retrieval system was the first mechanical thrombectomy device and functioned as a clot retriever [8]. The Merci® Retrieval System has 3 components: the Merci retriever, a Balloon Guide Catheter (BGC), and a microcatheter. The BGC is a 9 French catheter with a 2.1-mm lumen and a balloon located at its distal tip [9]. The Merci retriever is a tapered wire which has 5 helical loops of decreasing diameter (from 2.8mm to 1.1mm) at its distal end. The Merci Retriever is advanced through the microcatheter in its straight configuration and resumes its pre-imposed helical shape once it is delivered into the occluded intracranial vessel [9].

The *MERCI trial* (Mechanical Embolus Removal in Cerebral Ischemia) tested the safety and efficacy of the MERCI® device to restore patency of occluded intracranial vessels within the first 8 hours from beginning of symptoms [10]. Recanalization of occluded vessels was achieved in 68 of the 141 patients (48%) in whom the MERCI® device was deployed. Symptomatic intracranial hemorrhages were observed in 7.8% of patients (11/141). Also, the MERCI® device showed improvement in both mortality (32% vs 54%; 95% CI, 0.39 to 0.89; $P = 0.01$) and good neurological outcomes at 90 days (mRS 0-2, 46% vs 10%; 95% CI, 2.1-9.3; $P < 0.0001$) in patients with successful recanalization compared with patients with unsuccessful recanalization [10].

The Penumbra® System (Second Generation Device)

The second clot retriever launched was The Penumbra® System (Penumbra Inc.) in 2008 [11]. The Penumbra® System was designed to remove the thrombus in AIS due to a large vessel occlusion. The device provides two mechanisms to remove the thrombus: aspiration and extraction [12].

Most important components of the Penumbra® System are: the reperfusion catheter, the separator, and the clot removal ring. For the first mechanism (aspiration), the reperfusion catheter is used in parallel with the separator and an aspiration source to separate the thrombus and aspirate it from the occluded vessel. If residual thrombus remains after revascularization with aspiration, the thrombus removal ring is used to directly engage and remove the thrombus (extraction) [12].

The Penumbra Pivotal Stroke Trial was a prospective, multicenter, single-arm study, in which 125 patients were enrolled. The Penumbra® system was able to achieve revascularization of large cerebral vessels in 81.6% of people (a much higher proportion than the 48% of patients with Merci®). Although it was more effective at revascularization, the rate of symptomatic hemorrhage was higher with the Penumbra® system (11.2% vs. 7.8% with the Merci® retriever). Good neurological outcomes (mRS 0-2) at 90 days and all-cause mortality were 25% and 32.8%, respectively [11].

Stent Retrievers (the Solitaire® and Trevo® Devices)

Both Solitaire® (Solitaire MEDTRONIC) and Trevo® (Trevo-STRYKER) are third generation thrombectomy devices which function as stent retrievers [13, 14]. A microcatheter is inserted through the clot over a guidewire. Then, using fluoroscopy, the most distal part of the stent is visualized at the end of the microcatheter. When the stent is deployed, the device expands radially (distally, within and proximally to the clot), embedding itself completely within the clot. Once the stent is withdrawn in its unfolded state, the thrombus is extracted from the vessel [8]. Also, the fact that stent retrievers provide a radial traction force (which decreases the likelihood of clot fragmentation and enable for more consistent removal of the entire clot), give them a significant advantage over other devices [8].

The SWIFT trial was a multicenter, prospective, randomized trial in which the efficacy and safety of thrombectomy with Solitaire® was compared to the standard Merci® retriever. This trial enrolled a total of 144 patients and 113 of them were randomly assigned in two treatment groups (58 patients were treated with Solitaire® and 55 patients with Merci® retriever). The solitaire® stent retriever yield a greater recanalization rate (61% vs 24% in the Merci group). Furthermore, the Solitaire® device had improved rates of good neurologic outcome at 90 days (58% vs. 33% treated with Merci® retriever;

Odds Ratio 2.78 (CI 95; 1.25–6.22) and a lower 90-day mortality rate (17% vs. 38%) [13].

The TREVO 2 trial compared the safety and the recanalization rate of patients with AIS that underwent mechanical thrombectomy with two different retriever devices: the Trevo® Retriever and the Merci® Retriever. From a total of 178 patients enrolled, 88 of them were randomly assigned to be treated with Trevo® and 90 patients to be treated with to Merci®. Compared to Merci® device, the Trevo® stent retriever proved to have a superior rate of canalization (86% vs 60%; OR 4.22, 95% CI 1.92 – 9.69; $p < 0.0001$) and good neurological outcomes at 90-days (mRS 0 – 2,40% vs. 22%) [14].

Endovascular Therapy within 6 Hours from Beginning of Symptoms

In 2015, the paradigm of AIS treatment for patients who had a large vessel occlusion shifted definitely to endovascular therapy. Five multicenter randomized controlled trials (MR CLEAN, REVASCAT, ESCAPE, SWIFT PRIME and EXTEND-IA) demonstrated the efficacy of mechanical thrombectomy compared to intravenous thrombolysis alone in large artery occlusions within an early treatment window [15-20].

The MR CLEAN Trial

The first of the studies was the *MR CLEAN trial* (Multicenter Randomized Clinical Trial of Endovascular Treatment for Acute Ischemic Stroke in the Netherlands). In this trial, mechanical thrombectomy plus conventional care (intervention group) was compared with conventional care alone (control group) in patients with AIS caused by the occlusion of one of the arterial branches that forms the anterior circulation [15].

Eligibility criteria included occlusion of one of the arterial vessels of the anterior circulation: the intracranial carotid artery, the anterior cerebral artery or the middle cerebral artery (MCA) confirmed through computed tomography, angiography or magnetic resonance, within 6 hours of symptom onset [16]. The trial enrolled 500 patients at 16 medical centers in the Netherlands (233 assigned to intraarterial treatment and 267 to usual care alone). The mean age was 65 years (range, 23 to 96), and 445 patients (89.0%)

were treated with intravenous alteplase before randomization. Retrievable stents were used in 190 of the 233 patients (81.5%) assigned to intraarterial treatment [16].

The main outcome of the trial, the modified Rankin score (mRS) at 90 days, revealed a difference of 13.5% in the number of patients who were functionally independent (mRS 0–2) in favor of the mechanical thrombectomy group (32.6% vs. 19.1%, 95% CI 5.9 – 21.2), with no significant difference in complications or mortality [5, 16]. Furthermore, 2-year follow-up studies demonstrated similar findings, with lower mRS scores in mechanical thrombectomy compared to conventional treatment [5, 15].

The REVASCAT Trial

In the *REVASCAT trial* (Randomized Trial of Revascularization with Solitaire FR Device versus Best Medical Therapy in the Treatment of Acute Stroke Due to Anterior Circulation Large Vessel Occlusion Presenting within Eight Hours of Symptom Onset), 206 patients were enrolled and randomly assigned in two groups: the thrombectomy group and the control group. 103 patients were assigned to thrombectomy group and received either medical therapy (alteplase when eligible) and endovascular treatment with the Solitaire stent retriever. The 103 patients in control group received medical therapy alone [5, 17].

Patients were eligible if they had an occlusion of the proximal artery in the anterior circulation and were able to receive treatment within the first 8 hours after the symptoms started [5]. The principal exclusion criteria were the confirmation of a big ischemic core, which was evidenced by an Alberta Stroke Program Early Computed Tomography Score (ASPECTS) < 7 on computed tomography or a DW-magnetic resonance with a score < 6 (ASPECTS values vary from 0-10, and lower infarct burden is indicated by higher values) [17].

The REVASCAT trial demonstrated that mechanical thrombectomy reduced the severity of disability over the range of the mRS and led to higher rates of functional independence (score of 0 - 2) at 90 days (43.7% vs. 28.2%; adjusted OR: 2.1; 95% CI, 1.1 to 4.0). At 90 days, the rates of symptomatic intracranial hemorrhage were 1.9% in both the thrombectomy group and the control group (p = 1.00), and rates of death were 18.4% and 15.5%, respectively (p = 0.60) [17].

The ESCAPE Trial

The *ESCAPE trial* (Endovascular Treatment for Small Core and Anterior Circulation Proximal Occlusion with Emphasis on Minimizing CT to Recanalization Times) enrolled 316 patients who were assigned, in a 1:1 ratio, to receive endovascular treatment with guideline-based care (intervention group) or guideline-based care alone (control group) [18]. As in REVASCAT, the eligibility criteria of ESCAPE trial included patients with a proximal anterior circulation occlusion and the absence of a large infarct via ASPECTS criteria (CT 0–6, MRI 0–5), but within 12 hours of symptom onset [5, 18].

The ESCAPE trial was finished promptly due to the clear benefits of endovascular treatment. From the 316 patients enrolled, 238 received intravenous alteplase (120 in the intervention group and 118 in the control group). The rate of functional independence (90-day mRS of 0-2) was increased with the intervention (53.0%, vs. 29.3% in the control group; $p < 0.001$). Moreover, the intervention was associated with reduced mortality (10.4%, vs. 19.0% in the control group; $p = 0.04$) and the percentage of patients that experienced intracerebral hemorrhage was 3.6% in the intervention group and 2.7% in control group ($p = 0.75$) [18].

Factors that distinguish ESCAPE trial from MR CLEAN include the use of imaging to exclude participants with a large infarct core and poor collateral circulation, a shorter interval from symptom onset to treatment initiation, a low rate of general anesthesia (9% in ESCAPE vs. 38% in MR CLEAN), and a higher rate of successful reperfusion [18].

The SWIFT PRIME Trial

In the *SWIFT PRIME trial* (Solitaire with the Intention for Thrombectomy as Primary Endovascular Treatment), a total of 196 patients were enrolled. Eligible patients with stroke received intravenous t-PA and then were randomly assigned to continue with t-PA alone (control group) or to undergo mechanical thrombectomy with the use of a stent retriever (intervention group) [19]. Eligibility criteria included patients who had imaging confirmed occlusion of the intracranial segment of the internal carotid artery, the MCA, or both, in the absence of a big ischemic core, and who could receive endovascular treatment in the first 6 hours from symptom onset [19].

The study was stopped early due to its efficacy. All patients in the trial received intravenous alteplase prior to randomization. Thrombectomy with the stent retriever added to intravenous t-PA reduced disability at 90 days over the entire range of scores on the modified Rankin scale ($p < 0.001$). The rate of functional independence (mRS 0 to 2) was 60% in the mechanical thrombectomy group and 35% in control group, which represent a significant difference ($p < 0.001$). However, the 90-day mortality percentage (9% vs. 12%, $p = 0.50$) and the rate of symptomatic intracranial hemorrhage (0% vs. 3%, $p = 0.12$) were not significantly different between the intervention and control group [19].

The EXTEND-IA Trial

The last of the five 5 studies published in 2015, the *EXTEND-IA trial* (Extending the Time for Thrombolysis in Emergency Neurological Deficits - Intra-Arterial) was a multicenter, prospective and randomized trial, with a total of 70 patients enrolled. Patients with AIS received intravenous alteplase (0.9 mg/kg) and were randomly assigned in two groups. Half of the patients were assigned to receive endovascular therapy with Solitaire FR stent retriever, and the other half continued receiving intravenous alteplase treatment [20]. Patients were eligible if they were medical treated with alteplase in the first 4.5 hours after the beginning of symptoms and had occlusion of the middle cerebral artery or the internal carotid artery. In addition, the ischemic core had to be <70ml on CT perfusion [20].

Although EXTEND-IA was stopped early due to efficacy, the trial demonstrated a higher rate of reperfusion of ischemic territory at 24h in the thrombectomy group compared to the alteplase-only group. Mechanical thrombectomy, performed at a median of 3.5 hours after the beginning of symptoms, enlarged the percentage of neurologic improvement at 72h (80% vs. 37%, $p = 0.002$) and led to higher rates of functional independence at 90 days (mRS 0 - 2, 71% in thrombectomy group vs. 40% alteplase group; p value = 0.01). The rates of symptomatic hemorrhage or death were similar in both groups [20].

In 2016, a meta-analysis called HERMES (Highly Effective Reperfusion evaluated in Multiple Endovascular Stroke Trials) aimed to pool individual patient data from the MR CLEAN, REVASCAT, ESCAPE, SWIFT PRIME and EXTEND-IA trials, in order to address remaining questions about the effectiveness of mechanical thrombectomy [21]. By direct access to the trials databases, the HERMES collaborators analyzed data from 1287 patients: a total of 634 were assigned to endovascular therapy and the 653 left, to control).

They found that mechanical thrombectomy decreased the rate of disability at 90 days (Odds Ratio 2.49, 95% CI [1.76 – 3.53], $p < 0.0001$) [21].

Effect sizes favoring endovascular treatment over medical therapy were observed in various subgroups of special interest, such as patients ≥ 80 years (Odds Ratio 3.68, 95% CI [1.95 – 6.92]), patients randomized more than 5 hours after the beginning of symptoms (Odds Ratio 1.76, 95% CI [1.05 – 2.97]), and the subgroup of patients that were not eligible for intravenous alteplase (Odds Ratio 2.43, 95% CI [1.30 – 4.55]). The 90-day mortality rate and risk hemorrhage did not differ between populations [21].

Expanding the Treatment Window

As the efficacy of mechanical thrombectomy consolidated in literature, investigators questioned whether an extension of the treatment window would achieve similar results. In 2018, two major clinical trials (DAWN and DIFFUSE 3) disrupted the time window concept in AIS, showing the excellent outcomes of mechanical thrombectomy in patients treated up to 24 hours from symptom onset [22, 23].

The *DAWN trial* (DWI or CTP Assessment with Clinical Mismatch in the Triage of Wake-Up and Late Presenting Strokes Undergoing Neuro-intervention with Trevo) was a multicenter, prospective, randomized trial in which patients were randomly assigned to thrombectomy plus standard care (thrombectomy group) or to standard care alone (control group) [22]. Patients were enrolled if they had occlusion of the proximal MCA or the intracranial segment of internal carotid artery demonstrated on CT angiography or MR angiography, and had last been known to be well 6 to 24 hours earlier and a mismatch between clinical severity of neurologic deficit (NIH stroke scale) and infarct volume (automated software on diffusion-weighted MRI or CT perfusion permitted) [22].

A total of 206 patients were enrolled; 107 were assigned to the thrombectomy group and 99 to the control group. At 90 days, the rate of function independence favored the thrombectomy group over the control group (mRS 0 – 2.49% vs. 13%; 95% CI 24–44). The rate of symptomatic intracranial hemorrhage did not differ significantly between the two groups (6% vs. 3%) nor did the 90-day mortality (19% vs, 18%) [22].

The *DEFUSE 3 trial* (Endovascular Therapy Following Imaging Evaluation for Ischemic Stroke) compared endovascular treatment plus standard therapy with standard therapy alone. Patients were eligible if they had an occlusion of the carotid artery (cervical or intracranial segments) or the proximal MCA, and were last known well between 6 and 16 hours [23]. In addition, neuroimaging criteria included an initial infarct volume < 70 mL, a ratio of volume of ischemic cerebral tissue to volume of initial infarct ≥ 1.8, and a volume of potentially reversible ischemia (penumbra) ≥ 15 ml on MRI perfusion [23].

The trial enrolled 182 patients, 92 were assigned to the thrombectomy group and 90 to the control group. Similar to DAWN trial, the 90-day rate of functional independence was greater in the thrombectomy group, as compared with the control group (mRS 0-2, 45% vs. 17%, p < 0.001). The mortality rate at 90 days in the thrombectomy group was 14% and 26% in the control group (p value = 0.05), and the reports of symptomatic intracranial hemorrhage were 7% in thrombectomy group vs 4% in control group (p = 0.75; no significant difference) [23].

Table 1. AHA recommendations for mechanical thrombectomy (0 to 6 hours from onset) [24]

No	Mechanical Thrombectomy (0 to 6 hours from onset)	COR	LOE
1	Patients should receive mechanical thrombectomy with a stent retriever if they meet all the following criteria: 1- pre-stroke mRS score of 0 to 1; 2)- causative occlusion of the internal carotid artery or MCA segment 1 (M1); 3- age ≥18 years; 4- NIHSS score of ≥6; 5- ASPECTS of ≥6; and, 6- treatment can be initiated (groin puncture) within 6 hours of symptom onset.	I	A
	Although the benefits are uncertain, the use of mechanical thrombectomy with stent retrievers may be reasonable for carefully selected patients with AIS in whom treatment can be initiated (groin puncture) within 6 hours of symptom onset and who:		
3	Have causative occlusion of the MCA segment 2 (M2) or MCA segment 3 (M3) portion of the MCAs.	IIb	B-R
4	Have pre-stroke mRS score >1, ASPECTS <6, or NIHSS score <6, and causative occlusion of the internal carotid artery (ICA) or proximal MCA (M1).	IIb	B-R
5	Have causative occlusion of the anterior cerebral arteries, vertebral arteries, basilar artery, or posterior cerebral arteries	IIb	C-LD

Class of recommendation (COR): I (strong benefit), IIa (moderate benefit), IIb (weak benefit). Level of evidence (LOE): A (high quality), B-R (moderate quality randomized), C-LD (observation or registry with limited data).

Based on the eligibility criteria and results of the trials previously discussed, the American Heart Association (AHA) recommends that patients must receive endovascular treatment if they meet the requirements described in table 1 (0 to 6 hours from onset) and table 2 (6 to 24 hours from onset) [24]:

Table 2. AHA recommendations for Mechanical Thrombectomy (6 to 24 hours from onset) [24]

No	Mechanical Thrombectomy (6 to 24 hours from onset)	COR	LOE
1	In selected patients with AIS within 6 to 16 hours of last known normal who have LVO in the anterior circulation and meet other DAWN or DEFUSE 3 eligibility criteria, mechanical thrombectomy is recommended.	I	A
2	In selected patients with AIS within 16 to 24 hours of last known normal who have LVO in the anterior circulation and meet other DAWN eligibility criteria, mechanical thrombectomy is reasonable.	IIa	B-R

Class of recommendation (COR): I (strong benefit), IIa (moderate benefit). Level of evidence (LOE): A (high quality), B-R (moderate quality randomized).

Decompressive Hemicraniectomy

Patients with large ischemic strokes may develop uncontrollable, progressive brain edema that generates an increased intracranial pressure (ICP), placing the patient at risk for compression of brain parenchyma and cerebral herniation. In this situation there are a limited number of therapeutic options, but research has shown that operative procedures, such as decompressive hemicraniectomy (DHC), can decrease patient mortality [25]. Malignant infarction treated only by conservative approaches results in a mortality rate of 80% within the first week after the stroke onset. Thus, cerebral edema that does not respond to medical treatment may require DHC as a life-saving procedure [25]. Moreover, investigation has shown that DHC reduce the mortality rate to 30%, and if the surgery is performed within 24-48 hours of stroke onset, the mortality rate can decrease to 10% [26].

Decompressive hemicraniectomy is a surgical procedure in which the neurosurgeon removes a portion of the patient's skull in order to allow swelling brain tissue to expand outward to relieve compression against the skull [26].

The typical DHC performed is via a unilateral approach to remove a 12 to 14 cm bone flap. By removing the skull, the brain is allowed to expand, thereby normalizing ICP and reducing compression and/or midline shift. By reducing ICP, cerebral perfusion pressure and blood flow are restored [27].

The efficacy of DHC in malignant MCA infarction has been reinforced in several recent randomized controlled trials [28-30].

The DECIMAL Trial

The Decompressive Craniectomy In Malignant MCA Infarction trial was a multicenter, prospective, randomized study that compared DHC plus standard medical therapy versus standard medical therapy alone in patients with malignant MCA infarction [28].

Patients were eligible if they had between 18 - 55 years of age within the first 24 hours of a malignant MCA infarction defined by 3 criteria: a NIHSS score ≥16 (including a score ≥1 for item 1a -level of consciousness-); a CT with demonstrated ischemic signs involving >50% of MCA territory; and a DWI infarct volume >145cm^3.

Patients were excluded if they had preexisting significant disability defined by a mRS score ≥2, a significant contralateral infarction, a severe secondary hemorrhagic infarction involving >50% of the MCA territory, any known coagulopathy, life expectancy <3 years [28].

In this trial, a total of 38 patients were enrolled and randomized until the data safety monitoring committee recommended to stop enrollment due to the high disparity in mortality between the two groups across 3 trials, in favor of decompressive craniectomy.

In the craniectomy group, the percentage of patients with a mRS ≤ 3 at the 6-month follow-up was 25% and 50% at the 12-month follow-up. The proportion of patients in the medical therapy group with a mRS ≤ 3 were 5.6% in the 6 month and 22.2% in the 12-month follow-up ($p = 0.18$ and $p = 0.10$, respectively).

Moreover, Craniectomy had a huge life-saving effect represented by a 52.8% reduction of death after the surgery compared with those who only received medical therapy ($p < 0.0001$) [28].

The DESTINY Trial

The results of the DESTINY (Decompressive Surgery for the Treatment of Malignant Infarction of the Middle Cerebral Artery) trial were published in the same year as DECIMAL. This study was a prospective, multicenter, randomized, controlled, clinical trial in which 32 patients were randomly assigned into DHC or standard medical therapy [29].

Patients were enrolled if they met inclusion criteria such as age 18–60 years, clinical signs of infarction of the MCA territory with an NIHSS score >18, decrease in the level of consciousness (a score of ≥1 on item 1a of the NIHSS), a CT documented unilateral MCA infarction, and onset of symptoms >12 and <36 hours before a possible surgical intervention. Similar to DECIMAL, this study was stopped due to a high disparity of mortality in favor of DHC. After 30 days, 15 of 17 (88%) patients randomized to DHC survived, compared to 7 of 15 (47%) patients randomized to conservative therapy, representing a statistically significant reduction in mortality ($p = 0.02$). After 6 and 12 months, 47% of patients in the surgical group versus 27% of patients in the conservative treatment group had a mRS score ≤3 ($p = 0.23$) [29].

The HAMLET Trial

A third study, the HAMLET trial (Hemicraniectomy after Middle cerebral artery infarction with Life-threatening Edema Trial), investigated the efficacy of DHC through a randomized, open trial [30]. In this trial, adult patients ≤60 years of age with space-occupying hemispheric infarction were enrolled and randomized in a 1:1 ratio to receive surgical decompression or to receive the best medical treatment. Unlike the two studies before mentioned, HAMLET expanded the eligibility criteria to patients within 4 days of stroke onset. Patients also required a NIHSS score ≥16; a Glasgow coma scale score of ≤13 for right-sided lesions or a score ≤ 9 for left-sided lesions; and ischemic changes on CT that affect 2/3 of the MCA territory [31].

In HAMLET, DHC had no effect on the risk of poor functional outcome at 3 years (absolute risk reduction, 1%; 95% CI, 21 - 22), but it reduced case fatality (absolute risk reduction, 37%; 95% CI, 14–60). Moreover, quality of life improved between 1 and 3 years in patients treated with surgery [31].

Moreover, a 2016 meta-analysis of seven randomized controlled clinical trials (including DECIMAL, DESTINY and HAMLET) aggregated data among 338 patients and found that decompressive hemicraniectomy decreased death (69% in medical therapy group vs 30% in DHC group), and increased the amount of patients with a score of 2 to 3 in the modified Rankin score (mild to moderate disability: 14 in medical therapy group vs 27% in DHC group). On the other hand, the DHC group also had higher rates of severe disability (mRS 4.32% vs. 10%, $p < 0.001$) and very severe disability (mRS 5, 11% vs. 7%, $p < 0.001$), indicating that the large reduction in mortality result in higher disease burden [5, 32].

Conclusion

Fortunately, there is an exponential growth of evidence favorable to improved functional outcomes and survival in stroke management. However, many of the aforementioned devices and clinical trials are available and conducted, respectively, in high-income countries. Further progress is needed in the search for tools and solutions that are feasible and applicable in all social and economic contexts of global neurosurgery.

References

[1] Kasper Dennis L et al. *Harrison's Principles of Internal Medicine 20th Edition* (Vol. 1 & Vol. 2). McGraw Hill Professional, 2018.

[2] Feigin Valery L et al. Global, regional, and national burden of neurological disorders, 1990–2016: A systematic analysis for the Global Burden of Disease Study 2016. *The Lancet Neurology*, 2019, vol. 18, no 5, p. 459-480.

[3] GBD 2016 Lifetime Risk of Stroke Collaborators. Global, regional, and country-specific lifetime risks of stroke, 1990 and 2016. *New England Journal of Medicine*, 2018, vol. 379, no 25, p. 2429-2437.

[4] Tadi P, Lui F. *Acute Stroke*. [Updated 2021 Mar 24]. In: Stat Pearls [Internet]. Treasure Island (FL): Stat Pearls Publishing; 2021 Jan-. Available from: https://www.ncbi.nlm.nih.gov/books/NBK535369/.

[5] Koltz Michael T, Kohli Vikraant. *Indications for Surgical Intervention in the Treatment of Ischemic Stroke*. Exon Publications, 2021, p. 97-109.

[6] Silva Gisele S, Nogueira Raul G. Endovascular treatment of acute ischemic stroke. *CONTINUUM: Lifelong Learning in Neurology,* 2020, vol. 26, no 2, p. 310-331.

[7] Mathews S, De Jesus O. *Thrombectomy*. [Updated 2021 Feb. 7]. In: StatPearls [Internet]. Treasure Island (FL): StatPearls Publishing; 2021 Jan-. Available from: https://www.ncbi.nlm.nih.gov/books/NBK562154/.

[8] Withrow J, Todnem N, Rahimi S. The Evolution of the Neurosurgical Treatment of Ischemic Stroke. *Journal of Cerebrovascular and Endovascular Neurosurgery*, 2018, vol. 20, no 1, p. 53.

[9] Pierre Gobin Y, et al. MERCI 1: A phase 1 study of Mechanical Embolus Removal in Cerebral Ischemia. *Stroke,* 2004, vol. 35, no 12, p. 2848-2854.

[10] Smith Wade S, et al. Safety and efficacy of mechanical embolectomy in acute ischemic stroke: Results of the MERCI trial. *Stroke*, 2005, vol. 36, no 7, p. 1432-1438.

[11] Penumbra Pivotal Stroke Trial Investigators. The penumbra pivotal stroke trial: safety and effectiveness of a new generation of mechanical devices for clot removal in intracranial large vessel occlusive disease. *Stroke*, 2009, vol. 40, no 8, p. 2761-2768.

[12] Bose A et al. The Penumbra System: A mechanical device for the treatment of acute stroke due to thromboembolism. *American journal of Neuroradiology,* 2008, vol. 29, no 7, p. 1409-1413.

[13] Saver Jeffrey L et al. Solitaire flow restoration device versus the Merci Retriever in patients with acute ischaemic stroke (SWIFT): A randomised, parallel-group, non-inferiority trial. *The Lancet,* 2012, vol. 380, no 9849, p. 1241-1249.

[14] Nogueira Raul G et al. Trevo versus Merci retrievers for thrombectomy revascularisation of large vessel occlusions in acute ischaemic stroke (TREVO 2): A randomised trial. *The Lancet,* 2012, vol. 380, no 9849, p. 1231-1240.

[15] Van Den Berg Lucie A et al. Two-year outcome after endovascular treatment for acute ischemic stroke. *New England Journal of Medicine,* 2017, vol. 376, no 14, p. 1341-1349.

[16] Berkhemer Olvert A et al. A randomized trial of intraarterial treatment for acute ischemic stroke. *New England Journal of Medicine,* 2015, vol. 372, p. 11-20.

[17] Jovin Tudor G et al. Thrombectomy within 8 hours after symptom onset in ischemic stroke. *New England Journal of Medicine*, 2015, vol. 372, no 24, p. 2296-2306.

[18] Goyal Mayank et al. Randomized assessment of rapid endovascular treatment of ischemic stroke. *New England Journal of Medicine*, 2015, vol. 372, no 11, p. 1019-1030.

[19] Saver Jeffrey L et al. Stent-retriever thrombectomy after intravenous t-PA vs. t-PA alone in stroke. *New England Journal of Medicine*, 2015, vol. 372, no 24, p. 2285-2295.

[20] Campbell Bruce CV et al. Endovascular therapy for ischemic stroke with perfusion-imaging selection. *New England Journal of Medicine*, 2015, vol. 372, no 11, p. 1009-1018.

[21] Goyal Mayank et al. Endovascular thrombectomy after large-vessel ischaemic stroke: A meta-analysis of individual patient data from five randomised trials. *The Lancet,* 2016, vol. 387, no 10029, p. 1723-1731.

[22] Nogueira Raúl G et al. Thrombectomy 6 to 24 hours after stroke with a mismatch between deficit and infarct. *New England Journal of Medicine,* 2018, vol. 378, no 1, p. 11-21.

[23] Albers Gregory W et al. Thrombectomy for stroke at 6 to 16 hours with selection by perfusion imaging. *New England Journal of Medicine,* 2018, vol. 378, no 8, p. 708-718.

[24] Powers William J et al. Guidelines for the early management of patients with acute ischemic stroke: 2019 update to the 2018 guidelines for the early management of

acute ischemic stroke: A guideline for healthcare professionals from the American Heart Association/American Stroke Association. *Stroke*, 2019, vol. 50, no 12, p. e344-e418.

[25] Daou Badih et al. Decompressive hemicraniectomy: predictors of functional outcome in patients with ischemic stroke. *Journal of Neurosurgery,* 2016, vol. 124, no 6, p. 1773-1779.

[26] Karasin Beth et al. Decompressive Hemicraniectomy for Middle Cerebral Artery Stroke: Indications and Perioperative Care. *AORN Journal,* 2021, vol. 114, no 1, p. 34-46.

[27] Crudele Angela, Shah, Syed Omar, Bar, Barak. Decompressive hemicraniectomy in acute neurological diseases. *Journal of Intensive Care Medicine,* 2016, vol. 31, no 9, p. 587-596.

[28] Vahedi Katayoun et al. Sequential-design, multicenter, randomized, controlled trial of early decompressive craniectomy in malignant middle cerebral artery infarction (DECIMAL Trial). *Stroke,* 2007, vol. 38, no 9, p. 2506-2517.

[29] JüTtler Eric et al. Decompressive surgery for the treatment of malignant infarction of the middle cerebral artery (DESTINY) a randomized, controlled trial. *Stroke,* 2007, vol. 38, no 9, p. 2518-2525.

[30] Geurts Marjolein, et al. Surgical decompression for space-occupying cerebral infarction: Outcomes at 3 years in the randomized HAMLET trial. *Stroke,* 2013, vol. 44, no 9, p. 2506-2508.

[31] Hofmeijer Jeannette et al. Surgical decompression for space-occupying cerebral infarction (the Hemicraniectomy After Middle Cerebral Artery infarction with Life-threatening Edema Trial [HAMLET]): a multicentre, open, randomised trial. *The Lancet Neurology*, 2009, vol. 8, no 4, p. 326-333.

[32] Alexander Paul et al. Hemicraniectomy versus medical treatment with large MCA infarct: A review and meta-analysis. *BMJ Open,* 2016, vol. 6, no 11, p. e014390.

Chapter 9

Low-Grade Glioma

Rupant Kumar Das, MCh,
Aishik Mukherjee, MCh, MRCS
and Dibyendu Kumar Ray, MCh, FRCS
AMRI Hospitals, Salt Lake, Kolkata, India

Abstract

Gliomas as a group constitute the most common malignant primary CNS tumors. They are a heterogeneous group of pathological entities which vary in their behavior, natural history, and prognosis. "Low grade" glioma, though less common than their higher-grade cousins, offers a markedly different prognosis. Earlier, the standard practice had been to categorize these tumors on the basis of their microscopic characteristics. Since 2016 there has been a paradigm shift in the way they are classified. Tumor genetic characteristics are now a part of the tumor classification. There remain several unanswered questions regarding the role of chemotherapy and radiotherapy, particularly the timing of initiation and the agents used. In this chapter, the authors endeavor to give an overview of current classification paradigms and trends in the management of low-grade glioma.

Introduction

Gliomas are the most common primary malignant CNS tumors and encompass a variety of histological subtypes and grades based on the putative cell of origin and other histopathological characteristics. Among these, the low-grade gliomas, though less common than their higher-grade counterparts, offer a

In: Advances in Neurosurgery Research
Editors: Amit Agrawal, Pradeep Chouksey, Adesh Shrivastava et al.
ISBN: 978-1-68507-859-1

better prognosis in terms of long- or medium-term survival, and from this, it follows that treatment paradigms need to be carefully considered to minimize morbidity from respective interventions and maximize survival while affording a reasonable quality of life. This has been a subject of several studies. A revision of criteria for classifying CNS tumors as put forth in 2016 has also brought about a shift in how these tumors are assessed and the impact of genetic characteristics of tumor cells on prognosis.

What follows is a brief overview of the classification of gliomas with particular reference to low-grade gliomas and recent trends in the management of low-grade glioma.

Classification and Pathology

Traditionally, the term low-grade glioma has been used with reference to WHO Grade 1 and Grade 2 tumors, though the term 'low-grade' does not find mention in the formal WHO classification. These include diffuse tumors like diffuse astrocytoma, pilomyxoid astrocytoma, pleomorphic xanthoastrocytoma (WHO Grade II), and more benign forms like pilocytic astrocytoma and subependymal giant cell astrocytoma (WHO Grade I). Other types include low-grade tumors of an oligodendroglial lineage (oligodendroglioma) and glioneuronal lineage like dysembryoplastic neuroepithelial tumor, ganglioglioma, and infantile desmoplastic astrocytoma among others [1].

Post Haarlem consensus guidelines, there has been a shift in the way these entities are viewed and has brought in the concept of an "integrated diagnosis" which includes the histological type of tumor, the WHO grade of the tumor (both reliant upon traditional histopathologic criteria), and finally the molecular or genetic information regarding the tumor [2]. Furthermore, if there is a discordance between the conventional histological criteria and the genetic criteria, the genotype takes precedence over the microscopic phenotype [3].

One of the points of departure from the previous classification scheme is that while in the previous iteration of WHO (2007) all astrocytomas and oligodendrogliomas were considered independent entities based on their phenotypical characteristics, in the new scheme all diffuse tumors (astrocytic as well as oligodendroglial) are considered together under one group based on their genetic characteristics (IDH1/IDH2 mutations and 1p/19q codeletion) and includes all diffuse astrocytoma's (grade II/III/glioblastoma) and oligodendroglioma. Grading continues to be based on conventional histopathological criteria. The well-circumscribed tumors are now grouped as a separate independent entity that generally lacks IDH gene family mutations and may have other distinct genetic signatures like BRAF mutations (pilocytic astrocytoma, pleomorphic xanthoastrocytoma) and TSC1/TSC2 mutations (subependymal giant cell astrocytoma). Some of the previous subtypes are no longer a part of the classification, notably protoplasmic and fibrillary variants of diffuse astrocytoma, and only one distinct variant remains i.e., gemistocytic astrocytoma. Similarly, oligoastrocytoma remains uncertain and it is suggested that the term be used only for those tumors in which cell populations demonstrating both mutations are seen. Most tumors earlier labeled as oligoastrocytoma are now classified as either astrocytoma or oligodendroglioma based on genetic mutations found.

One distinct, primarily pediatric, diffuse glioma has been defined and designated as "diffuse midline glioma" and includes diffuse intrinsic pontine glioma. These tumors are characterized by K27M gene mutations and involve midline structures like the thalamus, brainstem, and spinal cord.

In addition to the biomarkers detailed above, there are others used for disease prognostication and classification like MGMT promoter region mutations, Rho A overexpression, ATRX mutations, EGFR mutations, and SND1 overexpression. These are mostly markers of high-grade glioma and are beyond the scope of the present discussion.

Isocitrate Dehydrogenase 1/2

These genetic anomalies were first described in 2008 and have now been formally included in the WHO classification scheme [4]. IDH mutations involve codon 132 / R 132H in isoform 1 and codon 172 in isoform 2 resulting in amino acid substitution. They frequently occur in low-grade diffuse gliomas as well as grade III gliomas and the so-called secondary GBM which evolve from their lower-grade counterparts and may also occur in oligodendrogliomas along with 1p/19q codeletion. In addition to being a diagnostic marker, patients with LDH 1/ 2 mutations are more responsive to treatment and consequently have a better prognosis.

Chromosome 1p/19q Codeletion

This is a defining genetic anomaly for tumors classified as oligodendroglioma and has a favorable prognosis when compared to phenotypically oligodendroglial tumors lacking this mutation (Oligodendroglioma NOS).

Micro RNA

miRNA is a short non-coding RNA that plays a role in post-transcriptional control of gene expression by base-pairing with complementary mRNA molecules resulting in 'silencing' of the mRNA. They are believed to play a role in controlling cell growth, angiogenesis, etc. Studies have shown some miRNA clusters to be predictors of overall survival in conjunction with the traditionally used biomarkers [5].

Radiology and Imaging

MRI

MRI studies for glioma typically include standard T1 weighted sequences with and without contrast, T2 sequences, FLAIR, DWI, and MR spectroscopy. While these studies provide a detailed anatomical map of the lesion, imaging features do not correlate very well with tumor histology. Low-grade gliomas are usually seen as T1 hypointense, T2/FLAIR hyperintense, non-enhancing masses with little or no perilesional edema, and anatomical distortion due to bulk mass effect. Some authors report the use of perfusion-weighted sequences (dynamic contrast susceptibility) in differentiating low grade from high-grade glioma but definitive evidence validating the role of imaging in diagnosing tumor grade is lacking [6, 7, 8].

fMRI

Functional MRI is a non-invasive modality for anatomical localization and mapping of eloquent cortical structures. It reflects changes in metabolic activity in regions of the brain when specific tasks are performed or stimuli are given. It is most accurate for mapping the motor cortex and related association areas and sensory cortex. fMRI relies on detecting changes in relative levels of oxyhemoglobin and deoxyhemoglobin levels in the metabolically active cortex, the so-called blood oxygen level-dependent contrast. It is a useful adjunct to preoperative evaluation of eloquent area gliomas and in formulating a surgical strategy. Different authors report varying sensitivity and specificity of motor mapping when compared to direct cortical stimulation (sensitivity ranging from 70 – 100% and specificity ranging from 68 – 100%) [9, 10, 11].

Localization of language areas using fMRI is less precise, presumably due to greater spatial dispersion of language-related functions. Bizzi et. al report a sensitivity of 80% and specificity of 78% when compared to direct cortical stimulation.

DTI

One of the determinants of overall survival in low-grade glioma is the extent of surgical resection [12]. MR tractography facilitates maximal safe removal of gliomas located in or near eloquent regions of the brain and aids preoperative assessment of the feasibility of complete resection. In addition to KPS and age, tumor size and proximity to the eloquent cortex have been shown to be a predictor of progression-free as well as overall survival [13]. DTI helps define the relationship of the tumor to important white matter tracts, especially in the context of distorted local anatomy on account of the tumor mass and edema which makes assessment difficult on routine preoperative anatomical imaging. The functionally significant tracts that are frequently evaluated in tractography are the corticospinal tract, the superior longitudinal fasciculus, the inferior fronto- occipital tract, cingulum, uncinate fasciculus, and the arcuate fasciculus. Most cases with infiltration of the tracts which subserve important motor or language-related functions are not suitable for aggressive maximal resection. It has been reported that the distance between the tumor mass and three of the tracts (corticospinal/superior longitudinal fasciculus /cingulum) is a predictor of adverse surgical outcomes (distance < 1 cm) [14].

DTI imaging has its drawbacks, particularly in the setting of peritumoral edema or actual infiltration of the tract by tumor cells, where delineating the tracts becomes difficult and imprecise. It is suggested that DTI imaging be used in conjunction with intraoperative brain mapping to optimize outcomes [12].

Role of Radiotracer Based Imaging

The use of PET scans using various tracers has been widely studied in the context of prognostication, gauging therapeutic response, diagnosis of recurrence, and its differentiation from sequelae of radiotherapy. PET using 18F fluorodeoxyglucose is a functional imaging modality that relies upon the metabolic activity of the tissue under study. Some studies suggest that hypometabolism correlates with a lower grade of malignancy and an increased uptake of FDG points toward a more aggressive lesion with correspondingly poor survival [15, 16].

A higher specificity has also been reported vis-à-vis MRI in the diagnosis of recurrence, (97% vs 23%). O-(2-(18)F-fluoroethyl)- L-tyrosine (FET) PET-CT has been used to predict the biological behavior of newly diagnosed brain tumors. The tracer is an artificial amino acid that provides a measure of the activity of large neutral amino acid transport pathways which is upregulated in malignant gliomas as compared to low-grade gliomas. Pichler et. al report a sensitivity of 94% in the diagnosis of high-grade tumors using this modality [17]. Another application of PET study is in identifying sites of biopsy in heterogeneous tumors thereby avoiding necrotic and metabolically inactive regions and increasing diagnostic yield. Some studies indicate a role for FDG PET and FET- PET in predicting treatment response to irinotecan and bevacizumab in recurrent tumors [18, 19].

A major limitation of FDG PET is that it is not tumor-specific and only reflects metabolic hyperactivity, which may result in false positives as in the case of inflammatory lesions.

Approach to Treatment

The tools available in the therapeutic armamentarium are surgery, chemotherapy, and radiotherapy. While the role of surgery is well defined it is by no means sufficient in and of itself. The protocols defining the use and timing of radiotherapy and chemotherapy are still being debated and a uniform consensus is yet to evolve. The following is a brief overview of the various treatment modalities available and the methodology for their application.

Surgery: Surgery is usually the first step in the treatment of low-grade glioma. The neurosurgeon should aim at gross total removal of the tumor mass where possible and maximal safe resection in more eloquent regions of the brain. It is generally held that the extent of tumor removal at initial surgery has a bearing on both the progression-free survival and overall survival. The potential for surgical morbidity can be reduced significantly and the extent of resection maximized using adjuncts like neuro-navigation, ultrasound, intraoperative brain mapping, MR tractography, tumor fluorescence, and finally intraoperative imaging like MRI and CT. Surgery is not sufficient and other complementary treatment modalities are also required in most patients.

Adjuvant Treatment

Though adjuvant treatment in the form of RT and chemotherapy are needed in most patients there is some degree of uncertainty as to the timing of when these interactions should be undertaken. Some authors have tried to identify subgroups of patients with poorer prognosis and the factors to be considered for this stratification are tumor size (> 4 cm), age > 40 years, absence of 1p/19q codeletion, astrocytoma, incomplete resection, and tumors crossing the midline [20, 21].

The RTOG observational study of adults under the age of 40 years with low-grade glioma (grade II astrocytoma, oligodendroglioma, oligoastrocytoma), supratentorial tumor, gross total resection at surgery, and KPS > 60, found that overall survival at 2 and 5 years were 99% and 92% respectively and progression-free survival was 82 and 48% respectively. These patients did not receive any form of adjuvant therapy. The authors concluded that the risk factors for poor progression-free survival were tumor size (> 4cm), residual tumor >1cm on post-operative MRI, and astrocytoma/oligoastrocytoma on histology [22].

Though there is a lack of clarity in the literature regarding the time of initiation of adjuvant treatment, one may take a wait and watch approach in the low-risk group with an aim to avoid the morbidity of radiotherapy and chemotherapy. These are those under 40 years of age, IDH mutant, 1p/19q co-deleted who have undergone complete resection without residual tumor on postoperative MRI.

For older patients, those with unfavorable genotypes and incomplete resection, early adjuvant treatment should be considered.

Chemotherapy

The role of chemotherapy following radiotherapy is now well established in the treatment of low-grade (WHO Grade II) glioma. Level I evidence was provided by Jan Buckner et. al in a 2016 study (RTOG 9802 trial). The study included 251 (from 1998 to 2002) patients with astrocytoma, oligodendroglioma, and mixed astrocytoma- oligodendroglioma type tumors. This group was further divided into two groups, those under 40 years of age who had undergone subtotal resection of the tumor and those above 40 years of age regardless of the extent of tumor removal. Further stratification was done on the basis of KPS, tumor histology, and radiological features. Patients were then randomly assigned to receive either radiotherapy or radiation followed by chemotherapy. After a median follow-up of 11.9 years, the authors reported a median survival of 13.3 years and progression-free survival of 10.4 years in the radiotherapy + chemotherapy arm as compared to 7.8 and four years respectively in the radiotherapy only arm. The regime used by the authors consisted of procarbazine, lomustine, and vincristine. The authors reported an increased incidence of hematologic toxicity but no incidence of secondary malignancy or deaths attributable to this. This survival benefit was seen among all histological tumor types but was most pronounced for oligodendroglioma [23].

Temozolomide

In the RTOG 0424 trial outcomes of chemoradiation with Temozolomide were compared with historical controls. 129 patients of high-risk low-grade glioma were included (risk factors: age > 40 years, astrocytoma histology, bi-hemispheric tumor, preoperative tumor diameter 6 cm, pre-operative neurological deficits) were included and compared with the EORTC 22845 [24]. At a median follow-up of 4.1 years, the 3-year overall survival was 73% compared to 54% in patients who had received only RT in the EORTC 22845 trial. The treatment regimen consisted of daily Temozolomide with RT followed by once-monthly Temozolomide [25]. Though the data available suggests that chemoradiation with Temozolomide may be efficacious in low-grade glioma, level 1 evidence is lacking and it is still not clear if Temozolomide chemoradiation should replace the traditional PCV regime, unlike high-grade glioma where its role is well established and has largely replaced PCV on account of a more favorable toxicity profile and ease of administration.

Combined Chemotherapy and Radiotherapy or Single Modality Treatment

Combined modality treatment versus single modality treatment of high-risk low-grade glioma is a subject of ongoing debate. Clear guidelines regarding this are lacking. One prospective randomized study on the outcomes of radiotherapy or chemotherapy when used as the only modality of treatment in high-risk low-grade glioma (defined as having any one of the following - aged > 40 years, progressive disease, tumor size > 5 cm, tumor crossing the midline, or neurological symptoms) is the EORTC 22033-26033 trial published in 2016. This was a multi-center trial involving 707 patients across 19 countries. The patients were stratified on the basis of neurological status, age, presence or absence of contrast enhancement on MRI, 1p/19q codeletion, and randomized on a 1:1 basis to either the radiotherapy arm or chemotherapy (Temozolomide) arm. At a median follow-up of 48 months, the authors reported a median progression-free survival was 39 months in the temozolomide group and 46 months in the radiotherapy group. Furthermore, in 318 patients for whom genetic studies were available, the study found a significant difference in survival among different groups (IDH mutant / IDH mutant + 1p/19q codeletion/ IDH wild type). To summarise their results

I. Patients with IDH-mutant, 1p/19q non-co deleted tumors had longer progression-free survival for patients randomized to receive radiation (55 versus 36 months)

II. Patients with 1p/19q co-deleted tumors (62 versus 55 months) and with IDH-wild type tumors (19 versus 24 months) had similar progression-free survival for both groups.

The collection of follow-up data in the trial is ongoing and the authors concluded that though there were no significant differences in outcomes of patients treated with either radiotherapy or Temozolamide alone, further data maturation is needed before recommendations can be made regarding individualizing therapy [26].

IDH Wildtype Low Grade Glioma

These tumors constitute a small proportion of low-grade gliomas. These tend to be more aggressive and often share mutations common to their higher-grade counterparts (TERT, MGMT, loss of heterozygosity of chromosome 10). Prognostically, they have been shown to have poorer outcomes more in line with grade III and grade IV tumors than grade II gliomas. There are no clear guidelines regarding chemotherapy/radiotherapy/ chemoradiation for these tumors. But in view of their close similarity to GBM, many authors are of the view that they should be treated in a similar fashion with concurrent chemoradiation (Stupp regimen).

Radiotherapy

The role of radiotherapy in the treatment of low-grade glioma is now well established, as with chemotherapy. Technological advancements in the field aim to optimize the benefits of radiotherapy while minimizing acute and long-term adverse effects of radiotherapy, an important facet of which is neurocognitive function.

Modalities like intensity-modulated radiation and proton therapy reduce radiation to the normal brain as compared to conventional and 3 D conformal radiotherapy, while maximizing the dose to the targeted region.

In a prospective study of 20 patients of low-grade glioma who were administered proton radiotherapy, cognitive function was evaluated at yearly intervals over a period of 5 years. The authors reported stable cognitive function over the period of observation. The 5-year progression-free survival was 40% and the 5-year overall survival was 84% [27]. Compare these results to the radiotherapy-only trial using conventional photon radiotherapy (5-year progression-free survival of 46% and 5-year overall survival was 63%) [28]. The sample size, however, was very small, and larger studies are required to draw definitive conclusions. Trials comparing conventional photon radiotherapy + Temozolomide with proton radiotherapy + Temozolomide are underway.

The dose and timing of radiotherapy have been a subject of scientific scrutiny, mainly to study the benefit vis-a-vis radiation toxicity to the brain. Shaw et. al reported the results of a randomized controlled trial by the NCCTG/ECOG/RTOG. In the study, it was concluded that higher doses of radiation (50.4Gy vs 64.8Gy) did not confer a survival benefit at 2 and 5 years.

The incidence of severe radiation toxicity was 2.5% and 5% in the low dose and high dose arms respectively. About 5% of patients showed deterioration in cognitive function as assessed by MMSE and most remained stable [29].

In a study comparing early radiotherapy to deferred radiotherapy (at progression) Karim et. al reported a similar overall survival in irradiated and non-irradiated patients. However, the progression-free survival at 5 years was significantly different and in favor of early radiation (44% for the radiotherapy group and 37% for the non-radiotherapy group) [30]. Neurocognitive outcomes of radiotherapy were not assessed in this trial.

Conclusion

Our understanding of tumor genetics has evolved immensely over the last few decades. Efforts are on, to correlate genetic changes with tumor behavior and outcome. Hopefully, as our understanding increases further, it shall be possible to tailor treatment based on the genetic profile of the tumor, and this along with technological advances in imaging, radiotherapy, and chemotherapy will improve survival and enhance post-treatment quality of life. Having said that, the optimal management of glioma is an ever-evolving subject and a work in progress.

References

[1] Louis D N, et al. The 2007 WHO Classification of Tumours of the Central Nervous System, *Acta Neuropathol.* 2007;114:97–109.

[2] Louis D N, et al. International Society of Neuropathology—Haarlem: International Society of Neuropathology—Haarlem consensus guidelines for nervous system tumor classification and grading. *Brain Pathol.* 24: 429–435, 2014.

[3] Louis D N, et al. The 2016 World Health Organization Classification of Tumors of the Central Nervous System: a summary. *Acta Neuropathol.* 2016 Jun;131(6):803-20.

[4] Parsons D W, et al. An Integrated Genomic Analysis of Human Glioblastoma Multiforme, *Science.* 2008 September 26; 321(5897): 1807.

[5] Qian Z, et al. Prognostic value of a microRNA signature as a novel biomarker in patients with lower-grade gliomas. *J. Neuro-Oncol.* 2018; 137:127 –37.

[6] Law M, et al. Glioma grading: sensitivity, specificity, and predictive values of perfusion MR imaging and proton MR spectroscopic imaging compared with conventional MR imaging. *Am. J. Neuroradiol.* 24:1989–1998.

[7] Nguyen T B, et al. Diagnostic accuracy of dynamic contrast-enhanced MR imaging using a phase-derived vascular input function in the preoperative grading of gliomas. *Am. J. Neuroradiol.* 33:1539–1545.
[8] Arvinda H R, et al. Glioma grading: sensitivity, specificity, positive and negative predictive values of diffusion and perfusion imaging. *J Neurooncol* 94:87–96.
[9] Bizzi A, et al. Presurgical functional MR imaging of language and motor functions: validation with intraoperative electrocortical mapping. *Radiology.* 2008;248 (2):579– 89.
[10] Bartos R, et al. Validity of primary motor area localization with fMRI versus electric cortical stimulation: a comparative study. *Acta Neurochir.* 2009;151(9):1071–80.
[11] Meier M P, et al. Validation of functional motor and language MRI with direct cortical stimulation. *Acta Neurochir.* 2013;155(4):675–83.
[12] Lus T, et al. Low-grade glioma surgery in eloquent areas: volumetric analysis of extent of resection and its impact on overall survival. A single-institution experience in 190 patients. *Journal of Neurosurgery*, 117(6), 1039–1052.
[13] Chang E F et al. Preoperative prognostic classification system for hemispheric low-grade gliomas in adults. *J. Neurosurg*. 2008; 109:817–824.
[14] Meyer E J, et al. The impact of intracranial tumor proximity to white matter tracts on morbidity and mortality: a retrospective diffusion tensor imaging study. *Neurosurgery* 80:193–200, 2017.
[15] Raman A, Rothrock J F, Liu H G, Mountz J M. Differentiation of benign vs. malignant mass in a post-irradiation cerebral arteriovenous malformation by 2-deoxy-2-[18F] fluoro-D-glucose positron emission tomography. *Mol. Imaging Biol.* 2004; 6:1-6.
[16] Santra A, et al. F-18 FDG PET-CT for predicting survival in patients with recurrent glioma: a prospective study. *Neuroradiology* 2011; 53:1017-24.
[17] Pichler R, et al. Is there a place for FET PET in the initial evaluation of brain lesions with unknown significance? *Eur. J. Nucl. Med. Mol. Imaging* 2010; 37:1521-8.
[18] Heinzel A, et al. Management of bevacizumab and irinotecan in patients with recurrent high-grade glioma: a cost-effectiveness analysis. *J. Nucl. Med.* 2013; 54:1217-22
[19] Colavolpe C, et al. FDG-PET predicts survival in recurrent high-grade gliomas treated with bevacizumab and irinotecan. *Neuro Oncol.* 2012; 14:649-57.
[20] Pignatti F, et al. Prognostic factors for survival in adult patients with cerebral low-grade glioma. *J. Clin. Oncol.* 2002;20(8):2076–84.
[21] Chang EF, et al. Preoperative prognostic classification system for hemispheric low-grade gliomas in adults. *J Neurosurg*. 2008;109(5):817–24.
[22] Shaw EG, et al. Recurrence following neurosurgeon-determined gross-total resection of adult supratentorial low-grade glioma: results of a prospective clinical trial. *J Neurosurg*. 2008;109(5):835–41.
[23] Buckner J C, et al. Radiation plus Procarbazine, CCNU, and Vincristine in Low-Grade Glioma. *N. Engl. J. Med.* 2016;374(14):1344–55.
[24] Karim A B, et al. Randomized trial on the efficacy of radiotherapy for cerebral low-grade glioma in the adult: European Organization for Research and Treatment of

Cancer Study 22845 with the Medical Research Council study BRO4: an interim analysis. *Int. J. Radiat. Oncol. Biol. Phys.* 2002 Feb 1;52(2):316-24.

[25] Fisher B J, et al. Phase 2 Study of Temozolomide-based Chemoradiation Therapy for High-risk Low-grade Gliomas: Preliminary Results of Radiation Therapy Oncology Group 0424. *Int. J. Radiat. Oncol. Biol. Phys.* 2015 March 1; 91(3): 497–504.

[26] Baumert B G, et al. Temozolomide chemotherapy versus radiotherapy in high-risk low-grade glioma (EORTC 22033–26033): a randomised, open- label, phase 3 intergroup study. *Lancet Oncol.* 2016;17(11):1521–32.

[27] Sherman J C, et al. Neurocognitive effects of proton radiation therapy in adults with low-grade glioma. *J. Neurooncol.* (2016) 126:157–164.

[28] Shaw E G, et al. Randomized Trial of Radiation Therapy Plus Procarbazine, Lomustine, and Vincristine Chemotherapy for Supratentorial Adult Low-Grade Glioma: Initial Results of RTOG 9802. *Journal of Clinical Oncology*, 30 Jul 2012, 30(25):3065-3070.

[29] Shaw E, et al. Prospective Randomized Trial of Low- Versus High-Dose Radiation Therapy in Adults with Supratentorial Low-Grade Glioma: Initial Report of a North Central Cancer Treatment Group/Radiation Therapy Oncology Group/Eastern Cooperative Oncology Group Study. *Journal of Clinical Oncology*, 20(9), 2267–2276.

[30] Karim A B, et al. Randomized trial on the efficacy of radiotherapy for cerebral low-grade glioma in the adult: European organization for research and treatment of cancer study 22845 with the medical research council study bro4: an interim analysis. *Int. J. Radiation Oncology Biol. Phys.,* vol. 52, no. 2, pp. 316–324, 2002.

Chapter 10

Insular Glioma

Manas Panigrahi[1,*], MCh and Shrut Doshi[2], MS, DrNB

[1]Department of Neurosurgery, Krishna Institute of Medical Sciences, Secunderabad, Telangana, India
[2]Department of Neurosurgery, Zydus hospital, Ahmedabad, Gujarat, India

Abstract

Insular gliomas are one of the most difficult neurosurgical pathologies to treat. The most common clinical presentation in low grade gliomas is intractable epilepsy, whereas those with high grade gliomas typically complain of symptoms of mass effects like headache, sensory and/or motor complaints etc. Berger Sanai classification system divides the insula into four zones, with giant lesions occupying all four zones. Recent advances in Neuro-radiology help in early diagnosis and better planning of surgery. Preoperative functional MRI & DTI tractography should be performed in all patients with insular glioma. Considering insula's anatomical proximity with eloquent area & its own functional complexity, safe maximal resection with appropriate surgical corridor should be the primary goal of surgery. Intra-operative subcortical stimulation for motor tracts or awake craniotomy for speech area should be used to achieve safe maximal resection with no morbidity. In case of displaced corticospinal tracts, near total excision whether in case of infiltrated tracts, subtotal excision should be performed to achieve maximum extent of resection with less chance of recurrence & morbidity. Whenever it is feasible, transopercular approach should be used.

[*] Corresponding Author's Email: manasp1966@gmail.com. Department of Neurosurgery, Krishna Institute of Medical Sciences, 1-8-31/1, Ministers Road, Secunderabad - 500003, Telangana, India; Phone: +91 9618117118. Fax: + 91-40-27814499,

In: Advances in Neurosurgery Research
Editors: Amit Agrawal, Pradeep Chouksey, Adesh Shrivastava et al.
ISBN: 978-1-68507-859-1

Prognosis is influenced by MIB index, WHO grade and requirement of post-operative chemotherapy and/or radiation.

Keywords: insular gliomas, surgical excisions, functional MRI, outcome

Introduction

By definition, a neoplasm of glial cells is called glioma. Insula (i.e., island) is the anatomical interface between limbic system and neocortex. Unlike other areas of the cerebrum, the insular cortex as well as lobe is found underneath the cerebral cortex, within the depth of sylvian fissure and covered by the opercula and important vascular structures. Recently, the insular cortex has been defined as an associative multimodal compensable secondary area in terms of eloquency[1]. Additionally, venous complex covering the sylvian venous distribution contains important drainage veins that have to be preserved; this further narrows surgical strategies for tumor removal. Due to all these diversities, insular gliomas are among the difficult neurosurgical pathologies to treat effectively.

Epidemiology

According to recent epidemiologic data, insular gliomas account for 10% and 25% of the number of all high-grade and low-grade brain gliomas, respectively[2] and exhibit properties that make them distinct from tumors located in other parts of the brain. According to epidemiological studies[3], there is a clear trend of low-grade tumor growth in the insula. Less aggressive tumor growth is observed in patients with low-grade tumor in the insula compared to patients with the same pathology at other sites. Some researchers[4] highlight cytoarchitectonic features of this area (mesocortex) and functional features of this lobe, but the exact cause of this phenomenon has not yet been fully understood.

---

[1] Sanai, Polley, and Berger, "Insular Glioma Resection: Assessment of Patient Morbidity, Survival, and Tumor Progression.," January 2010.

[2] Duffau et al., "The Insular Lobe: Physiopathological and Surgical Considerations."

[3] Yaşargil et al., "Tumours of the Limbic and Paralimbic Systems."

[4] Sanai, Polley, and Berger, "Insular Glioma Resection: Assessment of Patient Morbidity, Survival, and Tumor Progression.," January 2010.

Eloquency of Insula

The insula belongs to the paralimbic system, the part of the central nervous system serving as a link between the limbic system (allocortex) and the cerebral hemispheres (neocortex). It is represented by mesocortex, i.e., it has 3 to 5 layers of neurons. The function of the insula has long been a subject of debate among researchers. Even today there is no consensus on this issue. For example, clinical cases of ischemic infarctions localized only in the insula manifest as a variety of symptoms depending on the location and distribution of the pathological process. C. Cereda et al[5] distinguish the following 5 main symptom complexes of the insular cortex injury: somatosensory deficit (infarction in the posterior lobe of the right/left insula), ageusia (posterior lobe of the left insula), vestibular syndrome (posterior lobe of the left/right insula), cardiovascular disorders (infarction in the posterior lobe of the right insula) and neuropsychological symptoms (ischemic injury of the posterior parts of the left/right insula).

Results obtained by A. Afif et al.,[6] in a study of 25 patients with pharmacoresistant epilepsy, who were stereotactically implanted with electrodes into the insular lobe suggested that the insula is involved in processing of sensory impulses (smell and taste), control of autonomic functions (the sympathetic control of the cardiovascular system), emotional and behavioural responses, as well as voluntary swallowing and speech modulation process. The insula is probably a part of the neuronal system connecting supramarginal gyrus with Broca's area, and can participate (along with the premotor cortex) in phonetic planning of speech[7].

Anatomy and Relations

The insula is a well-defined cerebral cortex which has elliptic borders, arranged beneath the sylvian fissure, flattened superiorly & covered by the opercula. Insula is divided into anterior and posterior lobules which are separated by central sulcus. Lateral surface of the anterior lobule gets divided in the anterior, middle and posterior short insular gyri (Figure 1). Sometimes

---

[5] Cereda et al., "Strokes Restricted to the Insular Cortex."

[6] Afif et al., "Anatomofunctional Organization of the Insular Cortex: A Study Using Intracerebral Electrical Stimulation in Epileptic Patients."

[7] Shelley and Trimble, "The Insular Lobe of Reil--Its Anatamico-Functional, Behavioural and Neuropsychiatric Attributes in Humans--a Review."

middle gyrus may not be conspicuous,[8] whereas the smaller posterior lobule is divided into an anterior and a posterior long insular gyrus. The limen insulae is the white matter structure that extends from the anterior perforated substance medially to insular pole along and situated in parallel with lateral olfactory stria.[9] The extreme capsule, claustrum, external capsule and putamen with its subjacent globus pallidus, are the structures which are respectively arranged deep to central part of insula, in a lateral to medial direction.

Superiorly - the corticospinal tract, antero inferiorly - the uncinate fasciculus and posteriorly - the arcuate fasciculus make the important relations with insula. Short & medium-sized perforating vessels of second (M2) segment of the MCA supply blood to the insula. The first (M1) segment of the MCA courses laterally from the carotid bifurcation, parallel and 1 cm behind the lesser sphenoid ridge. It commonly (88%) bifurcates at these ridge. It is noted that most of the lenticulostriate branches arise in a nearly equal distribution from before and after the carotid bifurcation.

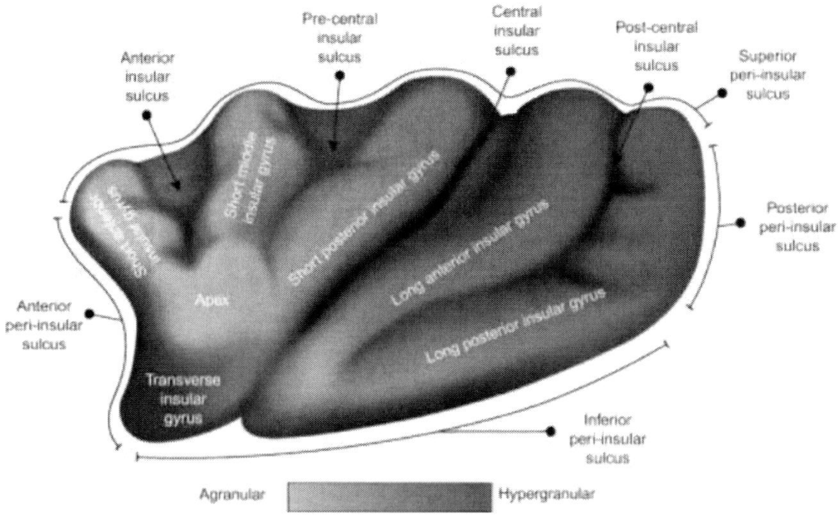

Figure 1. Insular cortex anatomy.

[8] Naidich et al., "The Insula: Anatomic Study and MR Imaging Display at 1.5 T."
[9] Vanaclocha, Sáiz-Sapena, and García-Casasola, "Surgical Treatment of Insular Gliomas."

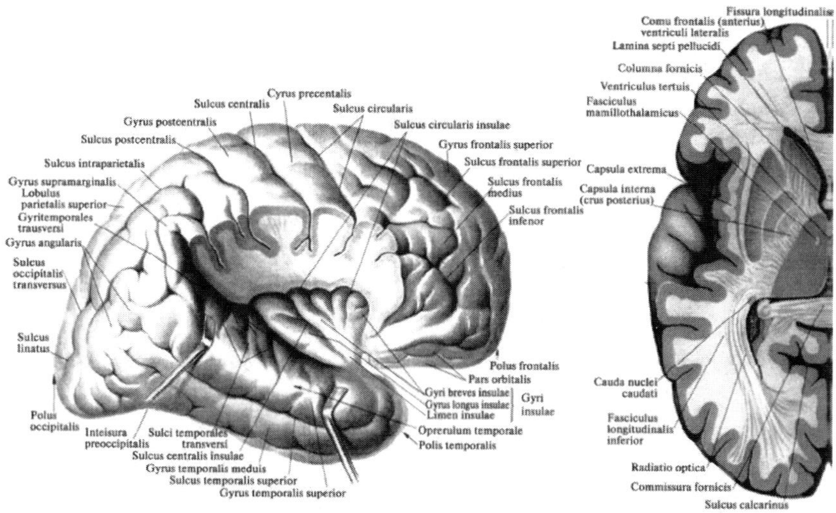

Figure 2. Relations of insula.

Classification

New classification was proposed in 2010 by N. Sanai et al.[10] According to Berger Sanai Classification System, the insula is divided into 4 zones, and tumor location is assigned to 1 or more of these zones (Figure 3). In the sagittal section - the insula is intersected along the sylvian fissure. In the coronal section - it is intersected at the level of the foramen of monro. The resultant antero superior, postro superior, postero inferior, and antero inferior quadrants are designated as Zones I, II, III, and IV, respectively. In case when the tumor occupies all four zones, it is categorized as "giant" insular glioma.

Symptomatology

The usual presentation of low grade insular gliomas is intractable epilepsy. As per available reports,[11] 64% to 98% of patients with insular tumors have presented as intractable epilepsy and the most common being simple and

[10] Sanai, Polley, and Berger, "Insular Glioma Resection: Assessment of Patient Morbidity, Survival, and Tumor Progression.," 2010.

[11] Sanai, Polley, and Berger; Yaşargil et al., "Tumours of the Limbic and Paralimbic Systems;" Simon et al., "Insular Gliomas: The Case for Surgical Management."

complex partial seizures (33% to 69%) and second most common are generalized seizures (23% to 29%). It may present as frontal or temporal lobe epilepsy as well.[12]

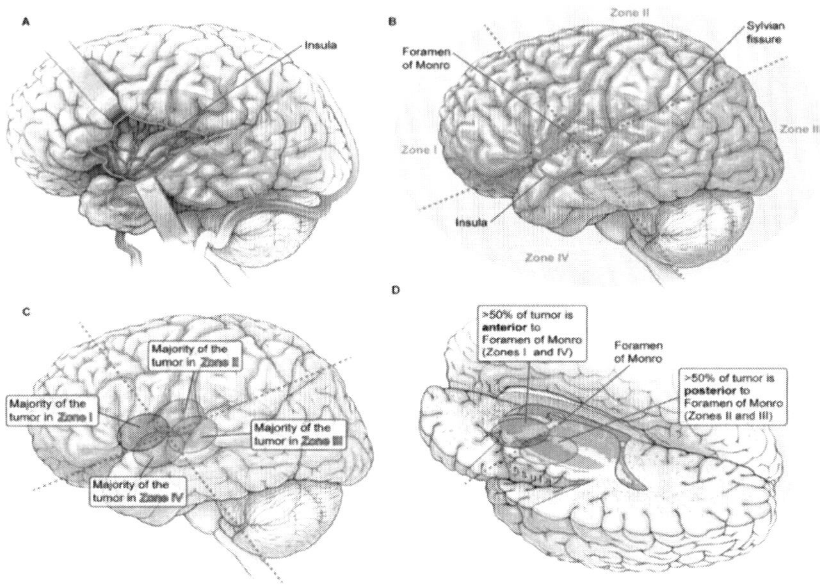

Figure 3. Berger Sanai classification for insular glioma. (Courtesy - Kenneth X. Probst. Published with permission).

The common presenting symptoms in high grade insular gliomas are headache, motor weakness, cognitive dysfunction or speech deficits that are associated with mass effects and peritumoral vasogenic oedema & electrophysiological abnormalities. In view of the functional complexity of the insula, various neurologic signs like memory & visual disturbance, attention deficits may manifest according surrounding extension of lesion beyond insula.

---

[12] Roux et al., "Methodological and Technical Issues for Integrating Functional Magnetic Resonance Imaging Data in a Neuronavigational System," Isnard et al., "Clinical Manifestations of Insular Lobe Seizures: A Stereo-Electroencephalographic Study;" MT et al., "Navigated Transcranial Magnetic Stimulation and Functional Magnetic Resonance Imaging: Advanced Adjuncts in Preoperative Planning for Central Region Tumors," Ostrowsky et al., "Functional Mapping of the Insular Cortex: Clinical Implication in Temporal Lobe Epilepsy."

Pathology

Gliomas' histological features, genetics, and locations are responsible for their heterogeneous nature. This is the reason why insular gliomas behave differently from tumors of a similar grade that are situated in other areas. It is to be noted that insular gliomas are associated with a prolonged clinical course characterized by comparatively longer intervals of overall survival which is encouraging for neurosurgeons & beneficial for patients.

In our case series of 100 patients, nearly two thirds (68.3%) patients had low grade glioma and one third (31.7%) patients had high grade glioma. The most common tumor was oligoastrocytoma, observed in 21.6% of patients, followed by glioblastoma observed in twelve 20% patients.

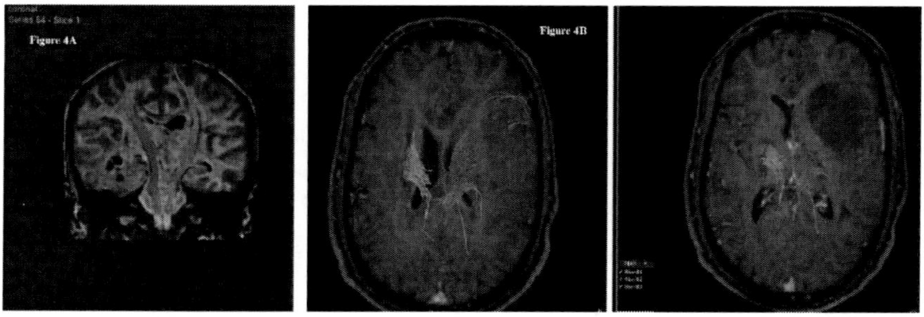

(A) (B)

Figure 4. (A) displaced tracts (B) infiltrated tracts.

Investigations

CT scan is first or emergency investigation which shows frontotemporal or temporal hyperdense lesion in sylvian fissure area according to anatomical distribution of insular glioma. MRI is the gold standard diagnostic investigation. It depicts the actual location and boundary of the tumor, the relationship between the tumor and adjacent vessels, presence of edema & mass effect. Moreover contrast scan gives us rough idea about high or grade glioma according to enhancement pattern.

Insular gliomas' proximity to functionally eloquent cerebral cortex, corticospinal tracts and basal ganglia make newly developed functional assessment tools really crucial to insular glioma surgery – its preoperative planning & intraoperative strategy. The first, Diffusion tensor imaging tractography (DTI) enables clinician to visualize the course of corticospinal tracts inside or around a tumor, and it provides important insights in planning a strategy for resection.[13] The presence of intact or displaced tracts are predictive of a better surgical outcome, because these category's cases have a higher probability of total resection than subtotal resection. Whereas the presence of infiltrated fascicles & tracts are predictive of a lower probability of total resection, especially for tumous with preoperative volume < 100 cm.[14] Thus DTI tractography can be considered to be a crucial investigation for estimating the degree of safe maximal resection pre operatively.

Functional MR Imaging (fMRI)

According to functional complexity of insula & its anatomical proximity with broca's area & corticospinal tract, we estimate the extent of involvement (uninvolved / abutment / partially or completely involved) of speech & motor area with this real time imaging. This information is crucial for decision on the requirement of subcortical stimulation during tumor removal in GA or to choose awake craniotomy for safe maximal tumor removal.

Nuances in Imaging

Magnetoencephalogram (MEG) is a non-invasive technique which does not depend upon traditional radiation, administration of contrast & hemodynamic changes to detect increased neuronal activity. It has an excellent temporal resolution. It is shown to be superior to fMRI in localizing the motor cortex and central sulcus. This can be merged to high-resolution MRI for

---

[13] Bello et al., "Intraoperative Use of Diffusion Tensor Imaging Fiber Tractography and Subcortical Mapping for Resection of Gliomas: Technical Considerations."

[14] Roux et al., "Methodological and Technical Issues for Integrating Functional Magnetic Resonance Imaging Data in a Neuronavigational System." Isnard et al., "Clinical Manifestations of Insular Lobe Seizures: A Stereo-Electroencephalographic Study"; Ostrowsky et al., "Functional Mapping of the Insular Cortex: Clinical Implication in Temporal Lobe Epilepsy;" Bello et al., "Intraoperative Use of Diffusion Tensor Imaging Fiber Tractography and Subcortical Mapping for Resection of Gliomas: Technical Considerations."

neuronavigation to include eloquent areas, giving the excellent intraoperative "functional neuronavigation."[15]

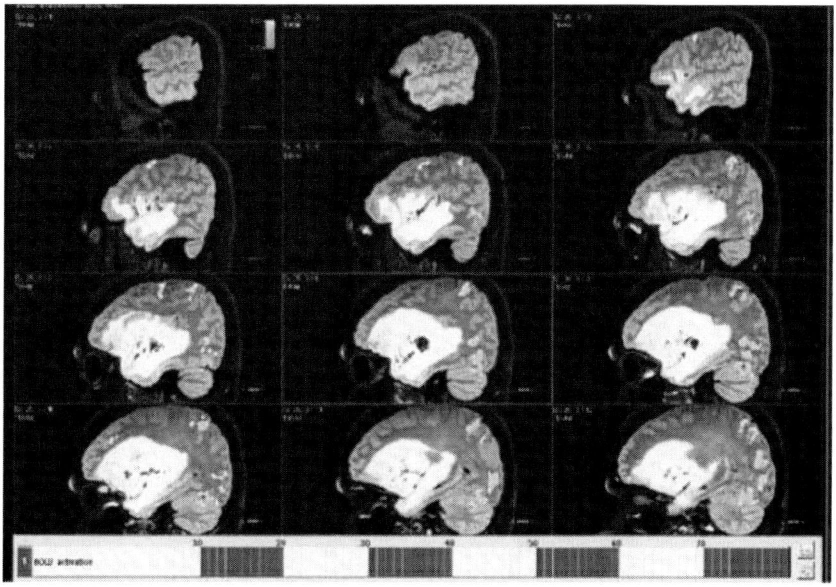

Figure 5. BOLD activities shown as yellow spots in fMRI.

Navigated Magnetic transcranial stimulation (nTMS) is a newer technique in which the system uses a magnetic stimulator with a biphasic TMS coil. Navigation device adjusts individual 3D MR imaging data to the patient's skull through infrared tracking using spheres coated with a retro-reflective surface.[16] This system can estimate the induced electric field strength concerning the patient's head shape. This electric field strength is then picked up from the cortex surface and then it is reconstructed by the MR imaging dataset. nTMS utility is being mentioned increasingly in the literature recently as the accuracy of nTMS is better than fMRI.[17]

---

[15] R et al., "Practicability of Magnetoencephalography-Guided Neuronavigation;" Nimsky, Ganslandt, and Fahlbusch, "Functional Neuronavigation and Intraoperative MRI."

[16] MT et al., "Navigated Transcranial Magnetic Stimulation and Functional Magnetic Resonance Imaging: Advanced Adjuncts in Preoperative Planning for Central Region Tumors."

[17] SM et al., "Utility of Presurgical Navigated Transcranial Magnetic Brain Stimulation for the Resection of Tumors in Eloquent Motor Areas."

Treatment

Near total resection is often preferred in glioma. Considering insula's anatomical proximity with eloquent area & its own functional complexity, safe maximal resection with appropriate surgical corridor should be the primary goal.

Preoperative Planning

A. planning of extent of resection & requirements of aids[18]

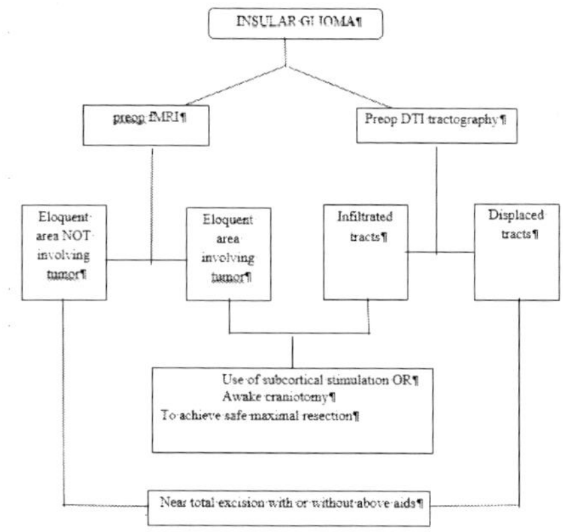

B. planning of operative approach[19]

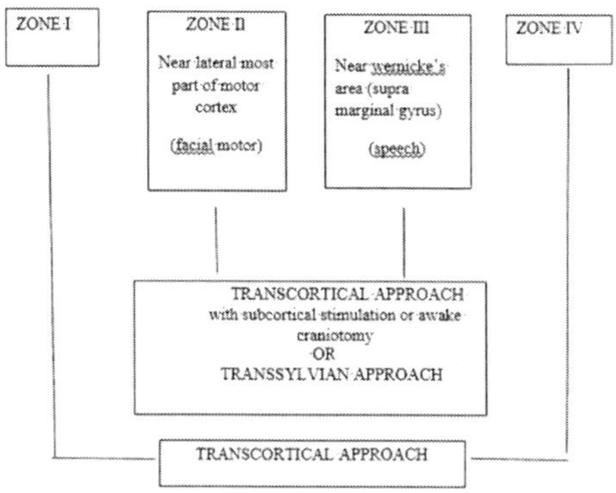

---

[18] M et al., "Surgical Resection of Insular Gliomas and Roles of Functional Magnetic Resonance Imaging and Diffusion Tensor Imaging Tractography-Single Surgeon Experience."

[19] Panigrahi et al., "Avoiding Complications in Surgical Resection of Insular Gliomas – Single Surgeon Experience."

Craniotomy and Tumor Excision

Excision of the tumor is the pinnacle of the all the process right from presentation of patient to the out-patient room till the operating room. All the preoperative planning, patient positioning and configurations of the craniotomy are aimed at putting the surgeon in the best position to safely excise the tumor.

Patient should be positioned for pterional craniotomy. The steps are 1. Head elevation – to promote venous drainage, 2. Head turn to contralateral side 30 degree – to minimize encroachment of temporal lobe in operative field, 3. Flexion of neck – to bring chin toward contralateral shoulder ensures floor of anterior cranial fossa is perpendicular to body & lastly, 4. Head is extended till maxillary prominence is set above orbital rim which makes sphenoid ridge axis parallel to operative surgeon's visual axis.

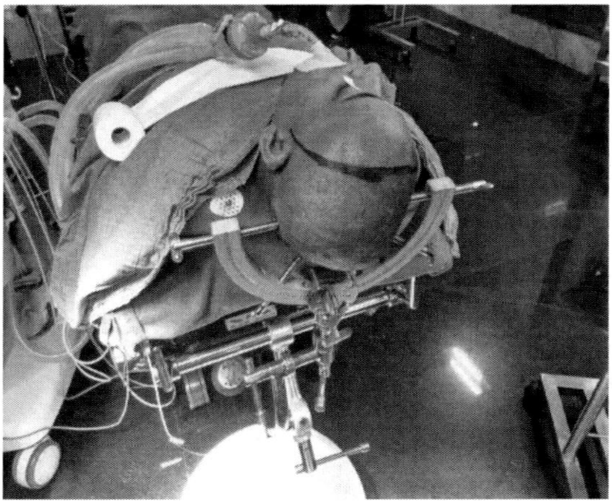

Figure 6. Operative position.

A wide frontotemporal craniotomy (pterional approach) which exposes the Sylvian fissure from the pars orbitalis of the inferior frontal gyrus (IFG) to the postcentral sulcus which gives proper visualisation of its anterior and middle parts.

Transsylvian approach expose a larger insular surface for a more direct approach to a tumor confined to the insular structure. After middle & posterior part of sylvian fissue dissection & identifying circular sulcus, tumor dissection should be started. Transopercular approach is more suitable when the tumor extends to opercula. After dissection of opercula respecting a subpial plane, tumor dissection should be started. Once entered, the tumor debulking reduces the need for retraction of related eloquent structures & avoids reactive edema or injury to eloquent tissue.

The medial side of insular tumors are supplied by lateral lenticulostriate arteries originating from the M1 trunk of MCA and the same vessels supply the internal capsule. As injury to these vessels results in a dense hemiplegia, defining the first lateral lenticulostriate artery is very crucial step while doing inferomedial dissection of the tumor. By keeping eye on their course, surrounded tumor removal can be done in piecemeal or with help of ultrasonic aspirator. Lenticulostriate arteries - M1 junction is limit of deep dissection (Figure 7E).

The resection of tumour infiltrating the posterior lobule, which is hidden by the subcentral gyrus is the most difficult part.[20] It is observed that usually the tumor displaces eloquent cortex at its periphery. That is why it is possible to resect a part of the frontoparietal operculum without leading any deficit.[21] Lateral ventricle's anterior extremity of the frontal horn corelates with the anterior periinsular sulcus. This is a useful landmark to judge the anterior extent of a tumor. It is to be noted that on the dominant side, subcortical area just lateral to the frontal horn is likely to disturb the initiation of spontaneous speech.

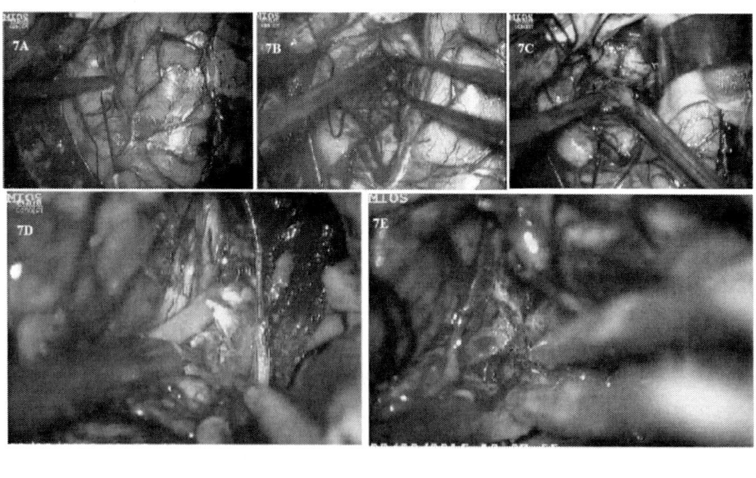

Figure 7. A) Exposure B) Circular sulcus C) Tumor dissection D) Lenticulostriate arteries E) Limits of deep dissection.

[20] Duffau et al., "The Insular Lobe: Physiopathological and Surgical Considerations."
[21] Duffau et al.

Table 1. Keypoints of approaches

Transsylvian approach	Transopercular approach
direct approach to a tumor confined to the insular structure	Wide corridor for surgery which helps in safe maximal resection
Less incidence of post operative seizures	Less incidence of arterial spasm of lateral lenticulostriate / perforators & venous injury

Subcortical Mapping

Subcortical mapping can be performed with MEP response. Also, a continuous free monopolar suction mounted subcortical mapping may help to avoid injury to the corticospinal tract. Such mapping will be helpful when approaching the the medial boundary of an insular glioma. One drawback of such dynamic subcortical mapping is that even when the proximal part of the corticospinal tract was damaged, stimulation of the portion of the CST distal to the damaged area may still elicit a normal response. However, continuous direct cortical stimulation in such a situation will be sensitive to any disruption of the corticospinal tract.

Awake Craniotomy

With the advent of newer & safer anaesthesia/analgesia techniques & fast acting hypnotic as well as sedative medications, awake craniotomy is considered as a safe and comfortable procedure for appropriate candidates. Insular glioma involving zone III may abut or infiltrate Wernicke's speech area (supramarginal gyrus). In fMRI if BOLD activity shows involvement of speech area, then awake craniotomy is preferred whereas in cases where speech area is not involved, tumor excision can be done under general anesthesia.

Complications

Although it is proven by evidence that maximal resection guarantees longer overall survival and progression free survival is convincing, since earlier neurosurgeons face number of obstacles in removing insular tumors radically as it can produce significant neurologic complications after surgery.

Table 2. Common complications and their causes

Type of complication	Due to injury to
Hemiparesis	Lateral lenticulostriate arteries and the long perforators of M2 vessels
Facial palsy	Lateral most strip of motor cortex
Broca's dysphasia with dysnomnia	Frontal operculum
Conduction aphasia	Horizontal fibers of the arcuate fasciculus
Semantic paraphasias	External capsule

In our case series of 100 patients, we have observed that.[22]

A) Using preoperarive fmri & DTI tractography help to decide which patient is appropriate for near total exicision of tumor and whether requirement of subcortical stimulation or awake craniotomy to achieve it with minimal complications.
B) Using transsylvian or transcortical approach judiciously according to tumor location helps in near total excision of tumor which minimizes the rate of complications & recurrence.

Illustrative Cases

Figure 8 and 9 summarize illustrative cases.

Adjuvant Therapy

In low grade glioma, near total resection is therapeutic without any adjuvant therapy. Oligodendroglima (grade II) are sensitive to chemotherapy whether in absence of oligodendroglioma, other pathology demands need of radiotherapy in presence of risk factors. Those risk factors are age > 40 years, left sided tumors, tumors crossing midline, subtotal resection & preoperative neurological deficits.

In high grade glioma[23] radical resection should be done whenever possible as it decreases the tumor load. Anaplastic astrocytoma & oligoastrocytoma

---

[22] Panigrahi et al., "Avoiding Complications in Surgical Resection of Insular Gliomas – Single Surgeon Experience."

[23] Stupp et al., "High-Grade Glioma: ESMO Clinical Practice Guidelines for Diagnosis, Treatment and Follow-Up."

(grade III) requires standard therapy consists of adjuvant radiotherapy upto 60 Gy after surgery while in glioblastoma (grade IV), concomitant & adjuvant temozolamide (TMZ) chemotherapy in addition to radiotherapy (TMZ/RT followed by TMZ) is current standard care. TMZ is administered daily (5 days a week) during radiotherapy & for 5 days every 4 weeks for 6 cycles as maintenance (adjuvant) treatment after radiation.

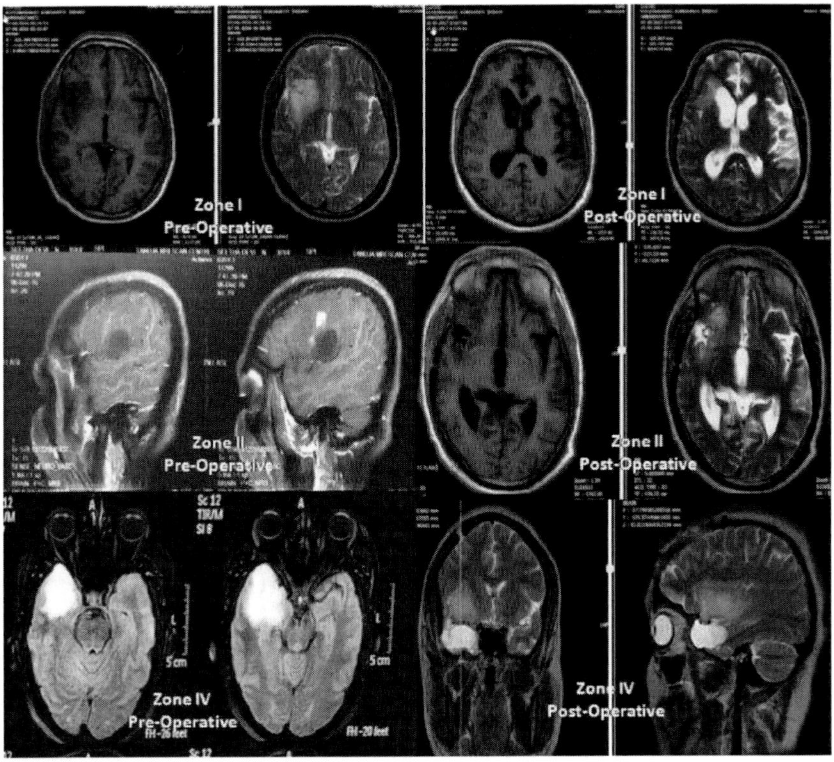

Figure 8. Pre and postoperative cases.

Prognosis

In our experience of 100 patients with insular gliomas, amongst various histopathological types, maximal overall survival was observed in patients with fibrillary astrocytoma (57.50 ± 4.04 month) followed by oligoastrosytoma (47.33 ± 2.75 month), whether it was least in glioblastoma (21.20 ± 03.54 month).

Overall, poor prognosis factors are

1. High MIB index (> 5%)
2. WHO grade IV tumors
3. requirement of post-operative chemotherapy and/or radiation

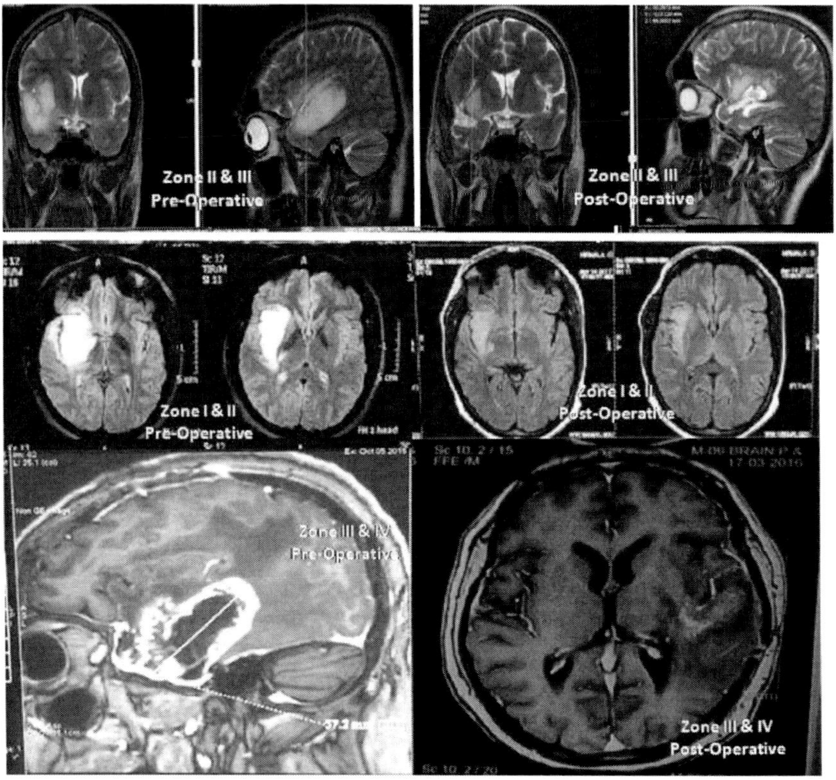

Figure 9. Pre and postoperative cases.

Conclusion

1. Preoperative functional MRI & DTI tractography should be performed in all patients of insular glioma.
2. In case of eloquent area lesions (detected with help of fMRI), intraoperative subcortical stimulation for motor tracts or awake craniotomy for speech area should be used to achieve safe maximal resection with no morbidity.

3. In case of displaced corticospinal tracts, near total excision whether in case of infiltrated tracts, subtotal excision should be performed to achieve maximum extent of resection with less chance of recurrence & morbidity.
4. Overall, transopercular approach provides better surgical corridor. Whenever it is feasible, transopercular approach should be used.

References

———. "Insular Glioma Resection: Assessment of Patient Morbidity, Survival, and Tumor Progression." *Journal of Neurosurgery* 112, no. 1 (January 2010): 1–9. https://doi.org/10.3171/2009.6.JNS0952.

Afif, Afif, Lorella Minotti, Philippe Kahane, and Dominique Hoffmann. "Anatomofunctional Organization of the Insular Cortex: A Study Using Intracerebral Electrical Stimulation in Epileptic Patients." *Epilepsia* 51, no. 11 (November 1, 2010): 2305–15. https://doi.org/10.1111/j.1528-1167.2010.02755.x.

Bello, Lorenzo, Antonella Castellano, Enrica Fava, Giuseppe Casaceli, Marco Riva, Giuseppe Scotti, Sergio Maria Gaini, and Andrea Falini. "Intraoperative Use of Diffusion Tensor Imaging Fiber Tractography and Subcortical Mapping for Resection of Gliomas: Technical Considerations." *Neurosurgical Focus* 28, no. 2 (2010): E6. https://doi.org/10.3171/2009.12.FOCUS09240.

Cereda, C, J Ghika, P Maeder, and J Bogousslavsky. "Strokes Restricted to the Insular Cortex." *Neurology* 59, no. 12 (December 24, 2002): 1950–55. http://www.ncbi.nlm.nih.gov/pubmed/12499489.

Duffau, H, L Capelle, M Lopes, T Faillot, J P Sichez, and D Fohanno. "The Insular Lobe: Physiopathological and Surgical Considerations." *Neurosurgery* 47, no. 4 (October 2000): 801–10; discussion 810-1. http://www.ncbi.nlm.nih.gov/pubmed/11014418.

Duffau, Hugues, Laurent Capelle, Manuel Lopes, Thierry Faillot, Jean-Pierre Sichez, and Denis Fohanno. *"The Insular Lobe: Physiopathological and Surgical Considerations."* Accessed August 25, 2017. https://pdfs.semanticscholar.org/e20b/1f44402f9 b4009f5e79b0ad8c21a9be017fa.pdf.

Firsching, R, Bondar I, Heinze H J, Hinrichs H, Hagner T, Heinrich J, and Belau A. "Practicability of Magnetoencephalography-Guided Neuronavigation." *Neurosurgical Review* 25, no. 1–2 (2002): 73–78. https://doi.org/10.1007/S101430100161.

Forster, M T, Hattingen E, Senft C, Gasser T, Seifert V, and Szelényi A. "Navigated Transcranial Magnetic Stimulation and Functional Magnetic Resonance Imaging: Advanced Adjuncts in Preoperative Planning for Central Region Tumors." *Neurosurgery* 68, no. 5 (May 2011): 1317–24. https://doi.org/10.1227/NEU.0B013E31820B528C.

Isnard, Jean, Marc Guenot, Marc Sindou, and Francois Mauguiere. "Clinical Manifestations of Insular Lobe Seizures: A Stereo-Electroencephalographic Study."

Epilepsia 45, no. 9 (September 1, 2004): 1079–90. https://doi.org/10.1111/j.0013-9580.2004.68903.x.

Krieg, S M, Shiban E, Buchmann N, Gempt J, Foerschler A, Meyer B, and Ringel F. "Utility of Presurgical Navigated Transcranial Magnetic Brain Stimulation for the Resection of Tumors in Eloquent Motor Areas." *Journal of Neurosurgery* 116, no. 5 (May 2012): 994–1001. https://doi.org/10.3171/2011.12.JNS111524.

Naidich, Thomas P, Eugene Kang, Girish M Fatterpekar, Bradley N Delman, S Humayun Gultekin, David Wolfe, Orlando Ortiz, Indra Yousry, Martin Weismann, and Tarek A Yousry. "The Insula: Anatomic Study and MR Imaging Display at 1.5 T." *AJNR. American Journal of Neuroradiology* 25, no. 2 (February 2004): 222–32. http://www.ncbi.nlm.nih.gov/pubmed/14970021.

Nimsky, C., O. Ganslandt, and R. Fahlbusch. "Functional Neuronavigation and Intraoperative MRI." *Advances and Technical Standards in Neurosurgery* 29 (2004): 229–63. https://doi.org/10.1007/978-3-7091-0558 0_6.

Ostrowsky, K, J Isnard, P Ryvlin, M Guénot, C Fischer, and F Mauguière. "Functional Mapping of the Insular Cortex: Clinical Implication in Temporal Lobe Epilepsy." *Epilepsia* 41, no. 6 (June 2000): 681–86. http://www.ncbi.nlm.nih.gov/pubmed/10840399.

Panigrahi, M, Chandrasekhar Y B, Vooturi S, Ram G A, and Rammohan V S. "Surgical Resection of Insular Gliomas and Roles of Functional Magnetic Resonance Imaging and Diffusion Tensor Imaging Tractography-Single Surgeon Experience." *World Neurosurgery* 98 (February 1, 2017): 587–93. https://doi.org/10.1016/J. WNEU. 2016.11.001.

Panigrahi, Manas, Shrut Doshi, Y. B. V. K. Chandrasekhar, and Sudhindra Vooturi1. "Avoiding Complications in Surgical Resection of Insular Gliomas – Single Surgeon Experience." *Neurology India* 69, no. 4 (July 1, 2021): 904. https://doi.org/10.4103/0028-3886.325334.

Roux, F E, D Ibarrola, M Tremoulet, Y Lazorthes, P Henry, J C Sol, and I Berry. "Methodological and Technical Issues for Integrating Functional Magnetic Resonance Imaging Data in a Neuronavigational System." *Neurosurgery* 49, no. 5 (November 2001): 1145–56; discussion 1156-7. http://www.ncbi.nlm.nih.gov/pubmed/11846909.

Sanai, Nader, Mei-Yin Polley, and Mitchel S Berger. "Insular Glioma Resection: Assessment of Patient Morbidity, Survival, and Tumor Progression." *Journal of Neurosurgery* 112, no. 1 (2010): 1–9. https://doi.org/10.3171/2009.6.JNS0952.

Shelley, Bhaskara P, and Michael R Trimble. "The Insular Lobe of Reil--Its Anatamico-Functional, Behavioural and Neuropsychiatric Attributes in Humans--a Review." *The World Journal of Biological Psychiatry : The Official Journal of the World Federation of Societies of Biological Psychiatry* 5, no. 4 (October 2004): 176–200. http://www.ncbi.nlm.nih.gov/pubmed/15543513.

Simon, Matthias, Georg Neuloh, Marec von Lehe, Bernhard Meyer, and Johannes Schramm. "Insular Gliomas: The Case for Surgical Management." *Journal of Neurosurgery* 110, no. 4 (April 2009): 685–95. https://doi.org/10.3171/2008.7.JNS17639.

Stupp, R., M. Brada, M. J. van den Bent, J.- C. Tonn, G. Pentheroudakis, and ESMO Guidelines Working Group. "High-Grade Glioma: ESMO Clinical Practice

Guidelines for Diagnosis, Treatment and Follow-Up." *Annals of Oncology* 25, no. suppl 3 (September 1, 2014): iii93–101. https://doi.org/10.1093/annonc/mdu050.

Vanaclocha, V., N. Sáiz-Sapena, and C. García-Casasola. "Surgical Treatment of Insular Gliomas." *Acta Neurochirurgica* 139, no. 12 (December 1997): 1126–35. https://doi.org/10.1007/BF01410972.

Yaşargil, M G, K von Ammon, E Cavazos, T Doczi, J D Reeves, and P Roth. "Tumours of the Limbic and Paralimbic Systems." *Acta Neurochirurgica* 118, no. 1–2 (1992): 40–52. http://www.ncbi.nlm.nih.gov/pubmed/1414529.

Chapter 11

Management of Eloquent Cortex Brain Tumors

Manas Panigrahi[1], MCh, FACS,
M. Manoranjitha Kumari[2], MCh
and R. Gopikrishnan[2], MS, MCh

[1]Krishna Institute of Medical Sciences, Secunderabad, Telangana, India
[2]Jawaharlal Institute of Medical Education and Research, Puducherry, India

Abstract

Tumors arising from the eloquent areas of the brain pose a challenge to the treating clinician. Resection of tumors in eloquent regions involves a compromise between the extent of resection and functional preservation. Radical resection of such lesions will result in severe neurological deficits that will significantly affect the quality of life and nullify the survival benefits. Various preoperative and intraoperative adjuncts have been developed to achieve maximum safe resection. Preoperative Functional Magnetic Resonance Imaging (MRI), Diffusion Tensor Imaging (DTI), intraoperative cortical and subcortical mapping of language and motor functions and intraoperative imaging help accomplish these goals. In addition, diligent surgical techniques like en-bloc tumor resection in a well-defined tumor and vessel preserving surgery help attain better resection with functional preservation in eloquent region tumors.

In: Advances in Neurosurgery Research
Editors: Amit Agrawal, Pradeep Chouksey, Adesh Shrivastava et al.
ISBN: 978-1-68507-859-1

Introduction

Eloquent cortex refers to any region of the brain in which injury causes motor or symptomatic cognitive deficits. Eloquent areas include the primary sensory-motor cortex, motor, premotor cortex, cingulate cortex, insular lobe, language cortex, visual cortex, and mesial temporal lobe. Any tumor in these eloquent areas always poses a challenge to the treating clinician. Gross total excision is considered the gold standard treatment for gliomas occurring in the supratentorial region (Frappaz et al. 2003). However, the extent of resection (EOR) is compromised in cases where there is a poor demarcation between the tumor and the brain, eloquent areas within and surrounding the tumor, and intricate vascular relationships. There is no clear consensus regarding treating low-grade glioma (LGG) presenting only with seizures in young patients. Choices vary from observation with periodic imaging, operation alone, only chemotherapy or radiation therapy, and surgical excision with chemoradiation (Jakola et al. 2014; Forst et al. 2014). At the same time, the standard treatment protocol for high-grade gliomas (HGG) is early treatment with maximal safe surgical excision with chemoradiation. With increasing advances in chemical components of chemotherapeutic agents and targeted molecular therapies with radiation, the outcomes are better in such tumors (Hervey-Jumper and Berger 2014; Bloch et al. 2012; Orringer et al. 2012). In Meningiomas and brain metastasis, gross total excision is usually possible as these tumors do not infiltrate instead push or compress the brain matter (De Witt Hamer et al. 2012). Surgical excision of highly eloquent cortex tumors always involves a trade-off between the EOR and preservation motor or linguistic function.

Furthermore, the variability of "Eloquent tumor location" has been found as the leading cause of incomplete resection and transient morbidities in 40-70% of the cases (Brell, Conesa, and Acebes 2003; Duffau et al. 2002; Pallud and Dezamis 2017). Many studies have demonstrated the association between radical excision of gliomas and progression-free survival (PFS). The EOR has a positive correlation with the survival rate, and studies have shown that EOR more than 90% was remarkably associated with PFS and overall survival in LGG (Eseonu et al. 2017; Tamura et al. 2015). However, severe language and motor functional deficits following radical excision of eloquent tumors will result in poor quality of life and may nullify the outcome benefits achieved from radical resection (Rahman et al. 2017; Molinaro et al. 2020; McGirt et al. 2009). And for this reason, various intraoperative neurophysiological monitoring methods have evolved to enhance the extent of resection by preserving functional areas and reducing surgery-related morbidities. The present-day notion is in "information-guided surgery" using multimodality pre and intraoperative adjuncts, which helps achieve maximum resection without deficits (Tamura et al. 2015). This chapter discusses various preoperative techniques and intraoperative modalities required to achieve a better resection in eloquent region tumors.

Factors to Consider in Eloquent Region Surgery

There could be some functional variability in the motor cortex. Even areas with the same anatomical landmarks may not harbor the same underlying function. The Brodmann area 4 may extend > 20 millimeter (mm) in front of the central sulcus. The "Hand knob" may represent area 4 or the premotor cortex. Stimulation in the precentral cortex can result in sensory and motor responses in > 1 motor group (Pouratian and Bookheimer 2010; Shinoura et al. 2009; Uematsu et al. 1992). Similarly, language areas can have a disparity of around 4 centimeters (cm) in intraoperative cessation of speech (Berger, Cohen, and Ojemann 1990). Apart from the typical functional variability, space-occupying lesions can also affect functional reorganization depending upon the duration and course of the disease (Lucas et al. 2008). Congenital lesions can have an unusual functional acquisition. For example, arteriovenous malformations can have a higher incidence of right-sided localization of language area (Pouratian and Bookheimer 2010).

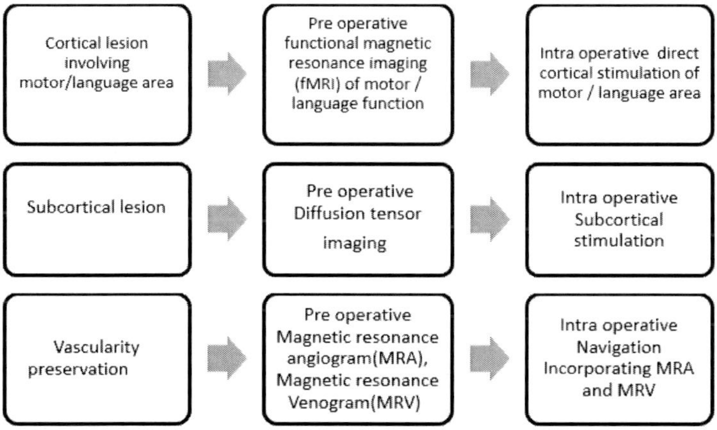

Figure 1. Flow chart of surgical planning.

Preoperative Workup

Proper preoperative planning yields better postoperative outcomes. Patients planned for eloquent region tumor surgery should undergo a thorough clinical psychological language evaluation, a battery of basic and advanced imaging. Some patients might require invasive preoperative brain mapping techniques. The Figure 1 flow chart depicts the essentials of surgical planning (Figure 1).

Preoperative Basic Radiological Imaging

Basic methods of Magnetic resonance imaging (MRI) consisting of T1, T2 weighted images, post-Gadolinium-T1- contrast sequences, fluid-attenuated inversion-recovery (FLAIR) sequences, and other diffusion-weighted sequences are mandatory to obtain general information about the operability and the expected possible extent of resection (Bello et al. 2008). These images give basic anatomical details on the number of regions affected, perilesional edema, subcortical white matter and deep nuclei, midline shifts, mass effects on the ventricle, the opposite side hemisphere's involvement, and concurrent lesions in the other parts of the brain. Post-contrast images show enhancement patterns, relationships with vessels, and contrast enhancement areas representing malignant transformation. The volumetric FLAIR and the volumetric post-contrast-T1-weighted images help evaluate the tumor volume in low and high-grade tumors, respectively (Rossi et al. 2019).

Advanced MRI Techniques

Functional MRI (fMRI) is an advanced method used to identify functional regions of the brain in a non-invasive manner. There are two types of fMRI, one is task-based, and the other is resting-state fMRI. In Task-based fMRI(tfMRI), patients do particular tasks. Variation in local blood flow in the brain occurs due to increased cerebral metabolism, which is detected using a blood oxygenation level-dependent (BOLD) signal. It has 87.5% to 100% sensitivity and specificity of 68.1% to 87.1% in identifying the motor cortex (Bizzi et al. 2008; Meier et al. 2013; Khanna et al. 2015) (Figure 2). For language function, the sensitivity is 59% to 78% and the specificity is 67.7% to 97% with fMRI (Bizzi et al. 2008; Meier et al. 2013; Xia et al. 2012; Roux et al. 2003; Brannen et al. 2001). The reliability is less in patients with significant infiltration or previous treatments (specificity < 35%). Resting-state fMRI(rs-fMRI) can acquire data in conscious, unconscious, or even sedated patients. A technician can do this rs-fMRI without the need for the physician for testing, and the patients do not have to perform the tasks. After the rs-fMRI is done, the data is processed using special software. A recently published study on rs-fMRI showed a 92% correlation with motor network detection and 42% in language networks with direct cortical stimulation (DCS) (Cochereau et al. 2016).

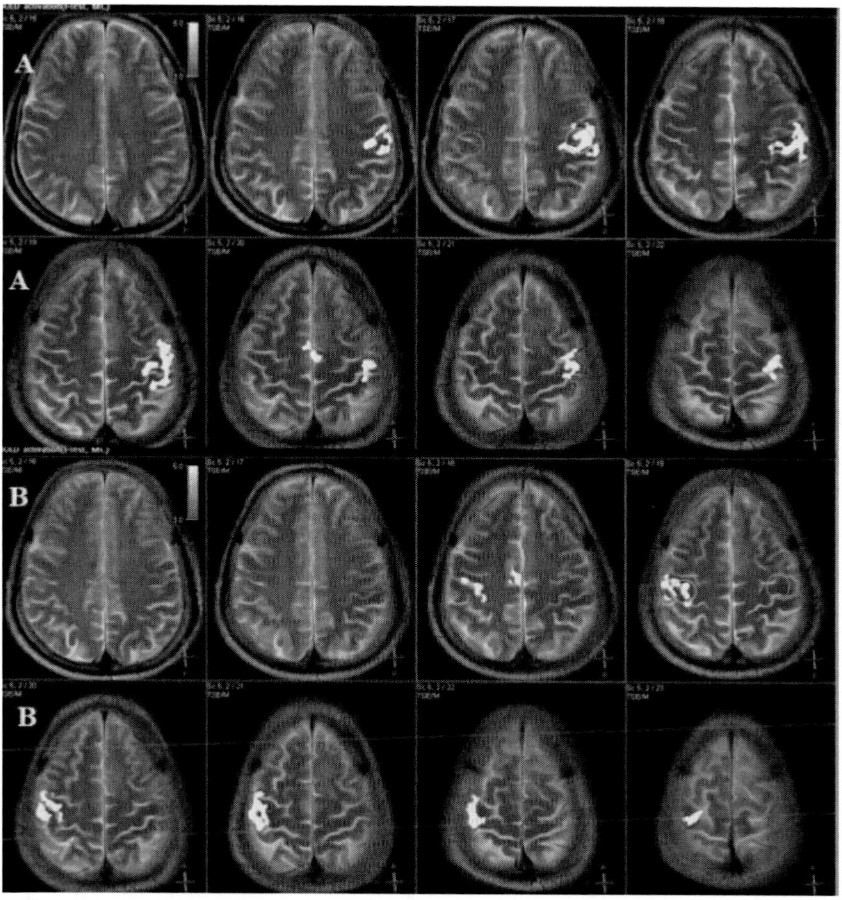

Figure 2. Task-based fMRI showing BOLD activation of the left motor cortex (A) and the right motor cortex (B) (yellow color).

Diffusion Tensor Imaging (DTI) is a non-invasive method of diffusion-weighted MRI that depends on physiological movement and direction of water molecules to delineate the white fiber tracts of the brain. DTI is used to visualize and reconstruct subcortical bundles or tracts at the subcortical level (Jellison et al. 2004; Alexander et al. 2007). (Figure 3). Studies have shown that white matter fibers are destroyed in malignant tumors and preserved within the lesion in low-grade tumors (Bello et al. 2008; Jellison et al. 2004; Assaf and Pasternak 2008; Witwer et al. 2002). DTI information can be used for 3 Dimensional (3D) reconstructions of tracts in relation to the tumor, which may help the surgeon intraoperatively avoid these structures during resection (Bello et al. 2008).

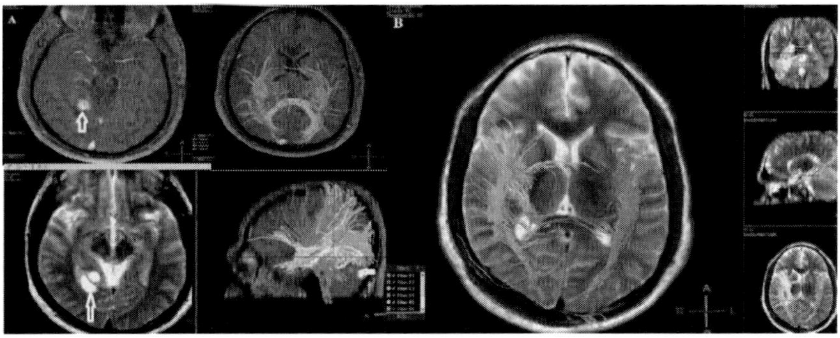

Figure 3. Diffusion tensor imaging (DTI) of (A)- right medial occipital lesion (yellow arrow) and its relation to the long fiber tracts, (B)- postoperative image showing preservation of long tracts without evidence of residual.

Magnetoencephalogram (MEG) is a non-invasive method with high resolution that does not need contrast agent injection and does not rely on BOLD activity. It is shown to be better than fMRI in localizing the motor area and central sulcus (Ottenhausen et al. 2015; Kirsch et al. 2007; Korvenoja et al. 2006). MEG can be merged to MRI for navigation to incorporate functional regions, giving the excellent intraoperative "functional neuronavigation" (Firsching et al. 2002; Nimsky, Ganslandt, and Fahlbusch 2004).

Navigated Magnetic transcranial stimulation (nTMS) is a newer technique in which the system uses a magnetic stimulator with a biphasic TMS coil. The infrared tracking retro-reflective spheres on the navigation system help adjust 3D MR imaging data to the patient's head (Forster et al. 2011). This device can evaluate and pick up the induced electric field strength from the brain surface, and it will be processed by the MR imaging data set. nTMS utility is being mentioned increasingly in the literature recently as the accuracy of nTMS is better than fMRI and correlates well with DCS (Krieg et al. 2012).

All these imaging modalities contribute to increasing preoperative planning results. The fMRI data is converted into digital imaging and communications in medicine (DICOM) format. The anatomical information obtained from 3 Tesla MRI is then merged with navigation and functional data. The plan and image incorporation into the navigation system are done on the day before surgery in the navigation systems' planning station. Established protocols are used to do image registration in the operating theater, mitigating registration errors and other brain shift-related errors during the surgery.

Preoperative Invasive Brain Mapping Techniques

Electrocortical frequency alteration mapping (EFAM) is an invasive brain mapping technique, which can be done in patients who cannot undergo awake craniotomy. The difference between DCS and EFAM is that EFAM does not require the passage of current into the brain. When the patient performs a particular task, a power fluctuation occurs in the brain at a specific frequency that will be projected in a spectrogram (Leuthardt et al. 2007). It records the intrinsic physiology passively and analyzes to conclude eloquent regions of the brain. For this procedure, patient participation is required. It can be done in a more convenient place and multiple times. It does not require electrical or magnetic stimulation and is considered a passive brain mapping technique (Roland, Hacker, and Leuthardt 2020). This passive brain mapping can be used in pediatric patients, aphasic patients as these techniques do not need patient cooperation or passage of current into the brain.

Stereo electroencephalography (SEEG) and Electrocorticography (ECoG) are the two techniques routinely used for invasive electrophysiological monitoring (Figure 4 A&B). In epilepsy surgery presurgical evaluation, these monitoring techniques are routinely used to localize ictal onset zones in patients with intractable seizures. Along with seizure monitoring, functional area mapping can also be done by stimulating those electrodes kept on the functional area with bipolar stimulation between adjacent invasive electroencephalogram (iEEG) electrodes in the pre-operative setting. The aim is to localize the functional area and mark it preoperatively in the navigation system to avoid the inclusion of the eloquent cortex during resection of the epileptic zone (Roland, Hacker, and Leuthardt 2020). During electrode stimulation, the physician should look for interruption of actions such as speech arrest or elicitation of involuntary movement of the opposite side limbs. Furthermore, if these kinds of interruption of action or elicitation of movements are reproducible with a lesser amount of current and repeated testing, then one can be sure about the underlying functional area stimulated. Since these methods have higher reliability and reproducibility, they are considered a gold standard method, especially for the patients who are uncooperative or not the candidate for awake craniotomy (Roland, Hacker, and Leuthardt 2020).

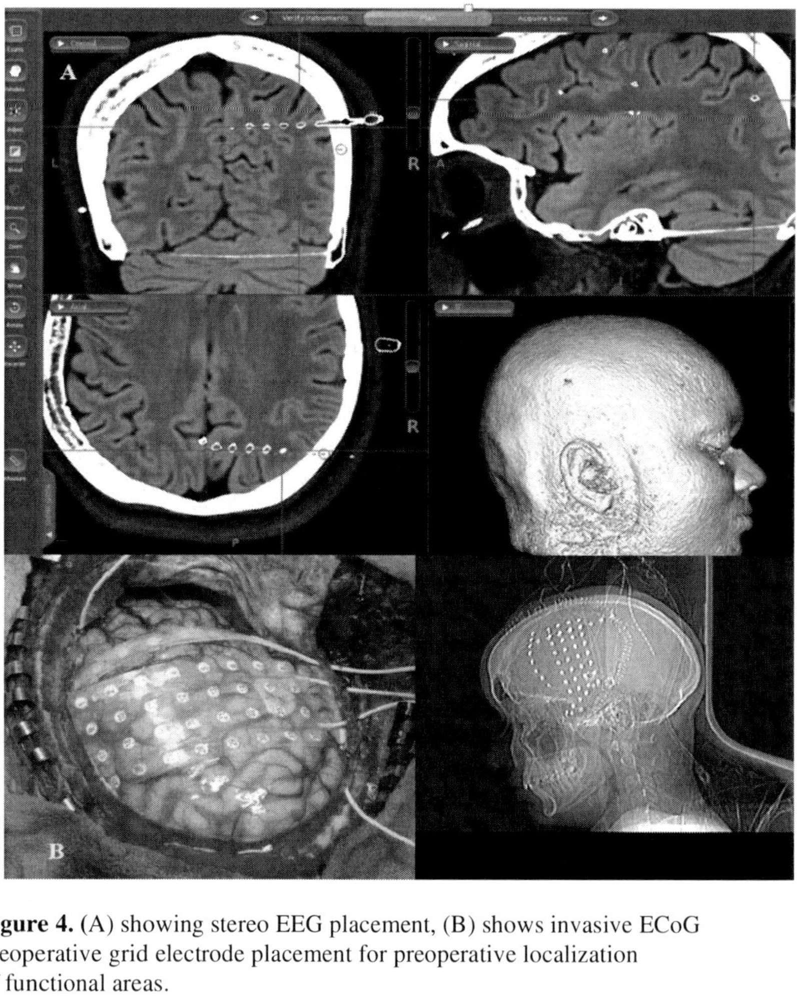

Figure 4. (A) showing stereo EEG placement, (B) shows invasive ECoG preoperative grid electrode placement for preoperative localization of functional areas.

Preoperative Patient Assessment and Neuropsychological Evaluation

The current gold standard treatment for eloquent region tumors, especially language area tumors, is awake surgery and intraoperative neuromonitoring using DCS. The treating physician is responsible for attending to patients' and relatives' queries and fears well ahead of the scheduled date for the operation. Good communication and understanding between the patient and the treating physician are mandatory to achieve a good outcome. A multidisciplinary approach composed of a neurosurgeon, neurologist, physiotherapist, intensive care physician, and neuropsychologist is vital for the best results. Each patient should be subjected to a detailed neurological evaluation at admission into the hospital. The clinical and complete CNS examination should cover handedness, language function, motor function, sensory function, coordination, cranial nerve examination, and preoperative Karnofsky performance status (KPS) score. Any preoperative neurological deficits should be noted for future reference in the postoperative period. Furthermore, the operating surgeon must assess every patient's level of concentration, cooperation, and ability to withstand an awake surgery. The neuropsychologist is responsible for performing presurgical neuropsychological evaluation and also counsels the patient about awake surgery.

Awake Craniotomy

With the advent of newer and safer anesthesia/analgesia techniques like laryngeal masks and fast-acting hypnotic and sedative medications, awake craniotomy is considered a safe and comfortable procedure for suitable candidates. With this technique, surgeons can be sure about radical resection without producing newer neurological deficits.

Preoperative Anesthetic Assessment and Patient Selection

Apart from regular pre-anesthetic workup, other essential factors that determine the outcome of surgery in awake craniotomy are choosing the right patient, preparing the patient mentally, and tailoring an appropriate anesthetic regime for each patient. Patients who cannot cooperate for surgery, do not understand the language, or patients with altered sensorium are not suitable for awake procedures. These categories of patients are considered as absolute contraindications for awake craniotomy. Other relative contraindications are morbidly obese patients with airway obstruction and breathing issues, patients with intractable seizures, suspected of having a difficult airway, bronchial asthma, gastroesophageal reflux disease, and patients who had had a delirium following anesthesia in history (Lee and Poon 2021). In addition to this, tumor characteristics, such as large lesions with increased intracranial pressure, deep-seated lesions where significant brain retraction is needed, and tumors with high vascularity may also pose challenges during surgery.

Anesthetic Techniques

Different anesthetic strategies have been described for awake surgery in the literature (Danks et al. 1998; Hervey-Jumper and Berger 2014; Olsen 2008). The "asleep-awake-asleep" technique using general anesthesia (GA) and "conscious sedation" technique using monitored anesthesia care (MAC) are the two anesthetic techniques practiced for awake craniotomy. In the "asleep-awake-asleep" technique, the patient is given general anesthesia for craniotomy until before intraoperative mapping is commenced. Then the patient will be awakened during mapping and testing of functional areas. Once the functional areas are reliably marked on the surface of the brain, then the patient will receive GA or sedation for tumor resection (Olsen 2008). In conscious sedation technique (MAC) the patient is sedated with mild to moderate, sometimes deep sedation, but can be aroused throughout the surgery (Danks et al. 1998; Hervey-Jumper and Berger 2014). While the patient is undergoing testing and resection, it is mandatory to have continuous support with communication and reassurance with the patient, which can help relieve the patient's fear. The addition of mild sedation will help to achieve patient cooperation during the procedure. The anesthetic agents commonly used in awake craniotomy are Midazolam, Propofol, Remifentanil, Dexmedetomidine (Grabert et al. 2019). For total intravenous anesthesia (TIVA), propofol and fentanyl are the preferred drugs. TIVA is preferred for cases with intraoperative neuromonitoring (IONM), as inhalation agents affect the amplitude and latency of Motor and Sensory Evoked Potentials (Kannabiran and Bidkar 2018). Local anesthesia of the scalp, by nerve blockade of supratrochlear nerves, facial nerve branches, and greater auricular and occipital nerve combined with local field infiltration along the scalp incision site reduces the need for more sedation and related complications.

In the authors' institution, for lesions in the motor cortex and the language area, awake craniotomy is done under local anesthesia (bupivacaine 2 to 3 mg/kg + 4 to 6 mg/kg of lignocaine). After the mapping is done, the patient is given sedation with Propofol (6 to 12 mg/kg/h) and Remifentanil (0.05 to 2 mg/kg/min) to complete the necessary resection and closure. Midazolam is used as an anxiolytic agent. General anesthesia is given for patients who cannot undergo awake procedures. In such scenarios muscle relaxant vecuronium is given only at the time of induction (0.08 to 0.1 mg/kg) and avoided until cortical stimulation is done..

Patient Positioning

The patient can be positioned in an MR-compatible table if an intraoperative MRI is planned. The table should be comfortable enough with regard to head position and appropriate padding of pressure points to allow cooperation throughout the procedure. The head is positioned at the required angle; if intraoperative MRI is used, the head fixator is avoided; otherwise, the head is fixed with a head fixator. The patient's face and contralateral limb must be kept visible to the physician to see the response during stimulation. Anaesthesiologists should also be able to reach the patient's airway and intravenous accesses. Positioning is done in such a way that there is no obstruction between the patient's navigation frame and the infrared camera of the navigation system (Figure 5).

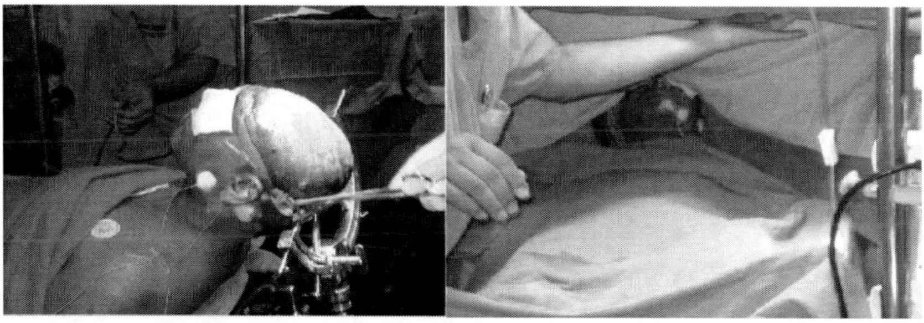

Figure 5. Positioning for awake craniotomy under local anesthesia.

Navigation Registration

Preoperative marking of eloquent regions and planning of extent of resection is done using a navigation workstation. The data from various MRI techniques is imported via a local area network or a magneto-optical disc. After aligning and merging the different MRI data sets, the tumor and the eloquent areas are marked and color-coded in the neuronavigation system, which will be projected as a multi-vision image on the navigation screen (Figure 6). Multiple reference points are identified on the images and are registered with a navigation wand. Once registration is done, lesion boundaries are marked over the scalp (Figure 7).

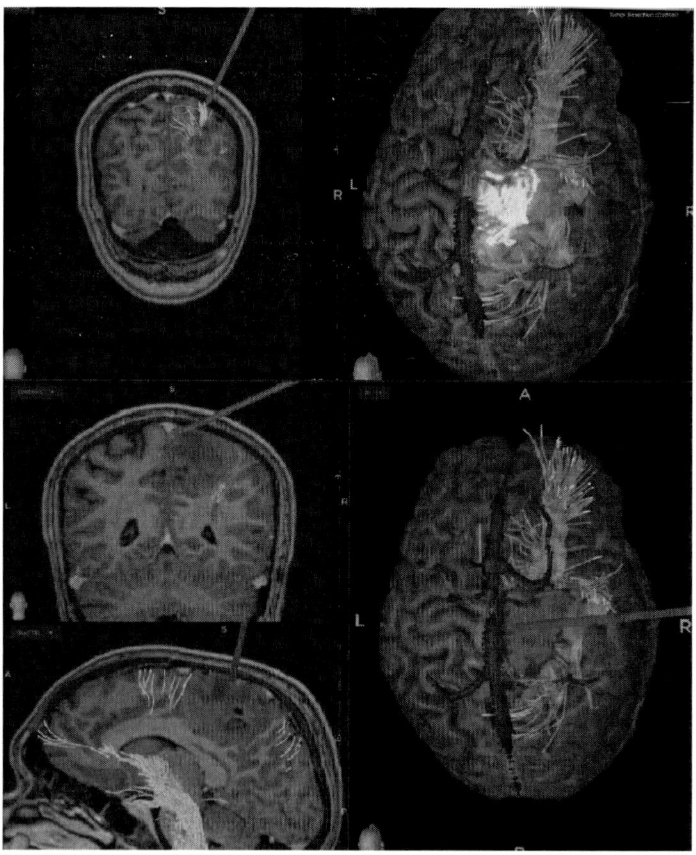

Figure 6. Multivision navigation image of a left motor cortex lesion incorporated with DTI with color coding for tumor (red) and corticospinal tract (green) and veins (violet).

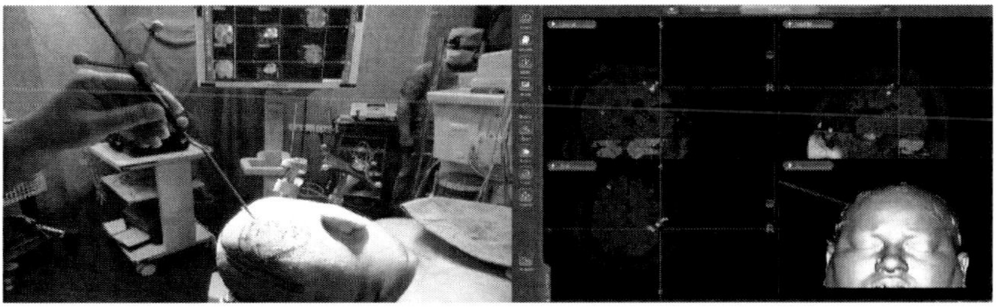

Figure 7. Navigation registration and surface marking.

Surgical Procedure

The scalp is prepared with antiseptics, and the skin flap incision and lesion are marked on the surface. The craniotomy is done, including the marked area, and the dural opening is made according to the surgeon's preference. The lesion is again confirmed with navigation. Multivision 3D images with different color codes for tumor and eloquent areas on the navigation system and image injection into the optics of the microscope's eyepiece will help the surgeon navigate in multiple planes without even looking at the navigation monitor during surgery. The main aim of surgery should be the recognition of tumor tissue and its resection. While doing tumor dissection, especially for low-grade tumors, it is preferred to go around the lesion and remove en-bloc rather than central decompression, as central decompression of the tumor would cause the collapse of the cavity resulting in brain shift related inaccuracies in navigation. If the tumor is removed en-bloc, there will not be any collapse of the tumor cavity at the beginning of surgery itself. Moreover, the relationship of the eloquent cortex and tracts could be relevant and accurate

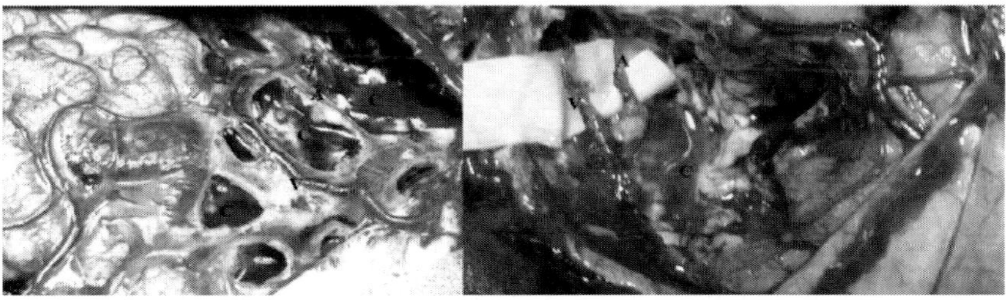

Figure 8. Intraoperative picture of tumor resection with vessel preservation.
A- arteries, V-veins C- tumor bed after resection.

on navigation during the procedure. It is crucial to preserve the surface-draining veins and sulcal arteries. And this is accomplished by doing vessel preserving surgery wherein the dissection should be carried out between the vessels without coagulating and cutting (Figure 8). The tumor might pass the vessel that might supply the distal eloquent cortex, which should be preserved to prevent ischemia-related neurological deficits. This can be achieved by doing a subpial dissection of the tumor.

Direct Cortical Stimulation and Motor Mapping

There is no defined standard method for DCS; different techniques of intraoperative brain mapping methods have been practiced by different centers. The strategy in doing the motor mapping should be personalized to the patient's general and clinical condition and the type of lesion. Two types of stimulation techniques have been described, low-frequency stimulation (LF), otherwise known as Penfield's technique, and the train of stimuli or high-frequency stimulation technique (HF). The technical difference between these two paradigms of stimulation has been enumerated in Table 1.

Low-Frequency Stimulation Mapping

This stimulation technique is used mainly for language mapping and also for motor mapping for low-risk tumors. In LF stimulation, the current delivers between the probe and the reference electrode fixed on the patient's scalp. Stimulation parameters have been described in the following table. The current is gradually increased in 1- to 2- milliampere (mA) until the evoked potentials are elicited. A visible movement of contralateral limbs or facial muscles or electromyography (EMG) recording is considered a positive response (Bello et al. 2008; A. Szelényi et al. 2011) (Figure 9). Further increased intensity of the current stimuli should be stopped. If the current stimulation produces seizures, the cortex is rinsed with cold saline or Ringer lactate solution (Sartorius and Berger 1998). LF stimulation is especially effective in picking up motor responses of low-risk tumors with sharp margins without infiltration of the corticospinal tract (CST) (Bello et al. 2014). In low-risk tumors with no tract infiltration or prolonged seizure history, the application of LF facilitates a high rate of EOR of more than 90%. Whereas, in complicated or high-risk tumors such as tract infiltration or prolonged history seizures, the EOR drops by less than 50% (Bello et al. 2014; A. Szelényi et al. 2011; Choi et al. 2012).

High-Frequency Stimulation Mapping

In HF stimulation techniques, the current passes between the two balls of the probe. It is given as a train of stimulus with the interstimulus interval of 2 to 4 milliseconds (ms) for every second, with a monopolar or bipolar probe. It is depicted as a monophasic-wave pulse of 0.5 ms in duration (Andrea Szelényi et al. 2010). The pattern of the Motor Evoked Potential (MEP) response is similar for cortical or subcortical stimulation. HF stimulation recordings give information regarding the amplitude, latency, and morphology of MEP waves. All this information enables the physician to exactly locate and map the eloquent cortex based on the type of evoked potentials obtained.

In most cases, HF stimulation using a monopolar probe is found to be very efficient in distinguishing the functional areas from the rest of the cortex. It helps elicit a response in high-risk cases like patients with preoperative neurological deficits, long history of seizures, infiltrating tumors with perilesional edema. The results are not influenced by the anesthesia regimen and the concurrent use of a CUSA (Han et al. 2018). And hence HF is considered to be the most efficient method for stimulating the motor cortex. It also gives insights regarding the extent between the stimulation area and primary motor tract when used subcortically with normal motor cortex excitability. In such situations, the current intensity is slowly brought down from 12 mA while approaching the CST. If the subcortical motor threshold of 3 mA is achieved, the stimulation area is very much near to the motor fibers, with a risk of producing a neurological deficit of less than 2% (Olsen 2008; Han et al. 2018; Schucht et al. 2017). In case of failed response, stepping up the train of pulses ranging from 7 - 9 mA, adjusting the pulse width ranging from 500 -800 ms may evoke desired motor responses. With the HF stimulation paradigm, motor mapping is possible in most cases, resulting in a higher percentage of EOR (>90%) and minimal post-surgical morbidity (2%) (Rossi et al. 2019; Bello et al. 2014; Raabe et al. 2014).

However, direct cortical stimulation does not always yield a positive mapping in all patients. Tailoring stimulation parameters for each patient might give a positive response in the majority of the cases. If the cortical exposure is limited in some patients, there is more probability that the surgeon may not get any positive motor mapping or speech arrest for that particular case. Nevertheless, this kind of negative mapping is a safe technique. This ensures that the eloquent area is far away from the lesion, and the surgeon can proceed with surgical excision without producing a new neurological deficit (Kim et al. 2009).

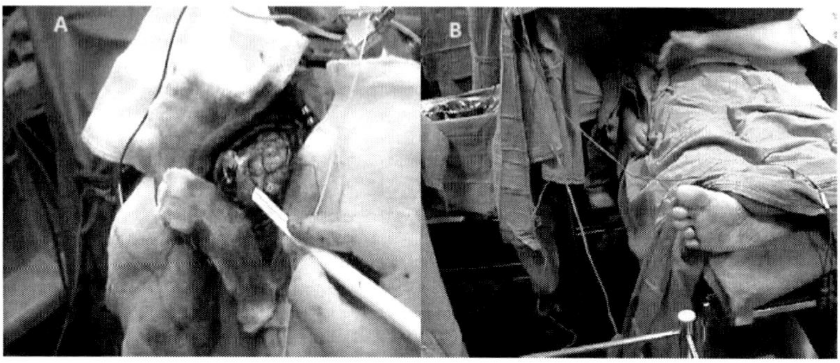

Figure 9. Direct cortical stimulation with the bipolar probe. (A) Motor cortex is being stimulated contralateral limbs are exposed to look for movements.

Table 1. Differentiation between LF stimulation and HF stimulation

Differentiating feature		Low-Frequency stimulation or (Penfield's technique)	High-Frequency stimulation or (train of stimuli)
Stimulation Parameters	Current delivery	continuously during the entire stimulation time every 20 ms	as a train with an interstimulus interval of 2 to 4 ms every second
	Current intensity required to elicit motor response	Awake patients - 2 to 7 (mA) Asleep patients - 7to16 (mA)	Awake patients - 2 to 7 mA Asleep patients- 5-15 mA
Wave patterns		biphasic square wave (0.5ms)	monophasic pulse wave (0.5ms)
Chances of seizure provocation		High (2-25% in various studies)	Low
Merits/Demerits		merits: 1. useful for language and motor mapping for low risk tumors demerits: 1. intraoperative seizure risk might result in negative mapping /aborting awake procedure 2. results might be influenced by concurrent usage of CUSA resulting in false-negative responses	merits: 1. useful in mapping for high risk tumors irrespective of seizure history 2. not influenced by concurrent usage of CUSA 3. can be used for continuous monitoring

Subcortical Mapping

Subcortical mapping can be performed using the exact parameters of cortical mapping with MEP response. Also, a continuous free monopolar suction mounted subcortical mapping may help avoid injury to the corticospinal tract. Such mapping will be helpful when approaching the posterior limit of a frontal glioma or the medial boundary of an insular or temporal glioma. One drawback of such dynamic subcortical mapping is that even when the proximal part of the CST was damaged, stimulation of the portion of the CST distal to the damaged area may still elicit a normal response. However, continuous Direct cortical stimulation in such a situation will be sensitive to detect any disruption of the CST.

Somatosensory Evoked Potential (SSEP) and Motor Evoked Potential (MEP)

Patients undergoing eloquent cortex tumor surgery under general anesthesia (GA) without muscle relaxants SSEP and MEP monitoring can be done. Use of SSEP phase reversal technique as the initial step to identify primary motor and sensory cortex. Continuous SSEP monitoring gives real-time information about sensorimotor function throughout the procedure. Thirumala et al., in their study done in 139 patients operated with intraoperative SSEP, showed 45.2% positive predictive value (FP, 4.3%), 99.2% negative predictive value (FN, 0.7%) for SEP (Thirumala et al. 2013). Continuous compound muscle action potential (CMAP) is used to record MEP of the opposite side of the limbs with DCS with a strip electrode. D waves recordings also have been shown to enhance the safety of resection of tumors in the motor cortex. However, there is a lack of adequate information about EOR and its effect on survival using SSEP and MEP (Tamura et al. 2015; Yamamoto et al. 2004). Triple motor mapping, including transcranial MEP, Bipolar, and Monopolar direct cortical mapping in asleep patients, is considered safer with low rates of deficits and better EOR (Gogos et al. 2020). EOR and neurological deficits are similar for motor mapping when using awake craniotomy or GA (Suarez-Meade et al. 2020).

Intraoperative Language Mapping

Unlike motor mapping, intraoperative language mapping requires an awake patient. Surgeons should be wary of the fact that language areas show a higher degree of variability compared to motor areas. Various protocols have been described for speech and language mapping. The Dutch Linguistic Intraoperative Protocol (DuLIP) is a valid method for preoperative, intra, and postoperative speech and language testing and helps intraoperative language area mapping in various domains of linguistic function (De Witte et al. 2015). A battery of language tasks should be tailored according to the patient's preoperative language function and the location of the lesion (Fernández Coello et al. 2013). Other tasks including cognitive functions or non-language tasks are also selected if relevant. All these tailored batteries of tests are practiced in the preoperative period. The tasks that the patient cannot perform in the preoperative language assessments correctly are omitted during intraoperative testing to make sure that the response, such as speech arrest during the procedure, is due to stimulation of the language area and not because of the pre-existing deficits (Jenkinson et al. 2018). Tasks are performed during direct cortical stimulation within a time frame of four seconds per item (Figure 10). Cortical stimulation is usually done with a bipolar stimulator using the Penfield method. During direct cortical stimulation, object naming (100 objects), repetition of words (phonology), reading, naming, sentence completion (semantic), syntax, and articulation are tested. When the cortex is not stimulated, the patient is tested for phonological sentence judgment and fluency, syntactic sentence judgment and fluency,

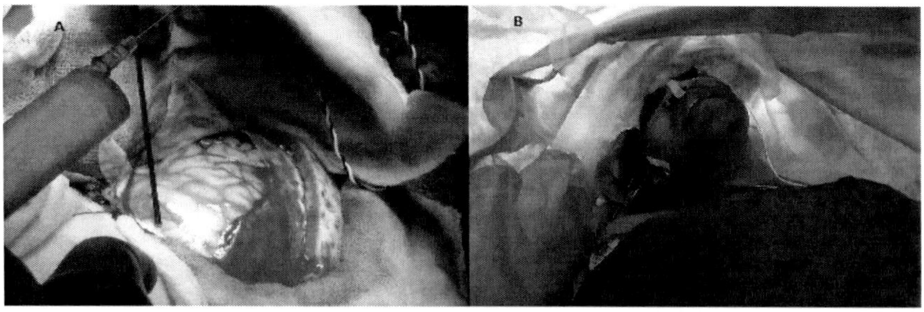

Figure 10. Direct cortical stimulation for language mapping for a tumor adjoining language area (A) Broca's area is being stimulated. (B) Patient is being tested for various components of language.

semantic sentence judgment, and verbal fluency. Transient language impairments occurring during three stimulations are widely recognized as sufficient evidence that the stimulated area is required for language processing (De Witte et al. 2015).

Intraoperative Imaging

Intraoperative MRI (iMRI) has the advantage over neuronavigation in terms of brain shift as it minimizes the error which happens due to brain shift during surgery. In addition, studies say that iMRI and 5-Aminolevulinic acid (ALA) maximize the extent of resection in high-grade gliomas. However, despite that fact, a Cochrane review by Jenkinson MD in 2018 concludes that the evidence on the intraoperative utility of iMRI is of low quality. Therefore, it is uncertain; the effect on long-term survival and PFS with iMRI is also unclear (Jenkinson et al. 2018). However, With the help of intraoperative fMRI and tractography, it is made accessible to determine the extent of residual tumor and its relation to the eloquent regions. The distance from intraoperative tractography of the CST to the motor evoked area has a positive correlation with the strength of stimulation, according to Maesawa and colleagues (Maesawa et al. 2010). Intraoperative tractography and diffusion-weighted imaging (DWI) were found to be more accurate than preoperative tractography in determining the site of the CST. If done combined, cortical mapping and intraoperative tractography improve the efficacy of eloquent region glioma surgery (Maesawa et al. 2010).

Histological Intraoperative Information

Intraoperative photodynamic diagnosis with 5-ALA fluorescence is a good example of a technology that has been developed for visualizing histological information about brain tumors. In this technique, the tumor cells "glow" in a particular pattern because of the metabolized porphyrin IX and are appreciable via microscope. The technique is beneficial for contrast-opaque glioblastoma; it has shown that in more cases, total excision is possible (65% vs. 36%) and also improved 6-month PFS (41% vs. 21%) when compared to excision under natural light (Level I evidence) (Xie et al. 2017). When these techniques are used along with other mapping modalities, they yield better EOR and survival rates.

Confocal laser endomicroscopy is a newer technique that uses a laser light wavelength that stimulates the tumor tissue fluorophores, which emits a photon that will be scanned and processed as a 3D image by software. The investigators who had utilized this technique found 90% sensitivity and 93% specificity in low-grade glioma, but the sample size was only ten (Eschbacher et al. 2012). Low-grade gliomas will not avidly take up 5ALA, unlike high-grade gliomas; hence using confocal microscopy might yield better results; however, more extensive trials are required to validate its utility.

Special Considerations

For patients with large tumors near the eloquent region, staged procedures can be tried in some exceptional circumstances. First, the initial tumor debulking from the non-eloquent area can be performed under general anesthesia. Then, in the second stage, careful removal of the tumor near the eloquent cortex can be done under awake craniotomy with mapping and other monitoring techniques. For smaller lesions, the options are, to wait and watch or stereotactic biopsy with chemoradiation. Studies demonstrate better outcomes with stereotactic biopsy and stereotactic placement of ^{125}I brachytherapy for small lesions on the eloquent cortex (Schnell et al. 2008).

Conclusion

Management of the eloquent cortex still poses a surgical challenge. There should be better anatomical and physiological knowledge to achieve a more significant resection with lesser additional neurological deficit. Preoperative functional imaging, intraoperative mapping, intraoperative imaging modalities, multi-vision 3 D Navigation play a vital role in identifying eloquent cortex in most cases. Furthermore, meticulous surgical techniques such as en-bloc tumor removal and vessel preserving subpial resections, achieving a better extent of resection preserving eloquent regions is possible.

References

Alexander, Andrew L., Jee Eun Lee, Mariana Lazar, and Aaron S. Field. 2007. "Diffusion Tensor Imaging of the Brain." *Neurotherapeutics: The Journal of the American*

Society for Experimental NeuroTherapeutics 4 (3): 316–29. https://doi.org/10.1016/j.nurt.2007.05.011.

Assaf, Yaniv, and Ofer Pasternak. 2008. "Diffusion Tensor Imaging (DTI)-Based White Matter Mapping in Brain Research: A Review." *Journal of Molecular Neuroscience: MN* 34 (1): 51–61. https://doi.org/10.1007/s12031-007-0029-0.

Bello, Lorenzo, Anna Gambini, Antonella Castellano, Giorgio Carrabba, Francesco Acerbi, Enrica Fava, Carlo Giussani, et al. 2008. "Motor and Language DTI Fiber Tracking Combined with Intraoperative Subcortical Mapping for Surgical Removal of Gliomas." *NeuroImage* 39 (1): 369–82. https://doi.org/10.1016/j.neuroimage.2007.08.031.

Bello, Lorenzo, Marco Riva, Enrica Fava, Valentina Ferpozzi, Antonella Castellano, Fabio Raneri, Federico Pessina, Alberto Bizzi, Andrea Falini, and Gabriella Cerri. 2014. "Tailoring Neurophysiological Strategies with Clinical Context Enhances Resection and Safety and Expands Indications in Gliomas Involving Motor Pathways." *Neuro-Oncology* 16 (8): 1110–28. https://doi.org/10.1093/neuonc/ not327.

Berger, Mitchel S., Wendy A. Cohen, and George A. Ojemann. 1990. "Correlation of Motor Cortex Brain Mapping Data with Magnetic Resonance Imaging." *Journal of Neurosurgery* 72 (3): 383–87. https://doi.org/10.3171/jns.1990.72.3.0383.

Bizzi, Alberto, Valeria Blasi, Andrea Falini, Paolo Ferroli, Marcello Cadioli, Ugo Danesi, Domenico Aquino, Carlo Marras, Dario Caldiroli, and Giovanni Broggi. 2008. "Presurgical Functional MR Imaging of Language and Motor Functions: Validation with Intraoperative Electrocortical Mapping." *Radiology* 248 (2): 579–89. https://doi.org/10.1148/radiol.2482071214.

Bloch, Orin, Seunggu J. Han, Soonmee Cha, Matthew Z. Sun, Manish K. Aghi, Michael W. McDermott, Mitchel S. Berger, and Andrew T. Parsa. 2012. "Impact of Extent of Resection for Recurrent Glioblastoma on Overall Survival: Clinical Article." *Journal of Neurosurgery* 117 (6): 1032–38. https://doi.org/10.3171/2012.9.JNS12504.

Brannen, J. H., B. Badie, C. H. Moritz, M. Quigley, M. E. Meyerand, and V. M. Haughton. 2001. "Reliability of Functional MR Imaging with Word-Generation Tasks for Mapping Broca's Area." *AJNR. American Journal of Neuroradiology* 22 (9): 1711–18.

Brell, M., G. Conesa, and J. J. Acebes. 2003. "[Intraoperative cortical mapping in the surgical resection of low-grade gliomas located in eloquent areas]." *Neurocirugia (Asturias, Spain)* 14 (6): 491–503. https://doi.org/10.1016/s1130-1473(03)70507-7.

Choi, Bryan D., Ankit I. Mehta, Kristen A. Batich, Allan H. Friedman, and John H. Sampson. 2012. "The Use of Motor Mapping to Aid Resection of Eloquent Gliomas." *Neurosurgery Clinics of North America* 23 (2): 215–25, vii. https://doi.org/10.1016/j.nec.2012.01.013.

Cochereau, Jérôme, Jérémy Deverdun, Guillaume Herbet, Céline Charroud, Anthony Boyer, Sylvie Moritz-Gasser, Emmanuelle Le Bars, et al. 2016. "Comparison between Resting State FMRI Networks and Responsive Cortical Stimulations in Glioma Patients." *Human Brain Mapping* 37 (11): 3721–32. https://doi.org/10.1002/hbm.23270.

Danks, R. A., M. Rogers, L. S. Aglio, L. D. Gugino, and P. M. Black. 1998. "Patient Tolerance of Craniotomy Performed with the Patient under Local Anesthesia and

Monitored Conscious Sedation." *Neurosurgery* 42 (1): 28–34; discussion 34-36. https://doi.org/10.1097/00006123-199801000-00006.

De Witt Hamer, Philip C., Santiago Gil Robles, Aeilko H. Zwinderman, Hugues Duffau, and Mitchel S. Berger. 2012. "Impact of Intraoperative Stimulation Brain Mapping on Glioma Surgery Outcome: A Meta-Analysis." *Journal of Clinical Oncology: Official Journal of the American Society of Clinical Oncology* 30 (20): 2559–65. https://doi.org/10.1200/JCO.2011.38.4818.

De Witte, E., D. Satoer, E. Robert, H. Colle, S. Verheyen, E. Visch-Brink, and P. Mariën. 2015. "The Dutch Linguistic Intraoperative Protocol: A Valid Linguistic Approach to Awake Brain Surgery." *Brain and Language* 140 (January): 35–48. https://doi.org/ 10.1016/j.bandl.2014.10.011.

Duffau, H., L. Capelle, M. Lopes, A. Bitar, J.-P. Sichez, and R. van Effenterre. 2002. "Medically Intractable Epilepsy from Insular Low-Grade Gliomas: Improvement after an Extended Lesionectomy." *Acta Neurochirurgica* 144 (6): 563–72; discussion 572-573. https://doi.org/10.1007/s00701-002-0941-6.

Eschbacher, Jennifer, Nikolay L. Martirosyan, Peter Nakaji, Nader Sanai, Mark C. Preul, Kris A. Smith, Stephen W. Coons, and Robert F. Spetzler. 2012. "In Vivo Intraoperative Confocal Microscopy for Real-Time Histopathological Imaging of Brain Tumors." *Journal of Neurosurgery* 116 (4): 854–60. https://doi.org/10.3171/ 2011.12.JNS11696.

Eseonu, Chikezie I., Karim ReFaey, Oscar Garcia, Gugan Raghuraman, and Alfredo Quinones-Hinojosa. 2017. "Volumetric Analysis of Extent of Resection, Survival, and Surgical Outcomes for Insular Gliomas." *World Neurosurgery* 103 (July): 265–74. https://doi.org/10.1016/j.wneu.2017.04.002.

Fernández Coello, Alejandro, Sylvie Moritz-Gasser, Juan Martino, Matteo Martinoni, Ryosuke Matsuda, and Hugues Duffau. 2013. "Selection of Intraoperative Tasks for Awake Mapping Based on Relationships between Tumor Location and Functional Networks." *Journal of Neurosurgery* 119 (6): 1380–94. https://doi.org/10.3171/ 2013.6.JNS122470.

Firsching, R., I. Bondar, H. J. Heinze, H. Hinrichs, T. Hagner, J. Heinrich, and A. Belau. 2002. "Practicability of Magnetoencephalography-Guided Neuronavigation." *Neurosurgical Review* 25 (1–2): 73–78. https://doi.org/10.1007/s101430100161.

Forst, Deborah A., Brian V. Nahed, Jay S. Loeffler, and Tracy T. Batchelor. 2014. "Low-Grade Gliomas." *The Oncologist* 19 (4): 403–13. https://doi.org/10.1634/ the oncologist.2013-0345.

Forster, Marie-Thérèse, Elke Hattingen, Christian Senft, Thomas Gasser, Volker Seifert, and Andrea Szelényi. 2011. "Navigated Transcranial Magnetic Stimulation and Functional Magnetic Resonance Imaging: Advanced Adjuncts in Preoperative Planning for Central Region Tumors." *Neurosurgery* 68 (5): 1317–24; discussion 1324-1325. https://doi.org/10.1227/NEU.0b013e31820b528c.

Frappaz, D., O. Chinot, A. Bataillard, M. Ben Hassel, L. Capelle, S. Chanalet, M. Chatel, D. Figarella-Branger, Y. Guegan, and J. Guyotat. 2003. "Summary Version of the Standards, Options and Recommendations for the Management of Adult Patients with Intracranial Glioma (2002)." *British Journal of Cancer* 89 (1): S73–83.

Gogos, Andrew J., Jacob S. Young, Ramin A. Morshed, Lauro N. Avalos, Roger S. Noss, Javier E. Villanueva-Meyer, Shawn L. Hervey-Jumper, and Mitchel S. Berger. 2020. "Triple Motor Mapping: Transcranial, Bipolar, and Monopolar Mapping for Supratentorial Glioma Resection Adjacent to Motor Pathways." *Journal of Neurosurgery*, June, 1–10. https://doi.org/10.3171/2020.3.JNS193434.

Grabert, Josefin, Sven Klaschik, Ági Güresir, Patrick Jakobs, Martin Soehle, Hartmut Vatter, Tobias Hilbert, Erdem Güresir, and Markus Velten. 2019. "Supraglottic Devices for Airway Management in Awake Craniotomy." *Medicine* 98 (40): e17473. https://doi.org/10.1097/MD.0000000000017473.

Han, Seunggu J., Ramin A. Morshed, Irene Troncon, Kesshi M. Jordan, Roland G. Henry, Shawn L. Hervey-Jumper, and Mitchel S. Berger. 2018. "Subcortical Stimulation Mapping of Descending Motor Pathways for Perirolandic Gliomas: Assessment of Morbidity and Functional Outcome in 702 Cases." *Journal of Neurosurgery* 131 (1): 201–8. https://doi.org/10.3171/2018.3.JNS172494.

Hervey-Jumper, Shawn L., and Mitchel S. Berger. 2014. "Role of Surgical Resection in Low- and High-Grade Gliomas." *Current Treatment Options in Neurology* 16 (4): 284. https://doi.org/10.1007/s11940-014-0284-7.

Jakola, Asgeir S., Geirmund Unsg\aard, Kristin S. Myrmel, Roar Kloster, Sverre H. Torp, Lisa M. Sagberg, Sigurd Lindal, and Ole Solheim. 2014. "Surgical Strategies in Low-Grade Gliomas and Implications for Long-Term Quality of Life." *Journal of Clinical Neuroscience* 21 (8): 1304–9.

Jellison, Brian J., Aaron S. Field, Joshua Medow, Mariana Lazar, M. Shariar Salamat, and Andrew L. Alexander. 2004. "Diffusion Tensor Imaging of Cerebral White Matter: A Pictorial Review of Physics, Fiber Tract Anatomy, and Tumor Imaging Patterns." *AJNR. American Journal of Neuroradiology* 25 (3): 356–69.

Jenkinson, Michael D., Damiano Giuseppe Barone, Andrew Bryant, Luke Vale, Helen Bulbeck, Theresa A. Lawrie, Michael G. Hart, and Colin Watts. 2018. "Intraoperative Imaging Technology to Maximise Extent of Resection for Glioma." *The Cochrane Database of Systematic Reviews* 1 (January): CD012788. https://doi. org/10.1002/14651858.CD012788.pub2.

Kannabiran, Narmadhalakshmi, and P. Bidkar. 2018. "*Total Intravenous Anesthesia in Neurosurgery*." https://doi.org/10.1055/S-0038-1673544.

Khanna, Nishanth, Wilson Altmeyer, Jiachen Zhuo, and Andrew Steven. 2015. "Functional Neuroimaging: Fundamental Principles and Clinical Applications." *The Neuroradiology Journal* 28 (2): 87–96. https://doi.org/10.1177/1971400915576311.

Kim, Stefan S., Ian E. McCutcheon, Dima Suki, Jeffrey S. Weinberg, Raymond Sawaya, Frederick F. Lang, David Ferson, Amy B. Heimberger, Franco DeMonte, and Sujit S. Prabhu. 2009. "Awake Craniotomy for Brain Tumors near Eloquent Cortex: Correlation of Intraoperative Cortical Mapping with Neurological Outcomes in 309 Consecutive Patients." *Neurosurgery* 64 (5): 836–45; discussion 345-346. https://doi.org/10.1227/01.NEU.0000342405.80881.81.

Kirsch, Heidi E., Zhao Zhu, Susanne Honma, Anne Findlay, Mitchel S. Berger, and Srikantan S. Nagarajan. 2007. "Predicting the Location of Mouth Motor Cortex in Patients with Brain Tumors by Using Somatosensory Evoked Field Measurements." *Journal of Neurosurgery* 107 (3): 481–87. https://doi.org/10.3171/JNS-07/09/0481.

Korvenoja, Antti, Erika Kirveskari, Hannu J. Aronen, Sari Avikainen, Antti Brander, Juha Huttunen, Risto J. Ilmoniemi, et al. 2006. "Sensorimotor Cortex Localization: Comparison of Magnetoencephalography, Functional MR Imaging, and Intraoperative Cortical Mapping." *Radiology* 241 (1): 213–22. https://doi.org/ 10.1148/radiol. 2411050796.

Krieg, Sandro M., Ehab Shiban, Niels Buchmann, Jens Gempt, Annette Foerschler, Bernhard Meyer, and Florian Ringel. 2012. "Utility of Presurgical Navigated Transcranial Magnetic Brain Stimulation for the Resection of Tumors in Eloquent Motor Areas." *Journal of Neurosurgery* 116 (5): 994–1001. https://doi.org/10. 3171/ 2011.12.JNS111524.

Lee, Chanhung Z., and Clara C. M. Poon. 2021. "An Update of Neuroanesthesia for Intraoperative Brain Mapping Craniotomy." *Neurosurgery*, February, nyab022. https://doi.org/10.1093/neuros/nyab022.

Leuthardt, Eric C., Kai Miller, Nicholas R. Anderson, Gerwin Schalk, Joshua Dowling, John Miller, Daniel W. Moran, and Jeff G. Ojemann. 2007. "Electrocorticographic Frequency Alteration Mapping: A Clinical Technique for Mapping the Motor Cortex." *Neurosurgery* 60 (4 Suppl 2): 260–70; discussion 270-271. https://doi.org/10.1227/ 01.NEU.0000255413.70807.6E.

Lucas, Timothy H., Daniel L. Drane, Carl B. Dodrill, and George A. Ojemann. 2008. "Language Reorganization in Aphasics: An Electrical Stimulation Mapping Investigation." *Neurosurgery* 63 (3): 487–97; discussion 497. https://doi.org/10. 1227/01.NEU.0000324725.84854.04.

Maesawa, Satoshi, Masazumi Fujii, Norimoto Nakahara, Tadashi Watanabe, Toshihiko Wakabayashi, and Jun Yoshida. 2010. "Intraoperative Tractography and Motor Evoked Potential (MEP) Monitoring in Surgery for Gliomas around the Corticospinal Tract." *World Neurosurgery* 74 (1): 153–61. https://doi.org/10. 1016/j.wneu.2010. 03.022.

McGirt, Matthew J., Kaisorn L. Chaichana, Muraya Gathinji, Frank J. Attenello, Khoi Than, Alessandro Olivi, Jon D. Weingart, Henry Brem, and Alf Redo Quiñones-Hinojosa. 2009. "Independent Association of Extent of Resection with Survival in Patients with Malignant Brain Astrocytoma." *Journal of Neurosurgery* 110 (1): 156–62. https://doi.org/10.3171/2008.4.17536.

Meier, M. P., J. Ilmberger, G. Fesl, and M. I. Ruge. 2013. "Validation of Functional Motor and Language MRI with Direct Cortical Stimulation." *Acta Neurochirurgica* 155 (4): 675–83. https://doi.org/10.1007/s00701-013-1624-1.

Molinaro, Annette M., Shawn Hervey-Jumper, Ramin A. Morshed, Jacob Young, Seunggu J. Han, Pranathi Chunduru, Yalan Zhang, et al. 2020. "Association of Maximal Extent of Resection of Contrast-Enhanced and Non-Contrast-Enhanced Tumor With Survival Within Molecular Subgroups of Patients With Newly Diagnosed Glioblastoma." *JAMA Oncology* 6 (4): 495–503. https://doi.org/10.1001/ jamaoncol.2019.6143.

Nimsky, C., O. Ganslandt, and R. Fahlbusch. 2004. "Functional Neuronavigation and Intraoperative MRI." *Advances and Technical Standards in Neurosurgery* 29: 229–63. https://doi.org/10.1007/978-3-7091-0558-0_6.

Olsen, K. S. 2008. "The Asleep-Awake Technique Using Propofol-Remifentanil Anaesthesia for Awake Craniotomy for Cerebral Tumours." *European Journal of Anaesthesiology* 25 (8): 662–69. https://doi.org/10.1017/S0265021508003633.

Orringer, Daniel, Darryl Lau, Sameer Khatri, Grettel J. Zamora-Berridi, Kathy Zhang, Chris Wu, Neeraj Chaudhary, and Oren Sagher. 2012. "Extent of Resection in Patients with Glioblastoma: Limiting Factors, Perception of Resectability, and Effect on Survival." *Journal of Neurosurgery* 117 (5): 851–59. https://doi.org/10.3171/ 2012.8. JNS12234.

Ottenhausen, Malte, Sandro M. Krieg, Bernhard Meyer, and Florian Ringel. 2015. "Functional Preoperative and Intraoperative Mapping and Monitoring: Increasing Safety and Efficacy in Glioma Surgery." *Neurosurgical Focus* 38 (1): E3. https://doi.org/10.3171/2014.10.FOCUS14611.

Pallud, J., and E. Dezamis. 2017. "Functional and Oncological Outcomes Following Awake Surgical Resection Using Intraoperative Cortico-Subcortical Functional Mapping for Supratentorial Gliomas Located in Eloquent Areas." *Neuro-Chirurgie* 63 (3): 208–18. https://doi.org/10.1016/j.neuchi.2016.08.003.

Pouratian, Nader, and Susan Y. Bookheimer. 2010. "The Reliability of Neuroanatomy as a Predictor of Eloquence: A Review." *Neurosurgical Focus* 28 (2): E3. https://doi.org/ 10.3171/2009.11.FOCUS09239.

Raabe, Andreas, Jürgen Beck, Philippe Schucht, and Kathleen Seidel. 2014. "Continuous Dynamic Mapping of the Corticospinal Tract during Surgery of Motor Eloquent Brain Tumors: Evaluation of a New Method." *Journal of Neurosurgery* 120 (5): 1015–24. https://doi.org/10.3171/2014.1.JNS13909.

Rahman, Maryam, Joseph Abbatematteo, Edward K. De Leo, Paul S. Kubilis, Sasha Vaziri, Frank Bova, Elias Sayour, Duane Mitchell, and Alfredo Quinones-Hinojosa. 2017. "The Effects of New or Worsened Postoperative Neurological Deficits on Survival of Patients with Glioblastoma." *Journal of Neurosurgery* 127 (1): 123–31. https://doi. org/10.3171/2016.7.JNS16396.

Roland, Jarod L., Carl D. Hacker, and Eric C. Leuthardt. 2020. "A Review of Passive Brain Mapping Techniques in Neurological Surgery." *Neurosurgery* 88 (1): 15–24. https://doi.org/10.1093/neuros/nyaa361.

Rossi, Marco, Federico Ambrogi, Lorenzo Gay, Marcello Gallucci, Marco Conti Nibali, Antonella Leonetti, Guglielmo Puglisi, et al. 2019. "Is Supratotal Resection Achievable in Low-Grade Gliomas? Feasibility, Putative Factors, Safety, and Functional Outcome." *Journal of Neurosurgery* 132 (6): 1692–1705. https://doi. org/10.3171/2019.2.JNS183408.

Roux, Franck-Emmanuel, Kader Boulanouar, Jean-Albert Lotterie, Mehdi Mejdoubi, James P. LeSage, and Isabelle Berry. 2003. "Language Functional Magnetic Resonance Imaging in Preoperative Assessment of Language Areas: Correlation with Direct Cortical Stimulation." *Neurosurgery* 52 (6): 1335–45; discussion 1345-1347. https://doi.org/10.1227/01.neu.0000064803.05077.40.

Sartorius, C. J., and M. S. Berger. 1998. "Rapid Termination of Intraoperative Stimulation-Evoked Seizures with Application of Cold Ringer's Lactate to the Cortex. Technical Note." *Journal of Neurosurgery* 88 (2): 349–51. https://doi. org/10.3171/jns. 1998.88.2.0349.

Schnell, O., K. Schöller, M. Ruge, A. Siefert, J.-C. Tonn, and F. W. Kreth. 2008. "Surgical Resection plus Stereotactic 125I Brachytherapy in Adult Patients with Eloquently Located Supratentorial WHO Grade II Glioma - Feasibility and Outcome of a Combined Local Treatment Concept." *Journal of Neurology* 255 (10): 1495–1502. https://doi.org/10.1007/s00415-008-0948-x.

Schucht, P., K. Seidel, A. Jilch, J. Beck, and A. Raabe. 2017. "A Review of Monopolar Motor Mapping and a Comprehensive Guide to Continuous Dynamic Motor Mapping for Resection of Motor Eloquent Brain Tumors." *Neuro-Chirurgie* 63 (3): 175–80. https://doi.org/10.1016/j.neuchi.2017.01.007.

Shinoura, N., Y. Suzuki, R. Yamada, Y. Tabei, K. Saito, and K. Yagi. 2009. "Precentral Knob Corresponds to the Primary Motor and Premotor Area." *The Canadian Journal of Neurological Sciences. Le Journal Canadien Des Sciences Neurologiques* 36 (2): 227–33. https://doi.org/10.1017/s0317167100006594.

Suarez-Meade, Paola, Lina Marenco-Hillembrand, Calder Prevatt, Ricardo Murguia-Fuentes, Alea Mohamed, Thannon Alsaeed, Eric J. Lehrer, et al. 2020. "Awake vs. Asleep Motor Mapping for Glioma Resection: A Systematic Review and Meta-Analysis." *Acta Neurochirurgica* 162 (7): 1709–20. https://doi.org/10.1007/s00701-020-04357-y.

Szelényi, A., C. Senft, M. Jardan, M. T. Forster, K. Franz, V. Seifert, and H. Vatter. 2011. "Intra-Operative Subcortical Electrical Stimulation: A Comparison of Two Methods." *Clinical Neurophysiology: Official Journal of the International Federation of Clinical Neurophysiology* 122 (7): 1470–75. https://doi.org/10.1016/ j.clinph.2010.12.055.

Szelényi, Andrea, Lorenzo Bello, Hugues Duffau, Enrica Fava, Guenther C. Feigl, Miroslav Galanda, Georg Neuloh, Francesco Signorelli, Francesco Sala, and Workgroup for Intraoperative Management in Low-Grade Glioma Surgery within the European Low-Grade Glioma Network. 2010. "Intraoperative Electrical Stimulation in Awake Craniotomy: Methodological Aspects of Current Practice." *Neurosurgical Focus* 28 (2): E7. https://doi.org/10.3171/2009.12.FOCUS09237.

Tamura, Manabu, Yoshihiro Muragaki, Taiichi Saito, Takashi Maruyama, Masayuki Nitta, Shunsuke Tsuzuki, Hiroshi Iseki, and Yoshikazu Okada. 2015. "Strategy of Surgical Resection for Glioma Based on Intraoperative Functional Mapping and Monitoring." *Neurologia Medico-Chirurgica* 55 (5): 383–98. https://doi.org/10. 2176/nmc.ra.2014-0415.

Thirumala, Parthasarathy, Daniel Lai, Jonathan Engh, Miguel Habeych, Donald Crammond, and Jeffrey Balzer. 2013. "Predictive Value of Somatosensory Evoked Potential Monitoring during Resection of Intraparenchymal and Intraventricular Tumors Using an Endoscopic Port." *Journal of Clinical Neurology (Seoul, Korea)* 9 (4): 244–51. https://doi.org/10.3988/jcn.2013.9.4.244.

Uematsu, S., R. Lesser, R. S. Fisher, B. Gordon, K. Hara, G. L. Krauss, E. P. Vining, and R. W. Webber. 1992. "Motor and Sensory Cortex in Humans: Topography Studied with Chronic Subdural Stimulation." *Neurosurgery* 31 (1): 59–71; discussion 71-72. https://doi.org/10.1227/00006123-199207000-00009.

Witwer, Brian P., Roham Moftakhar, Khader M. Hasan, Praveen Deshmukh, Victor Haughton, Aaron Field, Konstantinos Arfanakis, et al. 2002. "Diffusion-Tensor

Imaging of White Matter Tracts in Patients with Cerebral Neoplasm." *Journal of Neurosurgery* 97 (3): 568–75. https://doi.org/10.3171/jns.2002.97.3.0568.

Xia, Hechun, Wei Huang, Liang Wu, Hui Ma, Xiaodong Wang, Xuexin Chen, Shengyu Sun, and Xiaoxiong Jia. 2012. "Preoperative Functional MRI Localization of Language Areas in Chinese Patients with Brain Tumors: Validation with Intraoperative Electrocortical Mapping." *Neural Regeneration Research* 7 (20): 1563–69. https://doi.org/10.3969/j.issn.1673-5374.2012.20.006.

Xie, Yijing, Maria Thom, Michael Ebner, Victoria Wykes, Adrien Desjardins, Anna Miserocchi, Sebastien Ourselin, Andrew W. McEvoy, and Tom Vercauteren. 2017. "Wide-Field Spectrally Resolved Quantitative Fluorescence Imaging System: Toward Neurosurgical Guidance in Glioma Resection." *Journal of Biomedical Optics* 22 (11): 1–14. https://doi.org/10.1117/1.JBO.22.11.116006.

Yamamoto, Takamitsu, Yoichi Katayama, Takafumi Nagaoka, Kazutaka Kobayashi, and Chikashi Fukaya. 2004. "Intraoperative Monitoring of the Corticospinal Motor Evoked Potential (D-Wave): Clinical Index for Postoperative Motor Function and Functional Recovery." *Neurologia Medico-Chirurgica* 44 (4): 170–80; discussion 181-182. https://doi.org/10.2176/nmc.44.170.

Chapter 12

Intraoperative Ultrasonography and Multimodality Mapping/Monitoring in Supratentorial Glioma Surgery

Maruti Nandan, Kuntal Kanti Das, Aanchal Datta and Kamlesh Singh Bhaisora

Department of Neurosurgery, Sanjay Gandhi Postgraduate Institute of Medical Sciences, Lucknow, India

Abstract

Gliomas are the commonest primary central nervous system tumors. Recent years have seen massive advances in the understanding of these tumors from radiological and histo-molecular perspectives. As far as their management is concerned, surgical resection still plays a central role. The extent of resection (EOR) and residual tumor volumes have emerged as perhaps the strongest modifiable predictors of overall survival, malignant progression free survival and seizure control in gliomas irrespective of the histological grade. While an incremental survival advantage beyond 78% tumor volume resection has been observed in high grade gliomas, the similar threshold for low grade gliomas have been observed to be 90%. It is very well known that surgeon's intraoperative estimation of the EOR can be erratic and hence a lot of reliance is placed now a days on the postoperative confirmation of EOR using appropriate magnetic resonance imaging (MRI) studies. Thus, it is imperative to improve the EOR to these recommended degrees. A set of adjuncts have thus been developed to aid in the surgeon's intraoperative assessments. Intraoperative image guidance plays a vital role is visualizing the tumor while intraoperative electrophysiological monitoring and awake mapping ensures that such

In: Advances in Neurosurgery Research
Editors: Amit Agrawal, Pradeep Chouksey, Adesh Shrivastava et al.
ISBN: 978-1-68507-859-1

surgical endeavors do not impair the functional status after surgery. Thus, these two modalities are paramount to achieving the modern-day goal of glioma surgery i.e., maximal safe resection or the onco-functional balance. This chapter addresses the role of these two adjunctive modalities in glioma surgery focusing on intraoperative ultrasonography and intraoperative brain mapping and monitoring in supratentorial glioma resections.

Introduction

Gliomas are the most common primary neoplasms of the central nervous system [1, 2]. In the recent years, several key changes have taken place in their understanding. Despite advances in molecular diagnostics, better treatment options and a simultaneous emphasis on the quality of life, little has changed in the survival of the affected patients [3]. A host of prognostic variables have been suggested and many of them are well established now. Amongst these, the extent of resection (EOR) is an important factor and remains a surgeon modifiable variable in the overall equation [4]. Different resection thresholds have been suggested by various leading groups and it appears that a survival benefit is obtained with at least 78% (high grade) to 90% resection of the tumor mass (low grade gliomas) [1]. This had led to the emergence of several techniques and technologies to assist surgeons' intraoperative impression to increase the EOR. This ushered in an era of image guidance in glioma surgeries to allow more accurate intraoperative tumor border delineation. In this process, neurological deficits can occur if the tumor being resected has functioning areas either within or more commonly adjacent to it. Thus, preservation of these functional areas assumes an equally important goal in the resection of gliomas in functionally eloquent areas. Otherwise, a permanent neurological deficit can negate the survival advantage obtained by a painstaking tumor resection [5]. This requires elaboration of the functional map of the tumor in a particular patient using multi modal pre and intraoperative brain mapping and brain function monitoring. These two contrasting objectives need to be balanced in glioma surgery and has come to be known as the "onco-functional balance." In this chapter, we provide an overview of image guided glioma surgery focusing on the role of intraoperative ultrasound as well as multimodality mapping and monitoring of neurological functions during supratentorial glioma surgery.

Issues with Surgeon's Intraoperative Estimation of Extent of Tumor Resection

Gliomas are intrinsic tumors of the brain, arising from the glial supporting cells. Except for the grade 1 tumors which are well circumscribed and distinctly different biologically, grade 2-4 gliomas are often diffuse in their boundaries, despite their seemingly well demarcated outline on neuroimaging. This infiltrating periphery is exactly the place which is incriminated in recurrence, malignant progression and epileptogenesis [6]. Therefore, surgical resection must include this peripheral infiltrative zone as well [7]. There are, however, several issues with such a resection and include the possibility of resecting normal adjoining brain, albeit tumor infiltrated, and production of neurological deficit if functionally important areas flank the tumor.

It has been shown that surgeons' intraoperative assessment of the EOR is often sub optimal [8]. It lacks objectivity and the same has resulted in a progressive change in the neurooncological community to seek for a uniform reporting of EOR based on early postoperative MRI and volumetric assessment. The place where surgeons tend to err with respect to EOR is the tumor periphery where the color difference between tumor and normal brain tissue becomes very blur. Moiyadi et al. demonstrated that the use of intraoperative ultrasonography helps the surgical team to proceed with further tumor resections when their intraoperative assessment had indicated a complete tumor extirpation [9].

Intraoperative Image Guidance and Relative Role of Intraoperative Ultrasound (IOUS)

One of the challenges involved in complete resection of gliomas is the difficulty in visualizing the tumor borders if we leave aside the functional eloquence of the adjoining area. Traditional intraoperative cues like tumor consistency, bleeding pattern, color, collapsibility of the resection cavity etc. are often insufficient predictors as far as tumor-brain interface determination is concerned. Therefore, as the surgeon approaches the peripheral infiltrative zone and these standard cues become inadequate, the fear of producing a neurological deficit takes over, often leading the surgical team to stop further resections. Moreover, even if there are no adjoining functional areas, the near normal naked eye appearance of the infiltration zone gives a false impression of a complete tumor clearance. Most studies have demonstrated that tumor recurrence, malignant transformation and epileptogenesis tend to occur within 2 cm of the visible tumor margin [10]. Therefore, the surgeon needs to know two key elements here to obtain a "true" complete tumor resection namely: visualization of the infiltrating tumor margin and information on the functional importance of this area. Thus, modern adjuncts are necessary to assist the surgeons in clearing this area, we prefer to call as "critical area." While intraoperative frozen section, Raman spectroscopy or confocal microscopy are quite definitive in their roles, logistic reasons come in the way of their integration into the routine neurosurgical practice [11, 12]. Thus, image guidance to determine the tumor borders has emerged as a more practical method. As of now, we have two types of image guidance namely: radiological imaging (Neuronavigation based on preoperative imaging, intraoperative magnetic resonance imaging, MRI and intraoperative ultrasound, IOUS) and biological imaging (e.g., florescence guided tumor resection). Each of these have specific sets of pros and cons [13]. Here we focus on IOUS.

IOUS

IOUS is not new in neurosurgery and has been in use for decades. Its use has predated other intraoperative technologies and navigation systems. First introduced by Loomis and Wood in 1920s, the technology has been refined over the years [14]. Dussik brothers were the first to use IOUS in brain tumors, but it was not until 1978 that it was used as an aid in tumor resection [15]. Technological advances and improvements in the image quality have made IOUS as a valuable intraoperative tool in surgical neurooncology.

Basic Principles of IOUS

When a vibrating source comes in contact with a medium, the medium vibrates, and sound is created as a mechanical energy. The sound then travels through the medium causing compression and rarefaction. Depending on the density of the medium through which the sound waves travel, one of the three things may happen: reflection, absorption or scattering. These three effects are detected on the probe containing the vibrating source, captured as an image. The time taken for the sound to reflect determines the shape and position of the medium in space.

In medicine, the vibrating source is an array of piezo electric crystals of the probe and the medium is human body tissue. The sound wave created is beyond human hearing threshold (that is why it is called "ultra" sound, typically between 2 and 20 MHz). When lower frequency waves are used, deeper tissues are better seen but resolution drops while a higher frequency improves image quality at the cost of reduced penetration to deeper tissues (better for superficial lesions). This inverse relationship between frequency and depth is an important thing to remember[16.]

Echogenicity is a frequently used term in ultrasound imaging lexicon. It refers to the ability of a tissue to either reflect or transmit US waves with respect to the surroundings. If two different echogenic structures are present side by side, a visible contrast (black and white) is displayed on the ultrasound screen. The images displayed on an US monitor can be bright (hyperechoic), gray (hypoechoic), black (anechoic) or of same intensity of the surrounding areas (iso echoic).

The natural hyperechoic structures inside the brain are dural folds, choroid plexus, and pineal gland (depending on the extent of calcification). Normal brain is isoechoic while the ventricles and brainstem are anechoic structures.

Utility and Evidence in Glioma Resection

In brain tumor surgery in general and glioma surgery in specific, IOUS is used at following stages:

1. Before durotomy:

This is done to see if the lesion is adequately exposed through the craniotomy created and whether the craniotomy requires further enlargement to have adjoining transcortical windows, the baseline sonographic features (outline, echogenicity, cystic areas etc.) to know if IOUS would be of help and if it is, to have a reference for later comparisons. This step also helps in orienting the surgical team by visualizing normal adjoining insonable structures.

2. During tumor resection:

As tumor resection continues, IOUS may supplement surgeon's intraoperative assessment in determining areas where residual tumor may be remaining. In this situation, it acts as a resection control. If a navigable ultrasound is being used with preoperative MRI based navigation, intermittent scans may allow fine tuning to compensate for the brain shift. * Additional information may be obtained with advanced IOUS features like contrast enhanced US (CEUS), US elastography and power doppler.

3. After tumor resection:

To confirm final status of the resection cavity, any deep lying hematomas and to evaluate in detail the acoustic artefacts at resection margins.

Figure 1 shows IOUS pictures in a case of motor strip glioma.

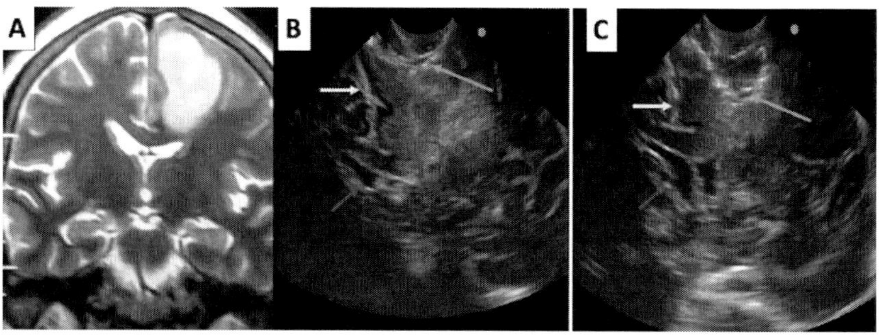

Figure 1. Shows IOUS appearance of a subcortical paramedial motor strip glioma. On MRI (coronal section), the mass is seen close to the flax cerebri and compressing the underlying lateral ventricle (A). Early IOUS during tumor resection (B), shows the residual tumor below the resection cavity (orange arrow), while falx cerebri (yellow arrow) and ventricles (red arrow) maintain orientation. A delayed scan (C) shows how the resection is proceeding and guides the surgeon regarding the extent and site of residual tumor.

Insonation Technical Details

Once it is decided to use intraoperative ultrasound, certain pre-requisites need to be ensured to have a good intraoperative ultrasound image. Gliomas are usually hyperechoic with respect to the surrounding brain. As the grade of the tumor increases, central necrotic areas may appear hypoechoic and thus the tumor may appear heterogenous in echogenicity [17]. The surrounding edema is usually seen as hypoechoic shadows.

Pre-Requisites to Obtain a Good Ultrasound Image

1. Patient position should be such that the resection cavity lies at the top and as horizontal as possible. This ensures that irrigation fluid can be retained in the cavity for a transcavitary ultrasound insonation.
2. A sufficiently sized craniotomy is necessary to allow the ultrasound probe to be applied on the brain/surgical cavity (30x12 mm, 7 MHz probe is the most used probe in neurosurgical cases). Moreover, the adjoining exposed cortex can allow both a transcortical ultrasonography and brain mapping. Also, the marker of the USG probe must be aligned to patient's anatomic right in cross sectional view and towards the vertex in a longitudinal view to maintain orientation [18].
3. Baseline image is to be obtained at two planes perpendicular to each other (in one of the three orthogonal planes). The best ultrasound image is obtained if the transducer is at a right angle to the reflecting or transmitting surface. Sometimes, an appropriate tilting of the ultrasound probe brings out the best image, the angle being called the angle of incidence.
4. The morphology of the image depends on how the probe is applied on the brain surface and one can obtain axial, coronal, or sagittal images. Many a times, depending on how the probe is placed, an image in between the orthogonal planes may be obtained and may confuse the surgeon due to the lack of familiarity. Navigated ultrasound can help in the image orientation and it is recommended for beginners if the facility is available.
5. Sometimes, a slight pressure on the probe applied on the brain may the improve image quality by reducing the distance for the waves to travel and by altering the echogenicity of the tissues [19].

Evidence for Ultrasonography Use in Glioma Surgery

A systematic review and metanalysis by *Gianluca* et al. was conducted in 2015 to validate the role of intraoperative USG in detecting the residual tumor volume after diffuse glioma surgery. They compared the diagnostic performance of intraoperative USG with that of early post-operative MRI and concluded that iUSG is an effective technique in assessment of diffuse low grade glioma resection with pooled sensitivity and specificity of 72.2% and

93.5% respectively. Diagnostic performance was higher in LGG and compared with the high-grade glioma surgery. Similarly, many other authors have validated the role of IOUS in glioma surgery [20].

n2DUS (Navigational 2D Ultrasonography)

If navigational 2DUS is available, scan is acquired with this system way like the 2D USG and navigation localizer is attached to the probe. Image thus acquired is displayed on the navigation screen and superimposed with the co-displayed MR brain scan. This adds in understanding the plane of insonation and necessary adjustment of the USG probe [17]. Thus, n2DUS system makes it easier to understand the anatomical landmarks on the US image as the same is superimposed on MR scan in the same plane.

n3DUS (Navigational 3D Ultrasonography)

A series of image is captured with n2DUS as described and used to reconstruct the 3D volume. This 3D image is fused with MR scan to produce 3D US-MR fusion image. MR image also provides information about functional areas of brain and therefore this fusion image provides functional information of brain which is lacking in US imaging [21].

Surgical resection is performed after obtaining the real time US scan under intraoperative neurophysiologic monitoring. Frequent US image is obtained during surgery for maximal resection of the lesion. Before obtaining the scan in between, hemostasis is achieved, and surgical debris is thoroughly rinsed with the normal saline. Surgical table is adjusted to make the surgical cavity vertical as much as possible, and cavity is filled with the saline. This image is compared with the image acquired preoperatively and extent of resection is estimated [9, 22].

Newer US Applications in Glioma Surgery

Contrast Enhanced Ultrasonography (CEUS)

When the conventional B mode ultrasonography, the insonated fields are depicted using a grey scale codification. Visualization and differentiation of LGG is quite difficult, operator dependent and requires long learning curve.

Contrast enhanced ultrasound when used leads to better differentiation between normal brain and tumor tissue especially in LGG. Contrast agent used for CEUS consists of microbubble of inert gas and a shell. Inert gas determines the solubility and acoustic property, whereas shell adds to the better viscoelastic property. Perfluorocarbon is commonly used inert gas and phospholipid is used to create a shell. Size of this microbubble ranges from 1-10 micron which can easily circumvent the pulmonary vasculature to reach the systemic circulation. Some study also showed that CEUS can evaluate the grade of glioma. Thus, CEUS can clearly add to the better visualization and differentiation between tumor and brain tissue, increasing the EOR and overall survival [22].

USG Elastography

This is newer ultrasonographic technique, way like that of fibro scan of liver which measures the elastogenic property of tissue and can differentiate between pathological from normal tissue. Real time USG elastography measures the relative hardness of tissue by evaluation local strain after external force is applied. Glioma has different elasticity as compared to brain and surrounding structures and therefore it can be differentiated from normal brain in real time intraoperatively to maximize the EOR [23].

Advantages of IOUS

The biggest advantage of IOUS as an intraoperative image guidance tool is its real time nature. This makes its use to make definitive decisions without worrying for brain shifts. Second advantage is its cost effectiveness compared to other adjuncts like intraoperative MRI. Portability, lack of need for specialized theatre and equipment and ability to be co-registered with neuronavigation make IOUS a very handy tool. Moreover, a rising number of publications support its utility is enhancing EOR as well as functional preservation in gliomas. With the advent of advanced technology and other modalities like CEUS, 3D nUS, the utility is only likely to increase in the future.

Limitations and Means to Reduce Them

The biggest limitation of USG is its operator dependence. Therefore, experienced teams find it very helpful while the reverse is seen with lesser experienced surgeons. Training at high volume centers, having a radiologist by the side in OR and using USG in all cases can be helpful.

The other disadvantage is the display images in all possible planes unlike the orthogonal planes. As neurosurgeons, this can be very disorienting as USG images depend on how the probe is applied on the brain. If available, using USG fused with preoperative MRI based navigation platforms in the initial cases can help [21]. If not, the operator must try changing angulation of the probe in such a way that an image close to the orthogonal planes are obtained for orientation. With an increasing experience, this limitation can be minimized.

Image quality can be a hurdle in USG usage. Using probes of appropriate frequency, ensuring acoustic gel coverage of USG probe, eliminating air/blood clots/cottonoids from the resection cavity, pressing slightly on the brain with the probe during examination and changes in the parameters like depth, time gain compensation etc. can improve image quality. Still, image quality remains a major limitation of IOUS.

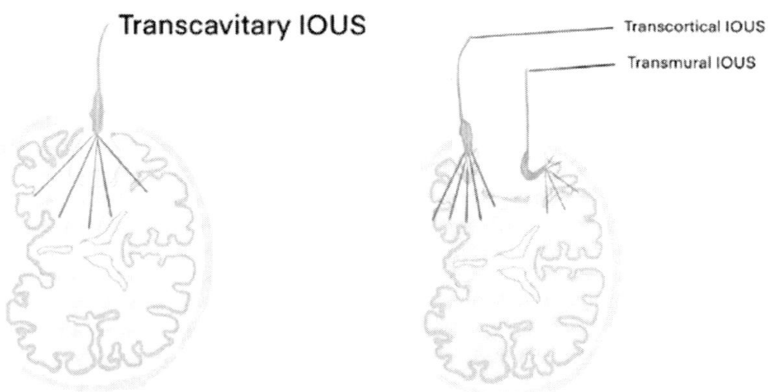

Figure 2. This cartoon shows insonation techniques. While transcavitary IOUS is most commonly applied (A), it can have acoustic artifacts beyond the walls of the cavity, sometimes defeating the purpose of its use. By using special techniques (B) like insonation through the adjoining normal cortex (transcortical US) and direct insonation of tumor cavity by specialized probes (trans mural US) can circumvent interface artifacts.

Another problem is interface artifact at the bottom/walls of the resection cavity. This is exactly where the IOUS is most critically required during glioma surgery. This artifact results from the difference in the acoustic properties of the fluid (generally normal saline) and the underlying brain. This can be minimized by insonating before application of hemostatic materials. Other solutions include transmural ultrasonography (probe is applied directly on the walls of the resection cavity) or a trans cortical ultrasound if sufficient cortex is available adjoining the resection cavity (that is why a large craniotomy is preferable) [24]. These methods are shown in Figure 2. New technology like acoustic coupling fluid, designed by a leading Norwegian group, offers a future solution [25]. Other practical solutions include comparison of the area compared to an earlier scan during the surgery, continuing resection of neuromonitoring parameters allow.

Intraoperative Neurophysiological Monitoring during Glioma Surgery

While intraoperative image guidance guides the surgeon as to what to resect, intraoperative patient monitoring acts as a checkpoint, indicating when to stop the surgery. These are a set of techniques where functionality of the tumor involved brain area and the neighborhood are determined intraoperatively to decide the "limit of tumor resection." Two important aspects of intraoperative patient monitoring include:

1. Awake patient monitoring where both clinical and electro-physiological monitoring can be performed.
2. Intraoperative electrophysiological monitoring under general anesthesia. Here, for obvious reasons, dynamic clinical patient monitoring is not performed, and language function monitoring cannot be performed.

In this section, we focus on intraoperative electrophysiological monitoring for functional preservation during supratentorial glioma surgery. We do not discuss about awake craniotomy per se but touch upon the differences in intraoperative monitoring between surgeries done in awake versus under general anesthesia.

The functions which a neurosurgeon aims to preserve during a supratentorial glioma surgery depends on the site of the lesions and the status of preoperative level of the function. The functions of interest under usual circumstances are:

1. Motor and sensory functions
2. Language functions

Cognitive functions and their preservation are equally important but not performed routinely in all centers. The common monitoring techniques employed for supratentorial glioma surgery include:

- Intraoperative eletroencephalography (EEG) and electrocorticography (ECOG).
- Somatosensory Evoked Potential (SSEP)/Motor Evoked Potential (MEP) monitoring.
- Direct electrical stimulation (DES).

A metanalysis conducted by De Witt et al. demonstrated late severe neurological deficit in 3.4% patient who underwent resection under neurophysiologic monitoring and 8.2% of the patient who underwent glioma resection without neuromonitoring. Radiologically confirmed GTR was 75% in monitoring group and 58% in non-monitoring group [26]. Brown et al. reviewed 8 studied comparing surgery under GA and awake craniotomy and found that EOR was similar in both the groups however incidence of post-operative deficits was less in awake craniotomy group as compared with patient who underwent surgery under GA [27].

Intraoperative EEG and ECOG, Methods and Its Role in Glioma Surgery

Intraoperative electroencephalography (EEG) is performed to localize the eloquent areas of the brain concerned with the executive function. It is also employed for localization and excision of the cortical areas having irritative activities responsible for seizure in LGG [28]. Intraoperatively cortical activities are recorded directly from the brain surface and is called ECOG.

Subsequently, electrical stimulation is given, and stimulation triggered seizure activity is determined relative to the site of stimulation. Intraoperatively with the help of Ecog we can determine whether these epileptogenic zones have completely been excised or not. With the help of

Ecog, we can also identify the cortical areas with larger amount of lesion to preserve the eloquent cortical areas with executive function with fewer lesions. Another use of Ecog is to detect after discharges following direct cortical stimulation [28].

Role of SSEP and MEP

Motor evoked potential MEP is used to detect integrity of motor pathway, SSEP is used for sensory pathway integrity, localization of Rolandic cortex and identification of central sulcus by phase reversal method under GA.

SSEP is the electrophysiological response of the nervous system to sensory stimulus. Thus, SSEP denotes the integrity of somatosensory pathway. Accurate localization of central sulcus may be difficult intraoperatively due to various reasons including distortion of brain by the tumor or brain shift. SSEP is a valuable tool to accurately localize the central sulcus intraoperatively by phase reversal method.

Median nerve on the contralateral side is stimulated as described earlier and is recorded from grid or strip electrode placed along the Rolandic fissure. The thalamocortical potential recorded from the postcentral gyrus have the characteristic of N19 and P22. Electrodes in precentral sulcus has the inverse polarity and has the latency of about 19ms post stimulus as compared with post central sulcus electrodes. This characteristic is employed to accurately localize the central sulcus during tumor resection around the eloquent areas. As depicted in picture below (Figure 3), strip electrodes are used to identify the central sulcus intraoperatively.

SSEP is also used for determining ischemia to the cerebral cortex [29]. The criterion for significant intraoperative SSEP change is an amplitude reduction of >50% or 10% increase in the latency as compared with the baseline. Hypothermia, hypoxia, and hypotension can result in global SSEP change bilaterally whereas unilateral significant SSEP change warns about possible mechanical compression, neurologic injury or ischemia and appropriate measures must be taken at that point to mitigate the risk of irreversible neurologic injury. It is also used in sensory function monitoring if required.

Motor evoked potential is continuous neurophysiologic monitoring technique performed by stimulation of the motor cortex using pairs of grid electrodes after motor cortex and its relation with the tumor is identified. MEP can also be recorded by transcranial stimulation of the motor cortex either by magnetic or electrical stimulation (Figure 4). MEP waves are most sensitive to anesthetic agent due to its effect on anterior horn cells in spinal cord.

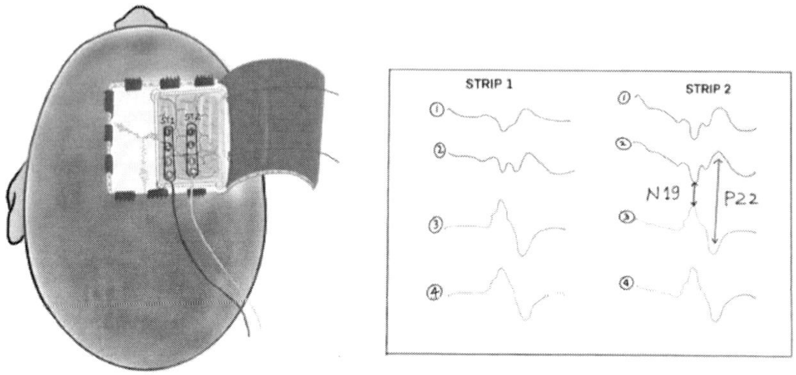

Figure 3. Schematic diagram depicting the strip electrode placement across the central sulcus. 1 and 2 in primary motor cortex (In blue) and 3, 4 in somatosensory cortex (in red). N19 and P21 wave with phase reversal between electrode 2 and 3.

Technique

Electrodes: For TcMEP 2 types of electrodes are used. Corkscrew electrode for stimulation and needle electrode for recording the compound muscle action potential cMAP. Electrodes are placed at C1/C2, C3/C4 of the 10-10 system and needle electrodes are placed in the desired muscle group on the opposite side. A baseline recording before the start of surgery is taken. High intensity multipulse 3-7 stimulus at 2-4ms interval is given and MEP is recorded. Stimulation is given continuously at some interval to assess the integrity of CST.

Parameters

Change in MEP as compared with baseline recording can be due to mechanical, thermal, or ischemic injury. Criteria for neurologic injury is >50% reduction of amplitude or >10% increase in latency. Where reversible decline of >50% denotes temporary motor deficits and irreversible MEP decline denotes the permanent motor deficits [28].

Fallacies of MEP

MEP is a reliable tool to determine the integrity of corticospinal tract during supratentorial glioma surgery, although false negative results where there was long lasting paresis despite of transient and reversible MEP changes, have been described in the literature [30]. There are also some instances, where postoperative power deteriorated without intact MEP during surgery. False negative results were studied by Neuloh G et al. may be correlated with postoperative edema, hemorrhage and tumor resected from SMA (supplementary motor area) [31]. Also, inadvertent high cortical stimulation current >30 mA can stimulate subcortical CST which has already been damaged. Planter flexor weakness can develop even if anterior tibial muscle group MEP is completely intact [32]. New paresis can also develop in muscle group which are not included in the monitoring during surgery. MEP recordings and interpretation is affected by several other factors which includes use of muscle relaxants, hypothermia, nerve compression during surgery.

MEP in Awake Surgery vs Surgery under GA

Under GA motor function is monitored through EMG recordings from the contralateral limb whereas in awake craniotomy patient is evaluated clinically and asked to perform a simple or complex task or asked to give indication if there is muscle contraction while eliciting the positive response. Cortical stimulation during awake craniotomy also let surgeon determine the safe area for corticectomy. *Paola* et al. conducted a systematic review and metanalysis comparing the EOR and postoperative morbidity and mortality between awake craniotomy and general anesthesia. They included 17 studies from 1983 to 2019 consisting of total 2351 glioma patients. According to this study mean percent of EOR for awake surgery and patient under GA was 90.1% and 81.7% respectively [33]. Although it was not statistically significant, there was a trend for achieving greater EOR during awake surgery. As we know, MEP is affected by several factors and value can decrease as compared with base line even if there is no neurologic injury and pose a risk of subtotal resection. Under awake craniotomy even if the MEP is decreased or absent, one can confirm voluntary movements and avoid under-resection.

Direct Electrical Stimulation

Direct cortical and subcortical stimulation is another neurophysiologic tool which can be employed for motor and language mapping during glioma surgery. Direct stimulation can be given either by monopolar or bipolar stimulating electrodes. For monopolar electrical stimulation, cathodic electrode is placed at the margin of resection cavity and reference electrode at the shoulder or forehead. In bipolar stimulation both cathodic and reference electrodes are adjacent 5 mm apart and are in direct contact of the brain. Therefore, current generated by monopolar electrode is more diffuse as compared with bipolar electrode in which the current is localized which is beneficial in patient with history of seizures.

Language Mapping

When tumor is located around the language area (e.g., insular glioma on the left side) and language preservation is the goal, neurophysiologic monitoring is performed during awake surgery by a trained neurophysiologist. A series of task which includes counting, naming, reading, repetition and semantic task is performed during the surgery. Also, direct cortical stimulation is done maximum for 4s by 1mm bipolar electrode positioned 5mm apart which delivers biphasic trains of 50Hz during the task. Initially low stimulus current with 1.5 mA square wave pulse is used and gradually increased up-to 6mA. Cortex is mapped every 5-10mm.

Task

Counting

First, the patient is asked to count from 1-30 and stimulus is given near tentative language areas and site of speech arrest is marked. Stimulation is then performed in a systematic manner every 8-10 mm along the cerebral cortex. Transient slurring of speech or speech arrest during stimulation signifies that language area is stimulated which is then marked and preserved during the surgery.

Naming/Reading

Location of language areas are reconfirmed by asking the patient to name the familiar objects shown through the pictures. Patient is also asked to read the simple and complex sentences. Tumor resection is started preserving those cortical areas which was marked earlier subserving the language function. This task is repeated during the surgery to confirm the functional integrity of language area throughout the procedure. Subcortical stimulation is done in the tumor cavity and resection is stopped when there is speech arrest or patient had difficulty in naming the pictured object [29].

Language mapping requires adequate cognitive function and emotional maturity. For patient to co-operate during surgery, he is counselled many times and every task performed during the surgery is explained and performed beforehand 1 day prior to the surgery.

Motor Mapping

Besides SSEP, direct cortical stimulation can be used to identify the primary motor cortex by using monopolar, bipolar, or subdural strip or grid electrodes.

Activation pathway is like that of MEP but in direct cortical mapping, relatively smaller cortical area is stimulated leading to focal activation of somatotopic axons. It can be utilized for both awake surgery as well as under general anesthesia. Generally, for awake surgeries, the requirement of current is lesser. The advantage of awake motor mapping is the ability to do map the inhibitory areas. For this purpose, certain activities like screw driving movement may be given to the patient. During electrical stimulation, if this complex activity gets halted then the excited area represents a supportive motor network and hence need to be preserved [34].

Technique

Under GA 2 stimulation technique can be used, Bipolar cortex stimulation (Penfield technique) and multiple train technique (Teniguchi method).

Multipulse Train Technique (Teniguchi Method)

Stimulation is performed using 4-6 pulse trains monophasic pulse 200-500 ms in duration with 2-4 ms interval are delivered via handheld probe or subdural grid. MEP is then assessed via subdermal needles placed 2 cm apart on contralateral muscle. Depending upon the tumor location following muscle can be employed for recording MEPs.

Bipolar Cortex Stimulation Technique (Penfield Method)

Here bipolar rectangular pulse with .5-1 ms duration are delivered via handheld probe or via subdural grid to the exposed cortex at 50-60 HZ for 1-4 s. To start with 3-5 mA current is used and increased by 0.5-2 mA to elicit threshold intensity. Generally, threshold amplitude for eliciting motor response is <10 mA [34, 35].

Cortical Stimulation

DCS is performed after central sulcus localization. Precentral sulcus with largest N25 peak is used as an ideal starting point for DCS. With the help of any of these methods cMAP can be recorded in facial, upper, and lower limb muscle groups, i.e., Orbicularis oculi, Orbicularis oris, deltoid, brachialis, biceps, Extensor digitorum, Abductor pollicis brevis (APB), Abductor digiti minimi, quadriceps, tibialis anterior and abductor hallucis. After localization of motor function, grid or strip electrodes are placed to stimulate and evoke CMAP response to ascertain functional integrity of CST. Under GA motor mapping can only be done for muscle group that are monitored with EMG or is visible, whereas in awake surgery feedback about entire muscle group can be obtained. It is always desirable to use threshold or near threshold stimulus to avoid activation of adjacent area. Study by Kombos et al. shown that when DCS is used as a monitoring tool, patient with significant signal deterioration or increased threshold had motor deficit 3-month postoperatively [36, 37].

Subcortical Stimulation

Subcortical stimulation during glioma surgery helps distinguish the corticospinal tract from the tumor tissue. Identification of motor pathway in white matter is assessed by stimulation intensity which is proportional to the distance between the corticospinal tract and the electrode [30]. Subcortical mapping is done like the direct cortical stimulation. Initially we use 15mA current and start resecting the tumor tissue. When cMAP is recoded via contralateral target muscle group with 15mA current, it means corticospinal tract is 15mm away from the stimulating electrode. Then we use 10 mA current and gradually decrease the current to 5mA. Further resection of tumor is avoided when corticospinal tract is stimulated and cMAP is recorded with

5mA current. Thus, it is an important tool in maximal safe resection of tumor without causing any neurological injury to the patient. There is associated risk of seizure during the cortical mapping which can be controlled with ice cold saline or Ringer lactate quickly applied to the cortical surface.

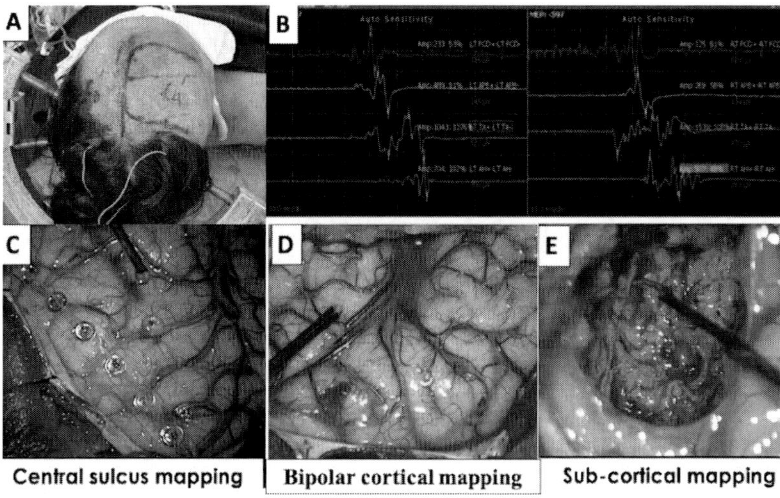

Figure 4. Shows the intraoperative monitoring and mapping techniques. Transcranial MEP (TcMEP) is obtained with corkscrew electrodes applied on the scalp over the anticipated location of the motor strip. Contralateral side stimulation acts as a control (A). Needle electrodes placed in various muscle groups of the upper, lower limbs as well as face allows compound muscle action potentials (cMAP, B) to be recorded on the screen for determining changes from the base line (loss, reduction of amplitude and increase in latency etc.). Strip electrodes placed across the anticipated location of the central sulcus to determine its exact location using cortical SSEP reversal (C). Cortical stimulation mapping for language/motor cortex is performed with bipolar stimulation, which provides focused current to determine accurately the patients functional map (D). Sub cortical stimulation (E) is being performed to determine the location of the corticospinal tract using the mA-mm rule (1 mA current activation = 1mm distance to target).

Figure 4 shows cortical and sub cortical stimulation in case of supratentorial gliomas.

Monopolar vs Bipolar Stimulation

As described earlier, current spread from monopolar and bipolar electrodes are distinct. In bipolar electrodes, current flows from one arm to another with a very limited current of spread to the surrounding structure and thus activates those tissue only which comes in between the two arms of the electrode. It is used for cortical mapping to identify the functional areas which need to be preserved and nonfunctional zone which can be utilized for safe corridor for glioma resection. In monopolar electrode, current flow is diffuse and discharges rapidly towards the reference electrodes. This spread allows surgeon to modulate the intensity of stimulating current to roughly localize the distance of CST from the margin of resection cavity. Szelényi et al. compared the monopolar and bipolar subcortical stimulation in 20 patients and revealed that stimulation was positive in 92% of cases with monopolar electrodes and only 54% while bipolar electrode was used for subcortical stimulation [38]. Similarly in a study by *Andrew j* et al. stimulation with monopolar probe was positive in 86.4% of case and with bipolar probe in only 30% cases [39].

Correlation between Distance and mA in Monopolar Stimulation

Identification of motor pathway in white matter is assessed by stimulation intensity which is proportional to the distance between the corticospinal tract and the electrode [5]. Previous study by several groups demonstrated that the current required to stimulate the CST mA roughly equals the distance from the CST in millimeter [30, 40]. Initially we use 15mA current and start resecting the tumor tissue. When cMAP is recoded via contralateral target muscle group with 15mA current, it means corticospinal tract is 15mm away from the stimulating electrode. Then we use 10 mA current and gradually decrease the current to 5mA. Further resection of tumor is avoided when corticospinal tract is stimulated and cMAP is recorded with 5mA current. Thus, it is an important tool in maximal safe resection of tumor without causing any neurological injury to the patient.

Combined Use of MEP and Motor Mapping

Fallacy of cortical and subcortical motor mapping is that it is practically cumbersome to ascertain the integrity of CST by continuous cortical or subcortical mapping during tumor resection. Monopolar or bipolar probe can only be use intermittently during surgical resection, and there is chance of neuronal damage when stimulation is not on. Advantage of MEP, either TcMEP or dcMEP, is that it can be used continuously during the surgical resection especially while resecting the tumor close to the motor pathway. Therefore, combining these two methods together is beneficial and reduces the risk of neuronal damage during surgery [41]. However, monopolar probe, attached to the suction device has provided an opportunity to perform stimulation mapping continuously.

Conclusion

Surgery for glioma has redefined itself. With mounting evidence clamoring for extensive resections in gliomas, it has put the surgeon in the limelight and pretty much in the driving seat in glioma management. A combination of image guidance and intraoperative monitoring has become a standard for modern day glioma surgery to strike an optimal onco-functional balance. Neurosurgeons embarking on glioma resection must quickly adapt to these technologies.

References

[1] Li YM, Suki D, Hess K, Sawaya R. The influence of maximum safe resection of glioblastoma on survival in 1229 patients: Can we do better than gross-total resection? *J Neurosurg*. 2016 Apr;124(4):977-88.

[2] Omuro A, DeAngelis LM. Glioblastoma and Other Malignant Gliomas: A Clinical Review. *JAMA*. 2013;310(17):1842–1850. doi:10.1001/jama.2013.280319.

[3] Raymond Liu, Margaretta Page, Karla Solheim, Sherry Fox, Susan M. Chang, Quality of life in adults with brain tumors: Current knowledge and future directions, *Neuro-Oncology*, June 2009;Volume 11, Issue 3, Pages 330–339, https://doi.org/10.1215/15228517-2008-093.

[4] Nader Sanai, M.D., Mitchel S. Berger, M.D., Glioma extent of resection and its impact on patient outcome, *Neurosurgery*, April 2008; Volume 62, Issue 4, Pages 753–766, https://doi.org/10.1227/01.neu.0000318159.21731.cf.

[5] Ius, T., Mazzucchi, E., Tomasino, B. et al. Multimodal integrated approaches in low grade glioma surgery. 2021; *Sci Rep* 11, 9964 https://doi.org/10.1038/s41598-021-87924-2.

[6] Friedrich K. Albert, M. D., Michael Forsting, M. D., Klaus Sartor, M. D., Hans-Peter Adams, D. I. M., Stefan Kunze, M. D., Early Postoperative Magnetic Resonance Imaging after Resection of Malignant Glioma: Objective Evaluation of Residual Tumor and Its Influence on Regrowth and Prognosis, *Neurosurgery*, January 1994;Volume 34, Issue 1, Pages 45–61, https://doi.org/10.1097/00006123-199401000-00008.

[7] Sébastien Boissonneau & Hugues Duffau. Identifying clinical risk in low grade gliomas and appropriate treatment strategies, with special emphasis on the role of surgery, *Expert Review of Anticancer Therapy*, 2017; 17:8, 703-716, doi: 10.1080/ 14737140.2017.1342537.

[8] Orringer, Daniel et al. "Extent of Resection in Patients with Glioblastoma: Limiting Factors, Perception of Resectability, and Effect on Survival." *Journal of neurosurgery*. 2012; 117.5 : 851–859.

[9] Moiyadi, A. V., Shetty, P. M., Mahajan, A. et al. Usefulness of three-dimensional navigable intraoperative ultrasound in resection of brain tumors with a special emphasis on malignant gliomas. *Acta Neurochir. 2017;* 155, 2217–2225.

[10] Fukuya, Y., Ikuta, S., Maruyama, T. et al. Tumor recurrence patterns after surgical resection of intracranial low-grade gliomas. *J Neurooncol. 2019;* 144, 519–528. https://doi.org/10.1007/s11060-019-03250-8.

[11] Chen D, Nauen DW, Park HC, Li D, Yuan W, Li A, Guan H, Kut C, Chaichana KL, Bettegowda C, Quiñones-Hinojosa A, Li X. Label-free imaging of human brain tissue at subcellular resolution for potential rapid intra-operative assessment of glioma surgery. *Theranostics*. 2021 May 24;11(15):7222-7234. doi: 10.7150/ thno.59244. PMID: 34158846; PMCID: PMC8210590.

[12] Riva, M., Sciortino, T., Secoli, R., D'Amico, E., Moccia, S., Fernandes, B., Conti Nibali, M., Gay, L., Rossi, M., De Momi, E., Bello, L. Glioma *biopsies* Classification Using Raman Spectroscopy and Machine Learning Models on Fresh Tissue Samples. *Cancers* 2021, *13*, 1073.

[13] Unsgård G., Solheim O., Lindseth F., Selbekk T. Intra-operative Imaging with 3D Ultrasound in Neurosurgery. In: Pamir M., Seifert V., Kiris T. (eds) Intraoperative Imaging. *Acta Neurochirurgica Supplementum*, 2011; vol 109. Springer, Vienna. https://doi.org/10.1007/978-3-211-99651-5_28.

[14] Wood RW, Loomis AL. The physical and biological effects of high frequency sound waves of great intensity. *Philos Mag Ser* 7 1927; 4 (22) 417-436.

[15] Dussik KT. On the possibility of using ultrasound waves as a diagnostic. *Aid Neurol Psychiatr*. 1942;174:153–68.

[16] Rantanen, N. and Ewing, R., III, Principles of ultrasound application in animals. *Veterinary Radiology*.1981; 22: 196-203.

[17] Yeole U, Singh V, Mishra A, Shaikh S, Shetty P, Moiyadi A. Navigated intraoperative ultrasonography for brain tumors: a pictorial essay on the technique, its utility, and its benefits in neuro-oncology. *Ultrasonography*. 2020 Oct;39(4):394-406.

[18] Hammoud MA, Ligon BL, elSouki R, et al: Use of intraoperative ultrasound for localizing tumors and determining the extent of resection: a comparative study with magnetic resonance imaging. *J Neurosurg*. 1996; 84:737–741.

[19] Munkvold BKR, Jakola AS, Reinertsen I, Sagberg LM, Unsgård G, Solheim O. The diagnostic properties of intraoperative ultra- sound in glioma surgery and factors associated with gross total tumor resection. *World Neurosurg*.2018; 115:e129–e136. https://doi.org/10.1016/j.wneu.2018.03.208.

[20] Trevisi, G., Barbone, P., Treglia, G. et al. Reliability of intraoperative ultrasound in detecting tumor residual after brain diffuse glioma surgery: a systematic review and meta-analysis. *Neurosurg Re.* 2020; *v* 43, 1221–1233.

[21] Tronnier VM, Bonsanto MM, Staubert A, et al. Comparison of intraoperative MR imaging and 3D-navigated ultrasonography in the detection and resection control of lesions. *Neurosurg Focus*. 2001; 10 (2):Article 3.

[22] ChengLG, HeW, ZhangHX, SongQ, NingB, LiHZ, HeY, LinS. Intraoperative contrast enhanced ultrasound evaluates the grade of glioma. *Biomed Res Int*. 2016; 2016:2643862.

[23] Cepeda S, Barrena C, Arrese I, Fernandez-Pérez G, Sarabia R, Intraoperative ultrasound elastography: a semi-quantitative analysis of brain tumour elasticity patterns and peritumoral regions., *World Neurosurgery*. 2019; doi: https://doi. org/ 10.1016/j.wneu.2019.11.133.

[24] Altieri R, Melcarne A, Di Perna G, Specchia FMC, Fronda C, La Rocca G, Cofano F, Sabatino G, Pepa GMD, Olivi A, Ducati A, Garbossa D. Intra-operative ultrasound: tips and tricks for making the most in neurosurgery. *Surg Technol* Int.2018; 33:353–360.

[25] Unsgård, G., Sagberg, L. M., Müller, S. et al. A new acoustic coupling fluid with ability to reduce ultrasound imaging artefacts in brain tumour surgery—a phase I study. *Acta Neurochir.*2019; 161, 1475–1486.

[26] De witt Hamer PC, Robles SG, Zwinderman AH, Duffau H, BergerMS: Impact of intraoperative stimulation brain mapping on glioma surgery outcome: a meta-analysis. *J Clin Oncol*. 2012; 30: 2559-2565.

[27] Brown T, Shah AH, Bregy A, Shah NH, Thambuswamy M, Barbarite E, Fuhrman T, Komotar RJ: Awake craniotomy for brain tumor resection: the rule rather than the exception? *J Neurosurg*. 2013; *Anesthesiol* 25:240-247.

[28] Vega-Zelaya L and Pastor J. Intraoperative Neurophysiological Monitoring Techniques for the Resection of Malignant Brain Tumors Located in Eloquent Cortical Areas. *Austin Neurosurg Open Access*. 2015; 2(4): 1038.

[29] Muzkya, I M., B Estephan, Somatosensory evoked potentials, Handbook of Clinical Neurology, Vol. 160 (3rd series) *Clinical Neurophysiology: Basis and Technical Aspects Ch* 35, 523-540.

[30] Kamada K et al. The motor-evoked potential threshold evaluated by tractography and electrical stimulation *J. Neurosurg.*2009; 111 785–95.

[31] Neuloh G, Pechstein U, Cedzich C et al. Motor evoked potential monitoring with supratentorial surgery. *Neurosurgery* 2004; 54: 1061–1070 discussion 1070-1062.

[32] Neuloh G, Schramm J. Are there false-negative results of motor evoked potential monitoring in brain surgery? *Cent Eur Neurosurg*. 2009 Nov;70(4):171-5.

[33] Paola S, Lina M, Calder P, Ricardo M, Alea M et al. Awake vs. asleep motor mapping for glioma resection: a systematic review and meta-analysis. *Acta Neurochirurgica*. 2020;162. 10.1007/s00701-020-04357-y.

[34] Berger MS, Kincaid J, Ojemann GA, et al. Brain mapping techniques to maximize resection, safety, and seizure control in children with brain tumors. *Neurosurgery*. 1989;25:786–92.

[35] Woolsey CN, Erickson TC, Gilson WE. Localization in somatic sensory and motor areas of human cerebral cortex as determined by direct recording of evoked potentials and electrical stimulation. *J Neurosurg*. 1979;51:476–506.

[36] Kombos T, Suess O, Ciklatekerlio O, Brock M. Monitoring of intraoperative motor evoked potentials to increase the safety of surgery in and around the motor cortex. *J Neurosurg*. 2001; 95:608–14.

[37] Seidel K, Beck J, Steiglitz L, Schucht P, Raabe A. The warning-sign hierarchy between quantitative subcortical motor mapping and continuous motor evoked potential monitoring during resection of supratentorial brain tumor: clinical article. *J Neurosurg*. 2013;118:287. (or 284)–296.

[38] Szelényi A, Senft C, Jardan M, et al. Intra-operative subcorti- cal electrical stimulation: a comparison of two methods. *Clin Neurophysiol*. 2011;122(7):1470–1475.

[39] Andrew J, Jacob S, Ramin A, Lauro N, Roger S. Javier E. Shawn L, Mitchel S. Triple motor mapping: transcranial, bipolar, and monopolar mapping for supratentorial glioma resection adjacent to motor pathways. *J Neurosurg*. 2021;134:1728–1737.

[40] Ohue S, Kohno S, Inoue A, et al. Accuracy of diffusion ten- sor magnetic resonance imaging-based tractography for sur- gery of gliomas near the pyramidal tract: a significant corre- lation between subcortical electrical stimulation and postoperative tractography. *Neurosurgery*. 2012;70(2):283–294.

[41] Moiyadi A, Velayutham P, Shetty P, Seidel K, Janu A, Madhugiri V, Singh VK, Patil A, John R. Combined Motor Evoked Potential Monitoring and Subcortical Dynamic Mapping in Motor Eloquent Tumors Allows Safer and Extended Resections. *World Neurosurg*. 2018 Dec;120:e259-e268.

Chapter 13

Brain and Spinal Tumors during Pregnancy

Ashutosh Kumar[1], Indubala Maurya[2], Balachandar Deivasigamani[1], Ved Prakash Maurya[1] and Jayesh Sardhara[1]

[1]Department of Neurosurgery, Sanjay Gandhi Postgraduate Institute of Medical Sciences, Lucknow, India

[2]Department of Anesthesiology, Kalyan Singh Super Speciality Cancer Institute, Uttar Pradesh, India

Abstract

Tumors of the central nervous system (CNS) diagnosed during pregnancy require a special set of care which includes diagnosis as well as treatment of these neuraxial lesions with proper care of fetus in utero. These modalities include unique imaging, obstetrical, neurosurgical as well as anaesthetic considerations, once this population of patients are diagnosed to have spinal or brain tumor. The mere diagnosis of pregnancy affects each and every aspect of management for these patients. The timing of surgery and the adjuvant therapy as well as their delivery get influenced by symptomatology of the neurological pathology and gestational age which affects their overall prognosis. There are factors which adversely affects the tumor growth which include hormone- mediated growth and a number of hemodynamic changes. Although there are limited studies which discuss the presence of brain tumors during pregnancy, no significant increase in incidence of these tumors is noticed during pregnancy as compared to the non-pregnant populations. The presence of headache, nausea, and vomiting which reflect the features of raised intracranial pressure are easily confused with pregnancy and pregnancy-related symptoms presenting an entirely different challenge to the treating physicians as well as the neurosurgeons. In this chapter, we intend to briefly discuss the CNS

In: Advances in Neurosurgery Research
Editors: Amit Agrawal, Pradeep Chouksey, Adesh Shrivastava et al.
ISBN: 978-1-68507-859-1

tumors which are encountered commonly during pregnancy as well as the anaesthetic implications specific in their management.

Introduction

The addition of ante-natal status to the clinical scenario of a patient with a brain tumor significantly affects the treatment protocols. From diagnostics to decision making and adjuvant therapy, every aspect of patient care needs individual customization, taking care of both the mother and fetus. Intervention-related complications due to drastic physiological changes in the mother, and those associated with fetal development are the key concerns in managing brain tumors during pregnancy. Due to limited data regarding the management of this cohort of patients, there exists a significant diagnostic and therapeutic challenge.

Common Brain Tumors during Pregnancy

Primary intracranial tumors rank fifth in the list of neoplasm-associated death in patients of the childbearing age group (20-39 years) (Dolecek et al. 2012). There is no specific tumor reported to have significantly more incidence during pregnancy as compared to the general population (Lambe, Coogan, and Baron 1997; J. F. Haas 1984; J. Haas, Jänisch, and Staneczek 1986). All types of tumors have been reported in ante-natal mothers. However, few common tumors diagnosed during pregnancy include pituitary adenoma, meningioma, and glial tumors, with their incidence not affected by the ante-natal status.

Clinical Presentation

Most of the tumors present with their characteristic clinical features similar to the general population. However, the hormonal and hemodynamic changes associated with pregnancy may sometimes affect the clinical course of these tumors. Normally, under the influence of elevated levels of estrogen, the pituitary gland increases in size by up to 45% due to an increase in the size and the number of lactotrophs (Friesen, Fournier, and Desjardins 1973; Scheithauer et al. 1990; Ylikorkala, Kivinen, and Reinilä 1979). Pituitary adenoma has been also reported to grow more rapidly during pregnancy, more so in the case of a macro than microadenomas (Wallach, Gemzell, and Wang 1979). Clinical features include symptoms and signs of local compression (optic apparatus, cavernous sinus) or endocrinological disturbance (hypo or hyperfunctioning adenomas). Incidence of pituitary apoplexy during pregnancy is rare (Grand'Maison et al. 2015). Few cases of pregnancy-associated aggravation of acromegalic features have been reported (Herman-Bonert, Seliverstov, and Melmed 1998).

Glial tumors also present with their usual symptoms including focal neurological deficits, seizures, or raised intracranial pressure (ICP). During pregnancy, there is a higher risk of clinical deterioration due to raised ICP because of the increased tendency for fluid retention leading to significant perilesional cerebral edema (Roelvink et al. 1987). The role of hormonal changes in accelerating tumor growth has not been validated yet. There is definite evidence of progression and relapse of meningiomas during pregnancy (Bickerstaff, Small, and Guest 1958; Hortobágyi et al. 2017). Though the overall risk for incidence of meningioma remains the same as the general population (Lambe, Coogan, and Baron 1997). Most of the meningiomas during pregnancy are diagnosed during the second or third trimesters (Roelvink et al. 1987; Kanaan, Jallu, and Kanaan 2003). Such incidences have been explained by the presence of progesterone receptors on the tumor, reversible hemodynamic changes associated with pregnancy, and prolactin modulated pathogenesis (Laviv, Ohla, and Kasper 2018). The location of meningiomas during pregnancy is similar to the general population, with similar clinical presentations.

Investigations

Radiological investigations are an important part of work up following clinical suspicion or after an incidental diagnosis of intracranial pathology. Computed tomography (CT) imaging and magnetic resonance imaging (MRI) are the most common investigations in evaluating these tumors. The radiation dose received by the fetus in the CT scan was reported to be less than 0.005 mGy, lesser than the maximum permissible dose of 0.5 mSv. Thus, the cranial CT of a mother poses a little risk for the fetus. Iodinated contrast agents are most commonly used with CT scans. There is a lack of evidence regarding their safety, and are recommended to be used only if essential.

MRI is considered safe during the second and third trimesters (Patenaude et al. 2014). Fetal abnormalities have been reported in only animal studies with the use of MRI in early pregnancy. However, its benefit in providing definitive diagnosis during early pregnancy outweighs the little risk, while repeat MRI scans during the first trimester should be avoided. Similarly, the use of gadolinium, as a contrast agent in MRI, should be restricted unless essential, given relative lack of safety evidence in humans. Despite the growing evidence suggesting the relative safety of these radiological investigations, most authors recommended that they should be avoided unless necessary. Due consideration should be given for ante-natal status while evaluating biochemical and endocrinological parameters because of significant physiological changes. This is more important while evaluating patients with pituitary adenoma. For example, it is difficult to diagnose acromegaly in pregnant women due to the presence of placental growth hormone (GH) and insulin-like growth factor-1 (IGF-1) along with maternal GH (Kasuki et al. 2012). Also in Cushing syndrome, a low-dose dexamethasone test is not recommended due to a high false positivity rate (Nieman et al. 2008).

Decision Making

The intervention in brain tumors associated with pregnancy is dependent on multiple factors like possible pathology based on radiological differential diagnosis, gestational age, clinical severity, patient choice, and availability of safe medical management options. Multiple studies have been reviewed retrospectively and their findings are summarized in Figure 1-3 as management algorithms (Peeters et al. 2018; Araujo, Neto, and Gadelha 2015; Laviv et al. 2018).

Most authors recommended medical therapy as the first option if it was available and not contraindicated in pregnancy. In case of stable disease, irrespective of the possible pathology and gestational age, it is recommended to continue pregnancy till fetal maturity is achieved, and do tumor resection post-partum (Laviv et al. 2018; Cohen-Gadol et al. 2009).

Nevertheless, surgery should not be denied in case of severe or rapidly progressive neurological symptoms, regardless of the gestational age. A decision to abort can be taken till the early second trimester in case of an advancing brain tumor or if symptoms are severe. In case the pregnancy cannot be continued till term, the second trimester is considered relatively safer for semi-urgent intervention for brain tumors due to fewer chances of preterm contractions and spontaneous abortions ('ACOG Committee Opinion No. 474: Nonobstetric Surgery during Pregnancy' 2011).

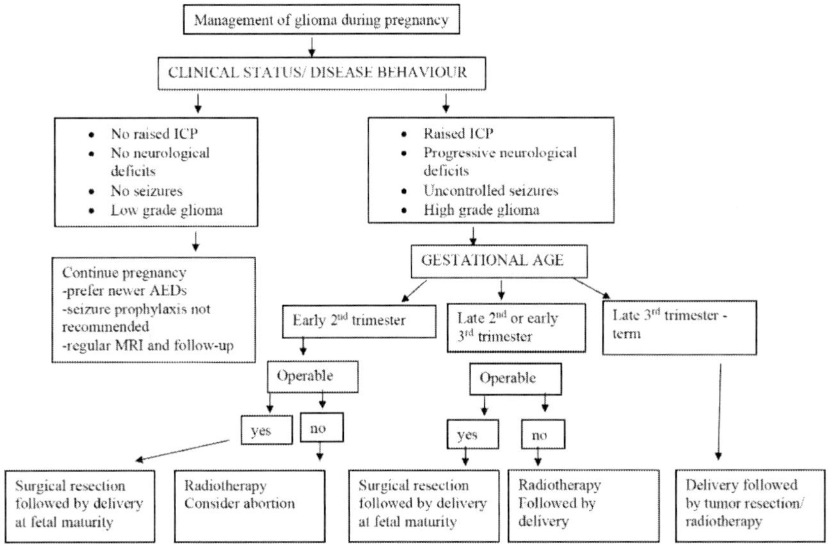

Figure 1. Algorithm for management of glioma during pregnancy (ICP-intracranial pressure, AED-anti epileptic drug) (Peeters et al. 2018).

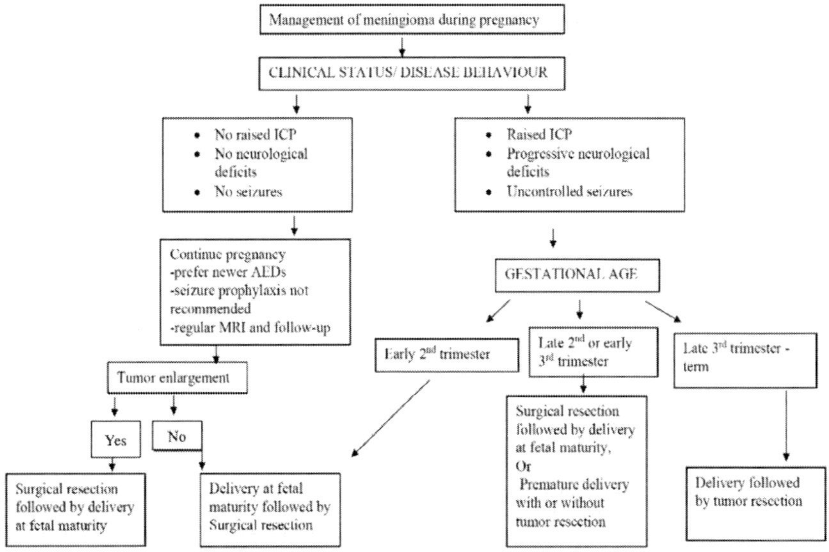

Figure 2. Algorithm for management of meningioma during pregnancy (ICP-intracranial pressure, AED-anti epileptic drug) (Laviv et al. 2018).

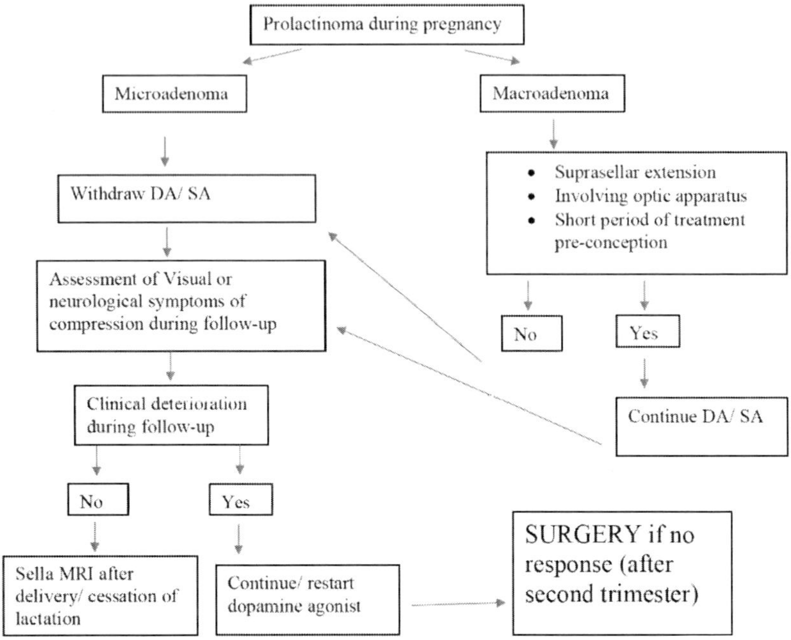

Figure 3. Algorithm for management of prolactinoma (DA-dopamine agonist) and acromegaly (DA-dopamine agonist/ SA-somatostatin analogue) during pregnancy (Araujo, Neto, and Gadelha 2015).

The Anaesthetic Implication of Neurosurgery during Pregnancy

The anaesthetic management needs to be individualized for pregnant patients undergoing neurosurgery while considering gestational age and need for surgery (Emergency vs. Elective). The general principles of neurosurgery and obstetric anaesthesia must be followed during planning and decision-making (Abd-Elsayed et al. 2013; Rodrigues et al. 2021).

Clinical Aspects of Pregnancy-Related Physiological Changes

Various pregnancy-related physiological changes such as high metabolic demand, mechanical effects of the gravid uterus, hemodynamic changes, etc. affect perioperative management and outcome (Kacmar and Gaiser 2019).

These physiological changes have an impact on anaesthesia care as shown in Table 1.

Table 1. Trimester wise physiological changes during pregnancy and its Implications

Physiological Changes	Implication
1st Trimester • Increased oxygen consumption • Respiratory alkalosis • Increased airway mucosal vascularity • Physiological anemia and increased blood volume • Decreased anaesthesia requirement	• Increased chance of hypoxia • Avoid hyperventilation • High incidence of difficult airway • Important for estimation of blood loss and replacement. • Dose titration
2nd and 3rd Trimester • Increased oxygen consumption & decreased Functional residual capacity • Respiratory alkalosis • Increased airway mucosal vascularity and edema • Decreased tone of lower esophageal sphincter, Increased intra gastric pressure • Aortocaval compression • Decreased anaesthesia requirement • Physiological anemia and increased blood volume • Hypercoagulable state	• Increased chance of hypoxia • Avoid hyperventilation • High incidence of difficult airway • Increased chance of aspiration, Consider aspiration prophylaxis • Chance of supine hypotension syndrome, consider left uterine displacement. • Dose titration • Important for estimation of blood loss and replacement. • Risk of thromboembolism, Consider early mobilization

Fetal Consideration

Perioperative Medication and Its Teratogenicity

There is no evidence of teratogenicity due to anesthetic agents if used during pregnancy in humans. Many retrospective studies did not show any increase in the incidence of congenital malformation in infants born to mothers who received anaesthesia during pregnancy (Mazze and Kallén 1989; Czeizel, Pataki, and Rockenbauer 1998; Visser et al. 2001).

The only drugs of concern are nitrous oxide, benzodiazepine and sugammadex. As Nitrous oxide inhibits methionine synthetase and impairing

DNA production, there is concern about its use during pregnancy. It has a weak teratogenic effect in animal models only. Thus, it is better to avoid nitrous oxide during the 1st trimester if possible. The sugammadex is a reversal agent for neuromuscular blockers. Sugammadex reduces the level of free progesterone levels in non-human studies which can be detrimental for pregnancy (Et et al. 2015).

Diazepam use during pregnancy may be associated with cleft palate, but most commonly used benzodiazepines during perioperative period is Midazolam. Midazolam use has not been found to be associated with development of congenital anomalies (Dolovich et al. 1998; Wikner et al. 2007). Though a single, brief exposure to anaesthesia does not affect the neurodevelopment of an unborn child. The peri-operative team must discuss the benefits, risks, and appropriate timing of surgery requiring anaesthesia that will take more than three hours (Sun et al. 2016).

Risk of Abortion/Preterm Labor/Intrauterine Growth Retardation/Stillbirth

Any intraoperative condition which can jeopardize uteroplacental perfusion can lead to fetal asphyxia. The most common causes of uteroplacental hypoperfusion during the perioperative period are difficulty during intubation, aspiration, hypoventilation, maternal hypercarbia/hypocarbia, inadequate analgesia, deeper/light plane of general anaesthesia, aortocaval compression, hypovolemia, hemorrhage, etc.

Anaesthesia Management

Preoperative Evaluation

All pregnant patients should be evaluated with detailed medical/obstetric history, physical examination, including airway assessment. The symptoms of raised intracranial tension such as headache, nausea/vomiting, the poor mental status might be confusing with eclamptic features. An anaesthesiologist must consider the impact of anti-epileptic drugs on peri-operative management. Always watch for side effects such as leukopenia, anemia, agranulocytosis, peripheral neuropathy in patients on antiepileptic medications. Few antiepileptics induce hepatic enzymes and accelerate the breakdown of opioids, neuromuscular blockers, and volatile anaesthetic agents. The preoperative investigation should be individualized based on patient factors and the planned procedure. Due to pregnancy-related physiological changes, all investigations must be interpreted accordingly.

Preoperative Preparation

a. Psychological preparation: All patients must be informed about the low risk of anaesthetic drugs on the fetus and the possible risk of fetal loss during the perioperative period. An obstetrician consultation must be taken if there is a need for tocolytic agents or the emergency cesarean section along with the neurosurgical procedure
b. Aspiration prophylaxis: All pregnant patients are at increased risk of aspiration during induction of general anaesthesia due to both anatomic and hormonal related physiological changes. Raised intracranial tension and decreased mental status may increase the risk of aspiration. The need for adequate preoperative fasting as standard adult fasting guidelines and uses of pharmacologic prophylaxis such as nonparticulate antacids/H2 receptor antagonists and/or prokinetics must be individualized as per the patient's condition and urgency of surgery.

Premedication

Preoperative anxiolysis is required to reduce the patient's psychological stress and endogenous catecholamines release. A small titrated dose of sedative (e.g., midazolam) can be given. Any type of sedative should be avoided in a patient with a difficult airway and depressed mental status.

Intraoperative Anaesthesia Management

Safe anaesthesia is more important than particular anaesthetic medication for a pregnant patient undergoing neurosurgical intervention (Shiro et al. 2021; Abd-Elsayed et al. 2013). We aim to provide maintenance of oxygenation, eucapnia, euglycemia, normotension and adequate surgical field. Optimal maternal blood pressure is important to maintain uteroplacental perfusion. Though anaesthetic drugs have minimal direct effects on the uterine blood flow, even though hypotension and vasodilation can lead to uteroplacental hypoperfusion.

All standard monitors (ECG, Non-Invasive Blood pressure, pulse oximeter, End-tidal CO2, Temperature) are used for all patients during anaesthesia. Advanced monitoring (e.g., continuous intra-arterial pressure monitoring, central venous pressure monitoring) may be required based on the type/duration of neurosurgery and the patient's comorbid condition. In selected cases intermittent/continuous fetal heart monitoring may be considered during surgery. The selection of the specific induction agent depends on patient factors and the anaesthesiologist's preference. As none of these agents has teratogenic/adverse effects on fetal brain development. The physiologic chronic respiratory alkalosis of pregnancy should be maintained during intraoperative ventilation with end-tidal CO_2 (30-32 mmHg). Patient's positioning during neurosurgery requires coordination between anesthesiologist and neurosurgeon. As prone position may not be achieved due to gravid uterus specially in $2^{nd}/3^{rd}$ trimester, alternate a lateral/rotated supine position can be achieved if possible. All precaution must be taken to prevent aortocaval compression throughout surgery. For anti-edema measure during intraoperative period, use of mannitol (0.25-0.5 g/kg) can be considered if necessary. It accumulates in the fetus and can lead to electrolyte disturbance and dehydration. Single dose dexamethasone may be safe to use. Loop diuretics should be avoided.

Post-Operative Care

During post-operative period both maternal and fetal monitoring should be done. Any airway and cardiovascular complications may occur during emergence or in the immediate postoperative period specially. The FHR should be monitored in the recovery room. Left lateral position or uterine displacement should maintained. Multimodal analgesia should be considered for postoperative pain control include acetaminophen, local anaesthetic infiltration and opioids Nonsteroidal anti-inflammatory drugs (NSAIDs) should not be used during pregnancy (Alon et al. 1993).

Safe Medications during Pregnancy

Most antiepileptic drugs (AED) are unsafe during pregnancy due to their teratogenic effect. Also, drugs like phenytoin, phenobarbitone, carbamazepine, primidone, and topiramate, can cause cytochrome P-450 enzyme induction, leading to hemorrhagic disease of a newborn as a result of vitamin K deficiency (Eadie 2014). Presently, levetiracetam is the only drug recommended during the antenatal period when indicated, preferably as a monotherapy (Mawhinney et al. 2013). Other newer AEDs include lamotrigine, carbamazepine and topiramate. Most studies do not recommend the use of prophylactic AEDs when there is no history of seizures in patients with a brain tumor in the antenatal period.

Corticosteroids group of drugs are also important in this cohort of patients, especially because of their role in disease stabilization. Dexamethasone and methylprednisolone are the most common drugs used in this category. However, there is no sufficient data regarding their safety and is recommended to be used with caution. Bromocriptine can be used for the medical management of prolactinomas with no increased risk of teratogenicity (Molitch 1985; De Wit and Bennink 1984). Cabergoline has also been shown to be safe, though data is inadequate for a definitive recommendation (Glezer and Bronstein 2014). It is recommended to discontinue octreotide (somatostatin analogue) during pregnancy for the treatment of acromegaly. Ketoconazole, metyrapone, amino glutethimide, and mitotane are contraindicated during pregnancy making medical management of Cushing syndrome less safe and compared to surgical intervention, in case there is clinical deterioration (Gadelha and Vieira Neto 2014).

Spinal Tumors during Pregnancy

The incidence of spinal tumors during pregnancy has been rarely reported. Due to a relative paucity of literature, definitive management protocols are lacking and treatment strategies are mainly based upon the finding of few case reports and case series. Meng et al. in their series of 21 cases of pregnancy-related spinal tumors (PRST), reported giant cell tumors, hemangioma, schwannoma, and neurofibroma to be the common pathologies (Meng et al. 2015). Their incidence was similar to that of the general population of the same age group.

The characteristic clinical presentation of these tumors remains the same irrespective of the antenatal status. Though it may lead to rapid clinical deterioration due to increased intravascular volume, increased intraspinal venous pressure, increased vascularity (estrogen and progesterone effect), and raised ICP because of compression of inferior vena cava by the gravid uterus (Hyuga et al. 2013; Divers, Hoxsey, and Dunnihoo 1978). Also, it significantly affects the management strategy. Similar to brain tumors during pregnancy, the treatment depends upon multiple factors like the nature of the pathology (benign or malignant), site (cervical, thoracic, lumbar, or sacral), clinical severity, gestational age, and most importantly patients' opinion regarding the continuation of gestation or otherwise. While most of the investigations that are performed majority of authors preferred deferring surgery till the term (Meng et al. 2015; Han et al. 2008). In case of clinical deterioration, induction of labor or cesarean section was preferred at fetal maturity, i.e., 32 to 36 weeks. In the case of expectant management, a close follow-up is essential for possible deterioration due to pregnancy-associated factors, as already mentioned. In the case of spinal tumors with rapid progression/malignant pathology, like metastatic lesions, an option of therapeutic abortion or premature delivery must be discussed with the patient and her partner. Elective cesarean section is considered relatively safer than parturition due to possible raised ICP secondary to raised intra-abdominal and intra-thoracic pressures in the latter (Meng et al. 2015).

Conclusion

The diagnosis and management of spinal and brain tumors in association with pregnancy require a multidisciplinary approach. The anaesthetic approach is significantly influenced by the physiological and pharmacodynamic alterations during pregnancy. Options regarding termination of pregnancy must be considered only if the aggressiveness of disease endangers the maternal safety. In case of neurologically stable patients, the neurosurgical intervention can be safely performed after delivery of the child.

References

Abd-Elsayed, Alaa A, Jose Díaz-Gómez, Gene H Barnett, Andrea Kurz, Maria Inton-Santos, Sabri Barsoum, Rafi Avitsian, Zeyd Ebrahim, Vesna Jevtovic-Todorovic, and Ehab Farag. 2013. 'A Case Series Discussing the Anaesthetic Management of Pregnant Patients with Brain Tumours.' *F1000Research* 2 (December): 92. https://doi.org/10.12688/f1000research.2-92.v2.

'ACOG Committee Opinion No. 474: Nonobstetric Surgery during Pregnancy.' 2011. *Obstetrics and Gynecology* 117 (2 Pt 1): 420-21. https://doi.org/10.1097/AOG.0b013e31820eede9.

Alon, Eli, Robert H. Ball, Mark H. Gillie, Julian T. Parer, Mark A. Rosen, and Sol M. Shnider. 1993. 'Effects of Propofol and Thiopental on Maternal and Fetal Cardiovascular and Acid-Base Variables in the Pregnant Ewe.' *Anesthesiology* 78 (3): 562-76. https://doi.org/10.1097/00000542-199303000-00020.

Araujo, Paula Bruna, Leonardo Vieira Neto, and Mônica R. Gadelha. 2015. 'Pituitary Tumor Management in Pregnancy.' *Endocrinology and Metabolism Clinics of North America* 44 (1): 181-97. https://doi.org/10.1016/j.ecl.2014.10.015.

Bickerstaff, Edwin R, JM Small, and IA Guest. 1958. 'The Relapsing Course of Certain Meningiomas in Relation to Pregnancy and Menstruation.' *Journal of Neurology, Neurosurgery, and Psychiatry* 21 (2): 89.

Cohen-Gadol, Aaron A., Jonathan A. Friedman, Jennifer D. Friedman, R. Shane Tubbs, James R. Munis, and Fredric B. Meyer. 2009. 'Neurosurgical Management of Intracranial Lesions in the Pregnant Patient: A 36-Year Institutional Experience and Review of the Literature.' *Journal of Neurosurgery* 111 (6): 1150-57. https://doi.org/10.3171/2009.3.JNS081160.

Czeizel, A. E., T. Pataki, and M. Rockenbauer. 1998. 'Reproductive Outcome after Exposure to Surgery under Anesthesia during Pregnancy.' *Archives of Gynecology and Obstetrics* 261 (4): 193-99. https://doi.org/10.1007/s004040050221.

De Wit, W, and HJT Coelingh Bennink. 1984. 'Prophylactic Bromocriptine Treatment during Pregnancy in Women with Macroprolactinomas: Report of 13 Pregnancies.' *BJOG: An International Journal of Obstetrics & Gynaecology* 91 (11): 1059-69.

Divers, Walter A, Rodney J Hoxsey, and Dale R Dunnihoo. 1978. 'A Spinal Cord Neurolemmoma in Pregnancy.' *Obstetrics and Gynecology* 52 (1 Suppl): 47S-50S.

Dolecek, Therese A, Jennifer M Propp, Nancy E Stroup, and Carol Kruchko. 2012. 'CBTRUS Statistical Report: Primary Brain and Central Nervous System Tumors Diagnosed in the United States in 2005-2009.' *Neuro-Oncology* 14 Suppl 5 (Suppl 5): v1-49. https://doi.org/10.1093/neuonc/nos218.

Dolovich, Lisa R., Antonio Addis, J. M. Régis Vaillancourt, J. D. Barry Power, Gideon Koren, and Thomas R. Einarson. 1998. 'Benzodiazepine Use in Pregnancy and Major Malformations or Oral Cleft: Meta-Analysis of Cohort and Case-Control Studies'. *BMJ* 317 (7162): 839-43. https://doi.org/10.1136/bmj.317.7162.839.

Eadie, Mervyn J. 2014. 'Treating Epilepsy in Pregnant Women.' *Expert Opinion on Pharmacotherapy* 15 (6): 841-50.

Et, Tayfun, Ahmet Topal, Atilla Erol, Aybars Tavlan, Alper Kılıçaslan, and Sema Tuncer Uzun. 2015. 'The Effects of Sugammadex on Progesterone Levels in Pregnant Rats.' *Balkan Medical Journal* 32 (2): 203-7. https://doi.org/10.5152/balkanmedj.2015.15502.

Friesen, HG, P Fournier, and P Desjardins. 1973. 'Pituitary Prolactin in Pregnancy and Normal and Abnormal Lactation.' *Clinical Obstetrics and Gynecology* 16 (3): 25-45.

Gadelha, Mônica R, and Leonardo Vieira Neto. 2014. 'Efficacy of Medical Treatment in C Ushing's Disease: A Systematic Review.' *Clinical Endocrinology* 80 (1): 1-12.

Glezer, Andrea, and Marcello D Bronstein. 2014. 'Prolactinomas, Cabergoline, and Pregnancy.' *Endocrine* 47 (1): 64-69.

Grand'Maison, Sophie, Florence Weber, Marie-Josée Bédard, Michele Mahone, and Ariane Godbout. 2015. 'Pituitary Apoplexy in Pregnancy: A Case Series and Literature Review.' *Obstetric Medicine* 8 (4): 177-83. https://doi.org/10.1177/1753495X15598917.

Haas, JF, W Jänisch, and W Staneczek. 1986. 'Newly Diagnosed Primary Intracranial Neoplasms in Pregnant Women: A Population-Based Assessment.' *Journal of Neurology, Neurosurgery & Psychiatry* 49 (8): 874-80.

Haas, Joanna F. 1984. 'Pregnancy in Association with a Newly Diagnosed Cancer: A Population-based Epidemiologic Assessment.' *International Journal of Cancer* 34 (2): 229-35.

Han, In-Ho, Sung-Uk Kuh, Jae-Hoon Kim, Dong-Kyu Chin, Keun-Su Kim, Young-Sul Yoon, Byung-Ho Jin, and Yong-Eun Cho. 2008. 'Clinical Approach and Surgical

Strategy for Spinal Diseases in Pregnant Women: A Report of Ten Cases.' *Spine* 33 (17): E614-19.

Herman-Bonert, Vivien, Maria Seliverstov, and Shlomo Melmed. 1998. 'Pregnancy in Acromegaly: Successful Therapeutic Outcome.' *The Journal of Clinical Endocrinology & Metabolism* 83 (3): 727-31.

Hortobágyi, Tibor, János Bencze, Balázs Murnyák, Mahan C Kouhsari, László Bognár, and György Marko-Varga. 2017. 'Pathophysiology of Meningioma Growth in Pregnancy.' *Open Medicine (Warsaw, Poland)* 12 (July): 195-200. https://doi.org/10.1515/med-2017-0029.

Hyuga, Shunsuke, Akiyuki Sakamoto, Tomoyuki Kawamata, Toshiyuki Shimizu, and Mikito Kawamata. 2013. 'Case of Parturient Who Underwent Resection of a Spinal Tumor.' *Masui. The Japanese Journal of Anesthesiology* 62 (5): 609-12.

Kacmar, Rachel M, and Robert Gaiser. 2019. 'Physiologic Changes of Pregnancy.' In: *Chestnut's Obstetric Anesthesia: Principles and Practice (6th Ed., pp. 13-37).* Elsevier, Philadelphia, PA.

Kanaan, Imad, Ashraf Jallu, and Huda Kanaan. 2003. 'Management Strategy for Meningioma in Pregnancy: A Clinical Study.' *Skull Base* 13 (04): 197-204.

Kasuki, Leandro, Leonardo Vieira Neto, Christina M. Takiya, and Mônica R. Gadelha. 2012. 'Growth of an Aggressive Tumor during Pregnancy in an Acromegalic Patient.' *Endocrine Journal* 59 (4): 313-19. https://doi.org/10.1507/endocrj.ej11-0306.

Lambe, Mats, Patricia Coogan, and John Baron. 1997. 'Reproductive Factors and the Risk of Brain Tumors: A Population-based Study in Sweden.' *International Journal of Cancer* 72 (3): 389-93.

Laviv, Yosef, Ahmed Bayoumi, Anand Mahadevan, Brett Young, Myles Boone, and Ekkehard M. Kasper. 2018. 'Meningiomas in Pregnancy: Timing of Surgery and Clinical Outcomes as Observed in 104 Cases and Establishment of a Best Management Strategy.' *Acta Neurochirurgica* 160 (8): 1521-29. https://doi.org/10.1007/s00701-017-3146-8.

Laviv, Yosef, Victoria Ohla, and Ekkehard M. Kasper. 2018. 'Unique Features of Pregnancy-Related Meningiomas: Lessons Learned from 148 Reported Cases and Theoretical Implications of a Prolactin Modulated Pathogenesis.' *Neurosurgical Review* 41 (1): 95-108. https://doi.org/10.1007/s10143-016-0762-3.

Mawhinney, Ellen, John Craig, Jim Morrow, Aline Russell, W Henry Smithson, Linda Parsons, Patrick J Morrison, Brenda Liggan, Beth Irwin, and Norman Delanty. 2013. 'Levetiracetam in Pregnancy: Results from the UK and Ireland Epilepsy and Pregnancy Registers.' *Neurology* 80 (4): 400-405.

Mazze, Richard I., and Bengt Kallén. 1989. 'Reproductive Outcome after Anesthesia and Operation during Pregnancy: A Registry Study of 5405 Cases.' *American Journal of Obstetrics and Gynecology* 161 (5): 1178-85. https://doi.org/10.1016/0002-9378(89)90659-5.

Meng, Tong, Huabin Yin, Zhenxi Li, Bo Li, Wang Zhou, Jing Wang, Lei Zhou, Dianwen Song, and Jianru Xiao. 2015. 'Therapeutic Strategy and Outcome of Spine Tumors in Pregnancy: A Report of 21 Cases and Literature Review.' *Spine* 40 (3): E146-53. https://doi.org/10.1097/BRS.0000000000000719.

Molitch, Mark E. 1985. 'Pregnancy and the Hyperprolactinemic Woman.' *New England Journal of Medicine* 312 (21): 1364-70.

Nieman, Lynnette K., Beverly M. K. Biller, James W. Findling, John Newell-Price, Martin O. Savage, Paul M. Stewart, and Victor M. Montori. 2008. 'The Diagnosis of Cushing's Syndrome: An Endocrine Society Clinical Practice Guideline.' *The Journal of Clinical Endocrinology & Metabolism* 93 (5): 1526-40. https://doi.org/10.1210/jc.2008-0125.

Patenaude, Yves, Denise Pugash, Kenneth Lim, Lucie Morin, Stephen Bly, Kimberly Butt, Yvonne Cargill, Gregory Davies, Nanette Denis, and Gail Hazlitt. 2014. 'The Use of Magnetic Resonance Imaging in the Obstetric Patient.' *Journal of Obstetrics and Gynaecology Canada* 36 (4): 349-55.

Peeters, Sophie, Mélanie Pagès, Guillaume Gauchotte, Catherine Miquel, Stéphanie Cartalat-Carel, Jean-Sébastien Guillamo, Laurent Capelle, et al. 2018. 'Interactions between Glioma and Pregnancy: Insight from a 52-Case Multicenter Series.' *Journal of Neurosurgery* 128 (1): 3-13. https://doi.org/10.3171/2016.10.JNS16710.

Rodrigues, Adrian J., Anne R. Waldrop, Sanaa Suharwardy, Maurice L. Druzin, Michael Iv, Jessica R. Ansari, Sarah A. Stone, et al. 2021. 'Management of Brain Tumors Presenting in Pregnancy: A Case Series and Systematic Review.' *American Journal of Obstetrics & Gynecology MFM* 3 (1): 100256. https://doi.org/10.1016/j.ajogmf.2020.100256.

Roelvink, Nico C. A., Wouter Kamphorst, H. August M. van Alphen, and B. Ramanath Rao. 1987. 'Pregnancy-Related Primary Brain and Spinal Tumors'. *Archives of Neurology* 44 (2): 209-15. https://doi.org/10.1001/archneur.1987.00520140069020.

Scheithauer, Bernd W, Toshiaki Sano, Kalman T Kovacs, William F Young Jr, Nancy Ryan, and Raymond V Randall. 1990. '*The Pituitary Gland in Pregnancy: A Clinicopathologic and Immunohistochemical Study of 69 Cases*.' In, 65:461-74. Elsevier.

Shiro, Reona, Kosuke Murakami, Masaharu Miyauchi, Yasuhiro Sanada, and Noriomi Matsumura. 2021. 'Management Strategies for Brain Tumors Diagnosed during Pregnancy: A Case Report and Literature Review.' *Medicina* 57 (6): 613. https://doi.org/10.3390/medicina57060613.

Sun, Lena S., Guohua Li, Tonya L. K. Miller, Cynthia Salorio, Mary W. Byrne, David C. Bellinger, Caleb Ing, et al. 2016. 'Association between a Single General Anesthesia Exposure before Age 36 Months and Neurocognitive Outcomes in Later Childhood.' *JAMA* 315 (21): 2312-20. https://doi.org/10.1001/jama.2016.6967.

Visser, Brendan C., Robert E. Glasgow, Kimberley K. Mulvihill, and Sean J. Mulvihill. 2001. 'Safety and Timing of Nonobstetric Abdominal Surgery in Pregnancy.' *Digestive Surgery* 18 (5): 409-17. https://doi.org/10.1159/000050183.

Wallach, Edward, Carl Gemzell, and Chun Fu Wang. 1979. 'Outcome of Pregnancy in Women with Pituitary Adenoma.' *Fertility and Sterility* 31 (4): 363-72.

Wikner, Birgitta Norstedt, Carl-Olav Stiller, Ulf Bergman, Charlotte Asker, and Bengt Källén. 2007. 'Use of Benzodiazepines and Benzodiazepine Receptor Agonists during Pregnancy: Neonatal Outcome and Congenital Malformations.' *Pharmacoepidemiology and Drug Safety* 16 (11): 1203-10. https://doi.org/10.1002/ pds.1457.

Ylikorkala, Olavi, Seppo Kivinen, and Matti Reinilä. 1979. 'Serial Prolactin and Thyrotropin Responses to Thyrotropin-Releasing Hormone throughout Normal Human Pregnancy.' *The Journal of Clinical Endocrinology & Metabolism* 48 (2): 288-92.

Chapter 14

Genetic and Stem Cell Therapies in the Treatment of Glioma

Balachandar Deivasigamani, Ved Prakash Maurya, Priyadarshi Dikshit and Awadhesh Kumar Jaiswal
Department of Neurosurgery, Sanjay Gandhi Postgraduate Institute of Medical Sciences, Lucknow, India

Abstract

Brain tumor stem cells and gene therapy for glioma are emerging as the main target in the treatment of glioma. Current treatment modalities, chemo and radiotherapy, are involved in indiscriminate targeting of tumor cells. Toxicity and side effects involved in this treatment take a toll on patients lifestyle. In patients with malignant glioma, life expectancy and quality of life are not satisfactory with current treatment modalities. Brain tumor stem cell therapy and gene therapy are all about focusing, targeting and destroying the tumor cells that have self-renewal and proliferating abilities and restoring the normal apoptotic pathway in them. In the present chapter, we would like to briefly discuss this very complex topic and focus on the issues of concern in stem cell and gene therapy in the management of glioma.

Introduction

Brain tumor stem cells are a minor group of cells found in many CNS malignancies which has all properties of stem cell and, when transplanted into

In: Advances in Neurosurgery Research
Editors: Amit Agrawal, Pradeep Chouksey, Adesh Shrivastava et al.
ISBN: 978-1-68507-859-1

phenotypically defined cells in a non-immune recipient, will reproduce the entire heterogeneous population of tumor cells found in humans (Singh et al., 2003; Singh, Hawkins, et al., 2004; Galli et al., 2004; Read et al., 2009; Galderisi, Cipollaro, and Giordano 2006; Quiñones-Hinojosa and Chaichana 2007). This observation supports the cancer stem cell hypothesis (CSC). The source of these cells is not clearly understood, but some say that it is formed due to the conversion of naturally occurring neural stem cells (NSCs) (Galderisi, Cipollaro, and Giordano 2006).

Cancer Stem Cell (CSC) – Hypothesis

It states that tumors are hierarchically organized like normal somatic cells. When transplanted into the recipient, not all cells in the tumor can produce disease, but a cancer stem cell (CSC) can produce all phenotypes observed in the donor. Tumors following this model are primary malignant brain tumors (Singh, Hawkins, et al., 2004; Galli et al., 2004) and acute myeloid leukaemia (Bonnet and Dick 1997).

Stochastic Model

It says that any cell in the tumor can obtain tumour-initiating functions without the need for a firm functional hierarchy inside the tumor (Shackleton et al., 2009). Tumors following this model are B-cell lymphoblastic leukaemia (Williams, den Besten, and Sherr 2007) and melanoma (Quintana et al., 2010).

Origin of Cancer Stem Cells

There are three conceivable descriptions for the origin of brain tumor stem cells.

(i) Brain tumors arise from dedifferentiation of a subset of adult brain cells and mutation accumulation over time (Nowell 1976). This makes the cells multiply and regenerate uncontrollably, eventually leading to the formation of CSCs – Clonal evolution hypothesis.
(ii) Abnormal dedifferentiation of NSCs (Nicolis 2007).

(iii) Single tumor precursor cells with unknown origin can attract normal quiescent neural progenitor cells and induce them to multiply in an uncontrolled manner by releasing local growth factors – Progenitor recruitment hypothesis.

Cancer Stem Cells (CSCs) in Glioma

A perfect example for explaining morphological heterogenicity would be glioblastoma (GBM). Glioblastoma is the most lethal brain tumor in which the cell population is so noticeably heterogeneous that the same feature was used to name it. GBM is a hierarchically organized tumor of the central nervous system. Gliomas tend to be more prevalent in the subventricular zone, a germinal centre containing adult NSCs and has a higher degree of cellular proliferation (Chaichana et al., 2008; Sanai, Alvarez-Buylla, and Berger 2005). In an experiment where rats' brains are implanted with carcinogenic hydrocarbons, it has been observed that the tumour-forming capacity is more in the subventricular zone compared with the cortex (Hopewell and Wright 1969). Another explanation for tumor formation is that CSCs may locally attract normal NSCs and liberate various growth factors. This turns the normal NSCs to multiply uncontrollably, which eventually forms a tumor mass. Nestin and CD 133 (prominin- 1) are the most sensitive markers available to identify NSCs and CSCs. Nestin positive brain tumors had enhanced migratory and infiltrative properties (Rutka et al., 1999). Wan and colleagues have found that increased tumor grade is associated with increased Nestin expression and poor survival (Wan et al., 2011). CD 133 positive cells successfully produced tumor in immunocompromised mice; however, CD133 negative cells failed to do it (Singh, Hawkins, et al., 2004).

There can be glioma formation if there is an absence of cell cycle regulator Ink4a-Arf in astrocytes (a critical genetic mutation). In the setting of overexpression of signal transduction protein Ras with deficient Ink4a-Arf, GBM formation can be stimulated (Bachoo et al., 2002). Platelet-derived growth factor (PDGF) – a molecule that regulates glial precursors in an undifferentiated state. Transfecting GFAP (Glial fibrillary acidic protein) positive cells with a viral vector delivering PDGF showed significant increase in glioma formation (Dai et al., 2001). This shows that even a differentiated cell can revert to a less differentiated state when it acquires a critical genetic mutation and contribute to tumorigenesis. Integrin α6 – a cancer stem cell marker in GBM, has been identified. Integrin α6 is the receptor for extracellular matrix protein laminin (Lathia et al., 2010).

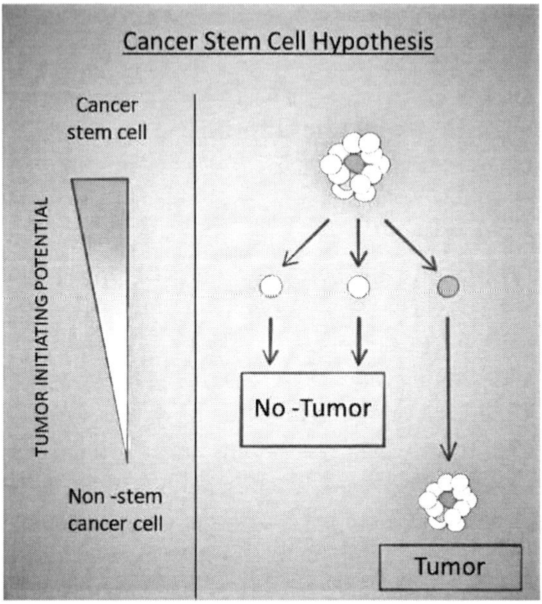

Figure 1. Shows the tumour initiating potential of various subcategory of tumor cells (Bernstein and Berger 2000).

A recent study demonstrated arrested proliferation and loss of tumorigenic potential in mouse recipients by turning off the SOX2 gene (Gangemi et al., 2009). Another research found that Wnt signalling (regulated by β-catenin) is fundamentally responsible for the self-renewal properties of CSC's in GBM (Reya et al., 2003; N. Zhang et al., 2011). So, turning β-catenin off reduced the tumorigenic potential by 80-90%. Due to rapidly proliferating tumor cells and their high metabolic needs, the CSCs promote angiogenesis by secreting high levels of Vascular endothelial growth factor (VEGF) (Bao, Wu, Sathornsumetee, et al., 2006), which makes them hyper vascular. Hence targeting angiogenesis can be a path for treating this tumor (Ricci-Vitiani et al., 2010; Soda et al., 2011). Bevacizumab, a VEGF neutralizing antibody, has resulted in a marked decrease in tumor growth in mice transplanted with GBM CSCs (Bao, Wu, Sathornsumetee, et al., 2006). Satisfying human trials are yet to come in this strategy (Lai et al., 2010).

Ephrin A2 (EPHA2) receptor is overexpressed on the cell surface of CSCs. EPHA1-Fc ligand causes loss of CSCs self-renewal capacity and induces cell differentiation, thereby losing tumour-initiating capacity. EPHA2 is also associated with increased angiogenesis. EPHA2 downregulation might be a future cell surface target for glioma treatment (Binda et al., 2012). BMP (Bone morphogenic protein) reduces the number of CD 133 positive cells causing tumor growth blocking. This improved mice survival by 80% (Piccirillo et al., 2006).

Pieces of evidence in literature say that CSCs are resistant to radiation (due to up-regulation of DNA damage response) and chemotherapy (due to downregulation of pro-apoptotic genes like BAX) (Bao, Wu, McLendon, et al., 2006; Liu et al., 2006) and might be the reason for recurrence (Chen et al., 2012). CSC hypothesis says that the tumor will regrow even if it is removed by surgical or reduced by chemical means if CSC'S are spared (Singh, Clarke, et al., 2004) (Figure 1) This clearly shows the need to target CSCs to control the disease and provide effective treatment. Indiscriminate targeting of cancer cells is not going to provide a lasting cure. So, emerging therapies should target the self-renewal capacity of the CSCs to fight against malignant brain neoplasms.

Cancer Stem Cells (CSCs) in Medulloblastoma

Like glioblastoma, medulloblastoma is also hierarchically organized. Transfer of medulloblastoma cells positive for CD 133 into a non-immune host caused tumor formation (Singh, Hawkins, et al., 2004).

Molecular pathways involved in medulloblastoma formation are SHH (Sonic hedgehog) and notch pathways (Lee et al., 2004; Varnum-Finney et al., 2000; Bhardwaj et al., 2001). This pathway maintains CSCs in an undifferentiated state, thereby controlling proliferation (Nicolis 2007). SHH pathway activation (SHH cell surface receptor activation by SHH activates transcription factors of the GLI complex) with loss of regulation is found be the cause for medulloblastoma formation in mice (i Altaba, Sánchez, and Dahmane 2002). Selective inhibition of SHH-GLI Pathway by cyclopamine (a plant-derived alkaloid) notably decreases the evolution of human medulloblastomas and gliomas (Bar et al., 2007; Dahmane et al., 2001). Notch signalling is vital for the development and maintenance of medulloblastomas (as shown by experimental evidence). Shutting down the notch pathway in medulloblastomas decreases rapid increase and increases neuronal differentiation of cells (Hallahan et al., 2004).

Gene Therapy in Gliomas

Inoculation of gene therapy vectors that shows an affinity for the central nervous system (CNS) is known as gene therapy. This may ideally be suited for brain tumors. Also, this avoids systemic toxicity due to current chemotherapeutic regimens (Aboody et al., 2000). Gene therapy for glioma is emerging due to the inadequacy of present-day care and encouraging preclinical studies.

Suicidal Gene Therapy

Initial gene therapy clinical trials began in the 1990s - vector to transfect glioma cells with the retrovirus vector herpes simplex virus type 1 (HSV1) gene thymidine kinase (TK) (suicide gene therapy) (Immonen et al., 2004). However, unfortunately, human trials showed no difference in survival rate (7.4 months) (Rainov 2000). This is due to the low transduction rate of HSV1-TK. LacZ-expressing adenovirus (AD), in comparison with HSV1-TK, was found to have high transduction rates (Puumalainen et al., 1998). AD with retrovirus vector was found to significantly increase in survival rate (15 months) (Sandmair et al., 2000). Cytosine deaminase (CD) -5FC, another suicidal gene that interrupts RNA and DNA synthesis, has proven effective in preclinical models (Pertschuk et al., 2012). Toca 511, another vector understudy found to have threefold effectiveness in infected cells (Perez et al., 2012).

Tumor Suppressor and Apoptotic Gene Therapy

Mutations occurring in the tumor suppressor genes (TP53, RB1, NF1 and PTEN) are the primary targets in this treatment modality. It aims in restoring normal cells cycle. Ad p53 vector (Zhu et al., 2010) and adenoviral vectors to transfer Rb tumor suppressor genes are under trial to repair and restore the apoptotic pathway (Fueyo et al., 1998; Jiang et al., 2009).

Non-Viral Vectors

This is a safe method of delivering genetic material as it is non-pathogenic and non-immunogenic (Thomas and Klibanov 2003). Various vectors ranging from naked DNA strands to complex chemical carriers have been used. Lipoplexes (DNA liposomal complexes) and antisense RNA molecule has been used widely and has been found to increase survival (Y. Zhang et al., 2004).

Neural and Mesenchymal Stem Cell Vectors

Neural stem cells were found to have tropism for gliomas, but it is challenging to obtain them (Aboody et al., 2000). Mesenchymal stem cells are easily collected (Doucette et al., 2011). Human mesenchymal stem cells derived from Bone marrow (BM-hMSCs) exhibit selective tropism for gliomas, and it has been proven to be a potent *in vivo* vector (Shinojima et al., 2013).

Oncolytic Viral Therapy

This works by selectively replicating viral vectors, set up to replicate in tumor cells. Amplification of therapeutic genes, the mechanism by which these vectors cause tumor cell lysis. Viruses presently being studied in anti-glioma clinical trials include oncolytic herpes simplex virus (oHSV), conditionally replicating Ad (CRAd), reovirus, poliovirus, vaccinia virus, measles virus (Tobias et al., 2013).

A genetically engineered HSV-1 that selectively multiplied in tumor cells was created using a virus built with two mutations (HSV -1 G207). This virus is hypersensitive to acyclovir and ganciclovir and has no significant toxicities. Preclinical studies demonstrated this virus to be safe and effective. The ad has produced the most comprehensive range and variety of selectively replicating oncolytic viruses for glioma therapy, including the ONYX-015, 01/PEME, and the previously mentioned Delta-24-RGD virus (Chiocca et al., 2004).

Conclusion

Stem cell therapy or Gene therapy unaided may or may not provide a remedy for malignant glioma. The morphological heterogeneity of these tumors and the whole milieu of the CNS make the annihilation of glioma by solo therapy improbable. However, the modalities mentioned above deliver an approach to glioma treatment that is selectively targeted at tumor cells and may induce cell death through multiple mechanisms with a single treatment, avoiding many of the present mechanisms of therapeutic resistance prevalent in glioma. If the cancer stem cell hypothesis is being correct, the strategy to vanquish this lethal disease will be dealt with by three steps they are (i) identify the cancer stem cell, (ii) find a way to destroy it and (iii) destroy it. The continuous development of vectors and incorporation of new delivery show great potential for improved outcomes and overall survival.

References

Aboody, K. S., Alice Brown, Nikolai G. Rainov, Kate A. Bower, Shaoxiong Liu, Wendy Yang, Juan E. Small, Ulrich Herrlinger, Vaclav Ourednik, and Peter McL Black. 2000. 'Neural Stem Cells Display Extensive Tropism for Pathology in Adult Brain: Evidence from Intracranial Gliomas.' *Proceedings of the National Academy of Sciences* 97 (23): 12846-51.

Altaba, A. R. I., Pilar Sánchez, and Nadia Dahmane. 2002. 'Gli and Hedgehog in Cancer: Tumours, Embryos and Stem Cells.' *Nature Reviews Cancer* 2 (5): 361-72.

Bachoo, R. M., Elizabeth A. Maher, Keith L. Ligon, Norman E. Sharpless, Suzanne S. Chan, Mingjian James You, Yi Tang, Jessica DeFrances, Elizabeth Stover, and Ralph Weissleder. 2002. 'Epidermal Growth Factor Receptor and Ink4a/Arf: Convergent Mechanisms Governing Terminal Differentiation and Transformation along the Neural Stem Cell to Astrocyte Axis.' *Cancer Cell* 1 (3): 269-77.

Bao, S., Qiulian Wu, Roger E. McLendon, Yueling Hao, Qing Shi, Anita B. Hjelmeland, Mark W. Dewhirst, Darell D. Bigner, and Jeremy N. Rich. 2006. 'Glioma Stem Cells Promote Radioresistance by Preferential Activation of the DNA Damage Response.' *Nature* 444 (7120): 756-60.

Bao, S., Qiulian Wu, Sith Sathornsumetee, Yueling Hao, Zhizhong Li, Anita B. Hjelmeland, Qing Shi, Roger E. McLendon, Darell D. Bigner, and Jeremy N. Rich. 2006. 'Stem Cell-like Glioma Cells Promote Tumor Angiogenesis through Vascular Endothelial Growth Factor.' *Cancer Research* 66 (16): 7843-48.

Bar, E. E., Aneeka Chaudhry, Alex Lin, Xing Fan, Karisa Schreck, William Matsui, Sara Piccirillo, Angelo L. Vescovi, Francesco DiMeco, and Alessandro Olivi. 2007. 'Cyclopamine-mediated Hedgehog Pathway Inhibition Depletes Stem-like Cancer Cells in Glioblastoma.' *Stem Cells* 25 (10): 2524-33.

Bernstein, M., and Mitchel S. Berger. 2000. *Neuro-Oncology: The Essentials*. Thieme.

Bhardwaj, G., B. Murdoch, D. Wu, D. P. Baker, K. P. Williams, K. Chadwick, L. E. Ling, F. N. Karanu, and M. Bhatia. 2001. 'Sonic Hedgehog Induces the Proliferation of Primitive Human Hematopoietic Cells via BMP Regulation.' *Nature Immunology* 2 (2): 172-80.

Binda, E., Alberto Visioli, Fabrizio Giani, Giuseppe Lamorte, Massimiliano Copetti, Ken L Pitter, Jason T Huse, Laura Cajola, Nadia Zanetti, and Francesco DiMeco. 2012.

'The EphA2 Receptor Drives Self-Renewal and Tumorigenicity in Stem-like Tumor-Propagating Cells from Human Glioblastomas.' *Cancer Cell* 22 (6): 765-80.

Bonnet, D., and John E. Dick. 1997. 'Human Acute Myeloid Leukemia Is Organized as a Hierarchy That Originates from a Primitive Hematopoietic Cell.' *Nature Medicine* 3 (7): 730-37.

Chaichana, K. L., Matthew J. McGirt, James Frazier, Frank Attenello, Hugo Guerrero-Cazares, and Alfredo Quinones-Hinojosa. 2008. 'Relationship of Glioblastoma Multiforme to the Lateral Ventricles Predicts Survival Following Tumor Resection.' *Journal of Neuro-Oncology* 89 (2): 219-24.

Chen, J., Yanjiao Li, Tzong-Shiue Yu, Renée M. McKay, Dennis K. Burns, Steven G. Kernie, and Luis F. Parada. 2012. 'A Restricted Cell Population Propagates Glioblastoma Growth after Chemotherapy.' *Nature* 488 (7412): 522-26.

Chiocca, E. A., Khalid M. Abbed, Stephen Tatter, David N. Louis, Fred H. Hochberg, Fred Barker, Jean Kracher, Stuart A. Grossman, Joy D. Fisher, and Kathryn Carson. 2004. 'A Phase I Open-Label, Dose-Escalation, Multi-Institutional Trial of Injection with an E1B-Attenuated Adenovirus, ONYX-015, into the Peritumoral Region of Recurrent Malignant Gliomas, in the Adjuvant Setting.' *Molecular Therapy* 10 (5): 958-66.

Dahmane, N., Pilar Sánchez, Yorick Gitton, Verónica Palma, Tao Sun, Mercedes Beyna, Howard Weiner, and Ariel Ruiz i Altaba. 2001. *'The Sonic Hedgehog-Gli Pathway Regulates Dorsal Brain Growth and Tumorigenesis.'*

Dai, C., Joseph C. Celestino, Yoshifumi Okada, David N. Louis, Greory N. Fuller, and Eric C. Holland. 2001. 'PDGF Autocrine Stimulation Dedifferentiates Cultured Astrocytes and Induces Oligodendrogliomas and Oligoastrocytomas from Neural Progenitors and Astrocytes *in Vivo*.' *Genes & Development* 15 (15): 1913-25.

Doucette, T., Ganesh Rao, Yuhui Yang, Joy Gumin, Naoki Shinojima, B. Nebiyou Bekele, Wei Qiao, Wei Zhang, and Frederick F. Lang. 2011. 'Mesenchymal Stem Cells Display Tumor-Specific Tropism in an RCAS/Ntv-a Glioma Model.' *Neoplasia* 13 (8): 716-25.

Fueyo, J., C. Gomez-Manzano, W. K. A. Yung, T. J. Liu, R. Alemany, Janet M. Bruner, S. K. Chintala, J. S. Rao, V. A. Levin, and A. P. Kyritsis. 1998. 'Suppression of Human Glioma Growth by Adenovirus-Mediated Rb Gene Transfer.' *Neurology* 50 (5): 1307-15.

Galderisi, U., M. Cipollaro, and A. Giordano. 2006. 'Stem Cells and Brain Cancer.' *Cell Death & Differentiation* 13 (1): 5-11.

Galli, R., Elena Binda, Ugo Orfanelli, Barbara Cipelletti, Angela Gritti, Simona De Vitis, Roberta Fiocco, Chiara Foroni, Francesco Dimeco, and Angelo Vescovi. 2004. 'Isolation and Characterization of Tumorigenic, Stem-like Neural Precursors from Human Glioblastoma.' *Cancer Research* 64 (19): 7011-21.

Gangemi, R. M. R., Fabrizio Griffero, Daniela Marubbi, Marzia Perera, Maria Cristina Capra, Paolo Malatesta, Gian Luigi Ravetti, Gian Luigi Zona, Antonio Daga, and Giorgio Corte. 2009. 'SOX2 Silencing in Glioblastoma Tumor-initiating Cells Causes Stop of Proliferation and Loss of Tumorigenicity.' *Stem Cells* 27 (1): 40-48.

Hallahan, A. R., Joel I. Pritchard, Stacey Hansen, Mark Benson, Jennifer Stoeck, Beryl A. Hatton, Thomas L. Russell, Richard G. Ellenbogen, Irwin D. Bernstein, and Phillip A. Beachy. 2004. 'The SmoA1 Mouse Model Reveals That Notch Signaling Is Critical for the Growth and Survival of Sonic Hedgehog-Induced Medulloblastomas.' *Cancer Research* 64 (21): 7794-7800.

Hopewell, J. W., and E. A. Wright. 1969. 'The Importance of Implantation Site in Cerebral Carcinogenesis in Rats.' *Cancer Research* 29 (11): 1927-31.

Immonen, A., Matti Vapalahti, Kristiina Tyynelä, Heleena Hurskainen, Anu Sandmair, Ritva Vanninen, Gillian Langford, Neil Murray, and Seppo Ylä-Herttuala. 2004. 'AdvHSV-Tk Gene Therapy with Intravenous Ganciclovir Improves Survival in Human Malignant Glioma: A Randomised, Controlled Study.' *Molecular Therapy* 10 (5): 967-72.

Jiang, H., Candelaria Gomez-Manzano, Frederick F. Lang, Ramon Alemany, and Juan Fueyo. 2009. 'Oncolytic Adenovirus: Preclinical and Clinical Studies in Patients with Human Malignant Gliomas.' *Current Gene Therapy* 9 (5): 422-27.

Lai, A., Anh Tran, Phioanh L. Nghiemphu, Whitney B. Pope, Orestes E. Solis, Michael Selch, Emese Filka, William H. Yong, Paul S. Mischel, and Linda M. Liau. 2010. 'Phase II Study of Bevacizumab Plus Temozolomide During and After Radiation Therapy for Patients With Newly Diagnosed Glioblastoma Multiforme.' *J Clin Oncol* 29: 142-48.

Lathia, J. D., Joseph Gallagher, John M. Heddleston, Jialiang Wang, Christine E. Eyler, Jennifer MacSwords, Qiulian Wu, Amit Vasanji, Roger E. McLendon, and Anita B. Hjelmeland. 2010. 'Integrin Alpha 6 Regulates Glioblastoma Stem Cells.' *Cell Stem Cell* 6 (5): 421-32.

Lee, H. Y., Maurice Kléber, Lisette Hari, Véronique Brault, Ueli Suter, Makoto M. Taketo, Rolf Kemler, and Lukas Sommer. 2004. 'Instructive Role of Wnt/ß-Catenin in Sensory Fate Specification in Neural Crest Stem Cells.' *Science* 303 (5660): 1020-23.

Liu, G., Xiangpeng Yuan, Zhaohui Zeng, Patrizia Tunici, Hiushan Ng, Iman R. Abdulkadir, Lizhi Lu, Dwain Irvin, Keith L. Black, and S. Yu John. 2006. 'Analysis of Gene Expression and Chemoresistance of CD133+ Cancer Stem Cells in Glioblastoma.' *Molecular Cancer* 5 (1): 1-12.

Nicolis, S. K. 2007. 'Cancer Stem Cells and "Stemness" Genes in Neuro-Oncology.' *Neurobiology of Disease* 25 (2): 217-29.

Nowell, P. C. 1976. 'The Clonal Evolution of Tumor Cell Populations.' *Science* 194 (4260): 23-28.

Perez, O. D., Christopher R. Logg, Kei Hiraoka, Oscar Diago, Ryan Burnett, Akihito Inagaki, Dawn Jolson, Karin Amundson, Taylor Buckley, and Dan Lohse. 2012. 'Design and Selection of Toca 511 for Clinical Use: Modified Retroviral Replicating Vector with Improved Stability and Gene Expression.' *Molecular Therapy* 20 (9): 1689-98.

Pertschuk, D., Timothy Francis Cloughesy, Susan Marina Chang, Manish K. Aghi, Michael A. Vogelbaum, Linda M. Liau, Bob B. Shafa, William H. Yong, Clark Chen, and Santosh Kesari. 2012. '*Ascending Dose Trials of the Safety and Tolerability of Toca 511, a Retroviral Replicating Vector Encoding Cytosine Deaminase, in Patients with Recurrent High-Grade Glioma.*'

Piccirillo, S. G. M., Brent A. Reynolds, Nadia Zanetti, Giuseppe Lamorte, Elena Binda, Giovanni Broggi, Henry Brem, Alessandro Olivi, Francesco Dimeco, and Angelo L.

Vescovi. 2006. 'Bone Morphogenetic Proteins Inhibit the Tumorigenic Potential of Human Brain Tumour-Initiating Cells.' *Nature* 444 (7120): 761-65.

Puumalainen, A. M., Matti Vapalahti, Reitu S. Agrawal, Maija Kossila, Johanna Laukkanen, Pauliina Lehtolainen, Helena Viita, Leo Paljärvi, Ritva Vanninen, and Seppo Ylä-Herttuala. 1998. 'β-Galactosidase Gene Transfer to Human Malignant Glioma *in Vivo* Using Replication-Deficient Retroviruses and Adenoviruses.' *Human Gene Therapy* 9 (12): 1769-74.

Quiñones-Hinojosa, A., and Kaisorn Chaichana. 2007. 'The Human Subventricular Zone: A Source of New Cells and a Potential Source of Brain Tumors.' *Experimental Neurology* 205 (2): 313-24.

Quintana, E., Mark Shackleton, Hannah R. Foster, Douglas R. Fullen, Michael S. Sabel, Timothy M. Johnson, and Sean J. Morrison. 2010. 'Phenotypic Heterogeneity among Tumorigenic Melanoma Cells from Patients That Is Reversible and Not Hierarchically Organized.' *Cancer Cell* 18 (5): 510-23.

Rainov, N. G. 2000. 'A Phase III Clinical Evaluation of Herpes Simplex Virus Type 1 Thymidine Kinase and Ganciclovir Gene Therapy as an Adjuvant to Surgical Resection and Radiation in Adults with Previously Untreated Glioblastoma Multiforme.' *Human Gene Therapy* 11 (17): 2389-2401.

Read, T. A., Marie P. Fogarty, Shirley L. Markant, Roger E. McLendon, Zhengzheng Wei, David W. Ellison, Phillip G. Febbo, and Robert J. Wechsler-Reya. 2009. 'Identification of CD15 as a Marker for Tumor-Propagating Cells in a Mouse Model of Medulloblastoma.' *Cancer Cell* 15 (2): 135-47.

Reya, T., Andrew W. Duncan, Laurie Ailles, Jos Domen, David C Scherer, Karl Willert, Lindsay Hintz, Roel Nusse, and Irving L. Weissman. 2003. 'A Role for Wnt Signalling in Self-Renewal of Haematopoietic Stem Cells.' *Nature* 423 (6938): 409-14.

Ricci-Vitiani, L., Roberto Pallini, Mauro Biffoni, Matilde Todaro, Gloria Invernici, Tonia Cenci, Giulio Maira, Eugenio Agostino Parati, Giorgio Stassi, and Luigi Maria Larocca. 2010. 'Tumour Vascularization via Endothelial Differentiation of Glioblastoma Stem-like Cells.' *Nature* 468 (7325): 824-28.

Rutka, J. T., Stacey Ivanchuk, Soma Mondal, Michael Taylor, Keiichi Sakai, Peter Dirks, Peter Jun, Shin Jung, Laurence E Becker, and Cameron Ackerley. 1999. 'Co-Expression of Nestin and Vimentin Intermediate Filaments in Invasive Human Astrocytoma Cells.' *International Journal of Developmental Neuroscience* 17 (5-6): 503-15.

Sanai, N., Arturo Alvarez-Buylla, and Mitchel S. Berger. 2005. 'Neural Stem Cells and the Origin of Gliomas.' *New England Journal of Medicine* 353 (8): 811-22.

Sandmair, A. M., Sami Loimas, Paula Puranen, Arto Immonen, Maija Kossila, Matti Puranen, Heleena Hurskainen, Kristiina Tyynelä, Marita Turunen, and Ritva Vanninen. 2000. 'Thymidine Kinase Gene Therapy for Human Malignant Glioma, Using Replication-Deficient Retroviruses or Adenoviruses.' *Human Gene Therapy* 11 (16): 2197-2205.

Shackleton, M., Elsa Quintana, Eric R. Fearon, and Sean J. Morrison. 2009. 'Heterogeneity in Cancer: Cancer Stem Cells versus Clonal Evolution.' *Cell* 138 (5): 822-29.

Shinojima, N., Anwar Hossain, Tatsuya Takezaki, Juan Fueyo, Joy Gumin, Feng Gao, Felix Nwajei, Frank C. Marini, Michael Andreeff, and Jun-Ichi Kuratsu. 2013. 'TGF-β

Mediates Homing of Bone Marrow-Derived Human Mesenchymal Stem Cells to Glioma Stem Cells.' *Cancer Research* 73 (7): 2333-44.

Singh, S. K., Cynthia Hawkins, Ian D. Clarke, Jeremy A. Squire, Jane Bayani, Takuichiro Hide, R. Mark Henkelman, Michael D. Cusimano, and Peter B. Dirks. 2004. 'Identification of Human Brain Tumour Initiating Cells.' *Nature* 432 (7015): 396-401.

Singh, S. K., Ian D. Clarke, Mizuhiko Terasaki, Victoria E. Bonn, Cynthia Hawkins, Jeremy Squire, and Peter B. Dirks. 2003. 'Identification of a Cancer Stem Cell in Human Brain Tumors.' *Cancer Research* 63 (18): 5821-28.

Singh, S. K., Ian D. Clarke, Takuichiro Hide, and Peter B. Dirks. 2004. 'Cancer Stem Cells in Nervous System Tumors.' *Oncogene* 23 (43): 7267-73.

Soda, Y., Tomotoshi Marumoto, Dinorah Friedmann-Morvinski, Mie Soda, Fei Liu, Hiroyuki Michiue, Sandra Pastorino, Meng Yang, Robert M. Hoffman, and Santosh Kesari. 2011. 'Transdifferentiation of Glioblastoma Cells into Vascular Endothelial Cells.' *Proceedings of the National Academy of Sciences* 108 (11): 4274-80.

Thomas, M., and A. M. Klibanov. 2003. 'Non-Viral Gene Therapy: Polycation-Mediated DNA Delivery.' *Applied Microbiology and Biotechnology* 62 (1): 27-34.

Tobias, A., Atique Ahmed, Kyung-Sub Moon, and Maciej S. Lesniak. 2013. 'The Art of Gene Therapy for Glioma: A Review of the Challenging Road to the Bedside.' *Journal of Neurology, Neurosurgery & Psychiatry* 84 (2): 213-22.

Varnum-Finney, B., Lanwei Xu, Carolyn Brashem-Stein, Cynthia Nourigat, David Flowers, Sonia Bakkour, Warren S. Pear, and Irwin D Bernstein. 2000. 'Pluripotent, Cytokine-Dependent, Hematopoietic Stem Cells Are Immortalized by Constitutive Notch1 Signaling.' *Nature Medicine* 6 (11): 1278-81.

Wan, F., Christel Herold-Mende, Benito Campos, Franz-Simon Centner, Christine Dictus, Natalia Becker, Frauke Devens, Carolin Mogler, Jörg Felsberg, and Niels Grabe. 2011. 'Association of Stem Cell-Related Markers and Survival in Astrocytic Gliomas.' *Biomarkers* 16 (2): 136-43.

Williams, R. T., Willem den Besten, and Charles J. Sherr. 2007. 'Cytokine-Dependent Imatinib Resistance in Mouse BCR-ABL+, Arf-Null Lymphoblastic Leukemia.' *Genes & Development* 21 (18): 2283-87.

Zhang, N., Ping Wei, Aihua Gong, Wen-Tai Chiu, Hsueh-Te Lee, Howard Colman, He Huang, Jianfei Xue, Mingguang Liu, and Yong Wang. 2011. 'FoxM1 Promotes β-Catenin Nuclear Localization and Controls Wnt Target-Gene Expression and Glioma Tumorigenesis.' *Cancer Cell* 20 (4): 427-42.

Zhang, Y., Yu-feng Zhang, Joshua Bryant, Andrew Charles, Ruben J. Boado, and William M. Pardridge. 2004. 'Intravenous RNA Interference Gene Therapy Targeting the Human Epidermal Growth Factor Receptor Prolongs Survival in Intracranial Brain Cancer.' *Clinical Cancer Research* 10 (11): 3667-77.

Zhu, J. X., Z. M. Li, F. Y. Geng, Qiang Fu, C. J. Guo, Y. L. Xiao, Z. T. Zhang, and Gang Li. 2010. 'Treatment of Recurrent Malignant Gliomas by Surgery Combined with Recombinant Adenovirus-P53 Injection.' Zhonghua Zhong Liu Za Zhi [*Chinese Journal of Oncology*] 32 (9): 709-12.

Chapter 15

Gamma Knife Radiosurgery for Brain Tumours: Contemporary Management

Ujwal Yeole and Nishanth Sadashiva
Department of Neurosurgery, National Institute of Mental Health and Neurosciences, Bengaluru, India

Abstract

"Everyone knows there is no such thing as Radiosurgery." That was the statement made by an editor when he rejected the seminal paper of Dr. Lars Leksell in 1951. Although many others contributed significantly to bringing it into reality, the surgical knife which works without opening the skull is a brainchild of 20 years of imagination and vision of Dr. Leksell. However, stereotactic device for lesion localisation in the brain was devised way before from 1908 through the work of Dr. Victor Horsley and Robert Clarke. In 1930, Leksell started his residency training under Olivercrona and saw frequent mortalities during open surgical procedures. Then he began developing techniques for minimal invasive intervention for treating neurosurgical ailments.

Introduction

The stereotactic devices use the three-dimensional Cartesian coordinate system for lesion localization. Leksell used rectilinear coordinate system with arc-centre principle in 1949 to deliver a probe to precise location and later changed it to an X-ray tube for delivering radiation in 1951. His initial interest was in treating functional disorders and his first attempt was made in a case of trigeminal neuralgia. There was complete pain relief at 5 months post

In: Advances in Neurosurgery Research
Editors: Amit Agrawal, Pradeep Chouksey, Adesh Shrivastava et al.
ISBN: 978-1-68507-859-1

procedure. As orthovoltage X-ray tubes were heavy and delivered low energy radiation, the procedure was tedious and time consuming to deliver required dose of radiation. Therefore, the search began for a high-energy source. The technical specifications for a prototype of gamma knife were finalised in 1967 with 179 sources of Cobalt-60. The first patient treated with this was in a factory at Studsvik, Sweden, who was suffering from craniopharyngioma. Gradually, gamma knife moved out of Sweden and reached Argentina, Italy, UK, US, and finally in Asia at Japan. Interest and acceptance of this technique came after multiple publications from different centres and especially Pittsburgh, USA, by Dr. Dade Lundsford after its establishment in 1987. Over the past 30 years, technological evolution with improved understanding of physics, radiobiology, and dose planning software has taken GKRS to higher echelons in the armamentarium of neurosurgeons worldwide. The number of Cobalt 60 sources increased from 179 to 192 in the latest version of machine ICON. Presently there are more than 340 functioning gamma knife centres treating more than 80,000 patients every year.

Functioning Unit of Gamma Knife Unit

Gamma knife uses radioactive source Cobalt 60. It decays to Nickel 60 to release gamma rays of 1.17 and 1.33 MeV for an average energy of 1.25 Mev. The Gamma Knife ICON, the latest version of the machine, harbours 192 sources of ^{60}Co. The typical half-life of ^{60}Co is 5.3 years, with an activity reduction rate of 1.1% per month. A single tungsten collimator allows beams of 4, 8, and 16mm in diameter in an eight-sliding-sector system design (Sahgal et al. 2009). Each source emits a beam of radiation that converges onto a focal point within the brain to deliver a "shot" of radiation. Multiple such shots of radiation cover the target volume and allow for sub-millimetre treatment accuracy and low-dose exposure beyond the target volume (Ma et al. 2011). As gamma rays are emitted continuously by the radioactive source, shielding is necessary when not in use. The 192 cobalt-60 sources are arranged into a conical shell and distributed within eight sectors, allowing for 2π geometry. Each sector has 24 sources, which can be blocked or positioned to 4-,8-, or 16-mm diameter collimators, resulting in converging beams of corresponding diameters at the centre. This source arrangement produces an ellipsoidal dose distribution with rapid three-dimensional (3D) falloff, which is the sharpest in the craniocaudal direction.

Mechanism of Action

Gamma rays are nothing but a packet of photons. These high energy photons interact with tissue by depositing energy through its path. They are called ionising radiation as their interaction with tissue leads to generation of ionised particles, electrons or free radicals. This is a cascading event as they interact with the lipids, proteins, nucleic acids, and water within cells causing damage by generation of further free radicals until energy in the photon becomes insufficient to cause further ionization.

Damage in the DNA is either seen as single stranded or double stranded breaks caused most frequently by hydroxyl (OH^-) free radicals generated by water ionisation. Once DNA damage occurs, cells either attempt to repair it by a series of steps, or if the damage is sufficient, cell death (apoptosis, necrosis) or growth arrest (senescence) occurs.

Radiobiology of Radiosurgery

Radiobiology is the study of normal tissue and target/tumour tissue response to ionizing radiation to maximise tumour response and minimize damage to normal tissue. Radiosurgery targets the lesion precisely due to use of stereotactic frame. Better localization eliminates the need to irradiate a 1-2 cm margin around a target/tumour tissue. It also exploits the ability of maximum radiation dosage to tumour tissue while minimizing spillage to surrounding tissue. Delivery of radiation dose through multiple small beams prevents exposure of normal tissue to full dose of radiation and it also reduces the radiation spilling into surrounding tissue beyond target volume. Cell death in tumour depends mainly upon the endothelial injury caused by high radiation doses, commonly used in excess of 8 Gy. Also, high dose of radiation delivered in single sitting impacts tumour cells directly, leading to cell necrosis. Radiopathology detected two types of changes: degenerative (in parenchyma) and proliferative (in connective tissue stroma or blood vessels of the lesion).

Technique of Gamma Knife Radiosurgery

Steps involved in GKRS:

1. Stereotactic frame placement.

2. Stereotactic brain imaging with MRI, CT, Angiography or any combination of these.
3. Coregistration of neurological images and importing to radio surgical outflow.
4. Treatment planning.
5. Dose prescription.
6. Dose limitations to critical structures.
7. Conformal dose planning.
8. Delivery of radiation to the target volume by positioning of the patient's head inside a collimator system.
9. Removal of stereotactic guiding device

Radiosurgery has other applications beyond brain tumours, but we are restricting our elaboration to brain tumours only to respect the editor's choice. Readers are advised to refer to other literature for different applications of radiosurgery in functional neurosurgery.

Tumours Treated with Radiosurgery (Figure 1)

Here we provide a brief overview of individual tumours treated with GKRS and available literature supporting it.

Table 1. The usual prescribed doses for single session gamma knife radiosurgery in commonly treated neurosurgical conditions

Diagnosis	Dose in Gy (median dose)
Vestibular schwannoma	11-13 (12)
Meningioma	10-20 (15)
Pituitary adenoma: non- secretory	12-17 (15)
Pituitary adenoma: secretory	22-28
Craniopharyngioma	10-15
Low Grade astrocytoma	12-15
High grade glioma	17-20
Metastatic tumour	16-24
Metastatic tumour plus Whole Brain RT	16-18
Glomus tumour	15
Other cranial schwannomas	12-14
Chordoma/Chondrosarcoma	17-22

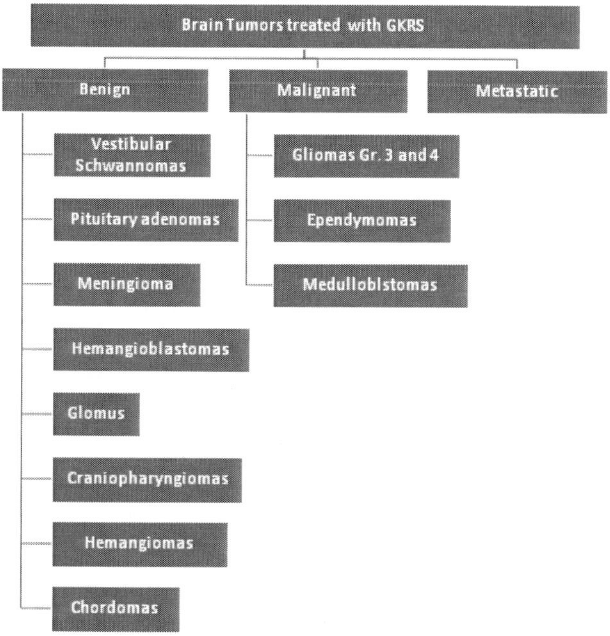

Figure 1. The list of commonly treated pathologies with gamma knife radiosurgery is as follows.

Vestibular Schwannoma

This is one of the biggest success stories of GKRS, with excellent tumour control rate of 98-99%, (A.R. et al. 2019) (Frischer et al. 2018) (Rueß et al. 2018) and facial nerve and trigeminal nerve preservation rate of 100% (J. C. Flickinger et al. 2001) (Régis et al. 2002)(Lobato-Polo et al. 2009) (Yang et al. 2009) and 96% (John C. Flickinger et al. 2004) (Marston et al. 2017) (Boari et al. 2014) respectively in different studies. GKRS is the preferred treatment for small and medium sized primary or residual VS. Long term follow-up form various series proved its efficacy over microsurgery or observation especially in functional preservation and excellent tumour control rates (Figure 2). The presently recommended marginal dose is 12-13Gy (Table 1) (John C. Flickinger et al. 2004).

By convention, most tumours are treated at around 50% isodose line, allowing the steepest dose falloff. Post gadolinium axial SPGR (Spoiled Gradient Recalled Acquisition in Steady State) imaging dataset is used for conformal dose planning. Hearing preservation primarily depends upon preprocedural hearing status, marginal dose, and the volume of tumour treated, along with dose received by cochlea. To a lesser degree, the radiation dose received by brainstem nuclei, cochlear nerve, and stria vascularis, considered to be the most sensitive area of the cochlea to ionizing radiation, also determine hearing preservation in the long-term. (Wackym et al. 2010) With advanced precision and dose reduction to cochlea to less than 4Gy, (Hasegawa et al. 2011)(Kano et al. 2013)(Baschnagel et al. 2013) hearing preservation rate has improved to more than 70% (A.R. et al. 2019) (Rueß et al. 2018).

Recently limits of GKRS expanded even beyond traditional limits of 3cm or 10cc tumour volume. Last decade showed multiple case series reporting successful treatment of larger tumours of more than 10cc or 3cm size with GKRS using similar dose of 12Gy with an acceptable tumour control rate of 82-92% (Yeole et al. 2021) (C. Huang et al. 2018)(Mezey et al. 2020). Functional outcome of facial nerve preservation following microsurgical resection is inversely proportional to size of the lesion (Iwai, Yamanaka, and Ishiguro 2003) (C.-K. Park et al. 2006). While GKRS has shown better preservation rate compared to microsurgery of 67% to 100%. (C. Huang et al. 2018)(Mezey et al. 2020) GKRS is also effective on other neurological symptoms associated with large VS like trigeminal pain or paresthesias (60%), gait disturbances (64%) at follow-up after reduction of lesion size (Yeole et al. 2021).

VSs in syndromic Neurofibromatosis type 2 (NF2) behaves more aggressively with a rapid growth rate and higher chances of recurrence and associated deafness. Morbidity associated with bilateral tumours is severe and hence GKRS provides a plausible option with tumour control rate of 50-88% (Sharma et al. 2010). Hearing preservation and facial or trigeminal neuropathy may occur more frequently than unilateral sporadic VS. Considering morbidity and mortality of microsurgery in bilateral VS, GKRS is a useful proactive measure available to neurosurgeons.

SRS has demonstrated reasonable tumour control for residual tumour after surgery, with an overall median growth control rate of 94% (range, 75–100%) at a median follow-up of 69 months. Follow-up imaging after secondary SRS demonstrate reduction in tumour size in 36 to 80% of cases, typically observed within 12 months of treatment (Mindermann and Schlegel 2014)(Pollock 2006) (Nagano et al. 2010) (Nagano et al. 2008). Tumour control after secondary SRS was not significantly different between patients being treated for progression and those being treated for recurrence (Pollock and Link 2008) (Bailo et al. 2017)(H.-C. Pan et al. 2012)(M. J. Huang et al. 2017). These results are favourable when compared to repeat MS, rendering SRS as the preferred secondary modality after primary MS for most cases of recurrent/progressive VS.

Meningioma

The gold standard treatment for meningiomas is Simpson's Gr. 0 microsurgical excision. But sometimes it is not feasible due to topographical location of tumour or its proximity to vital neurological structures like in skull base, cavernous sinus, or superior sagittal sinus. In such situations GKRS can be utilised either as primary form of treatment or as second line therapy after maximal microsurgical resection (Figure 3).

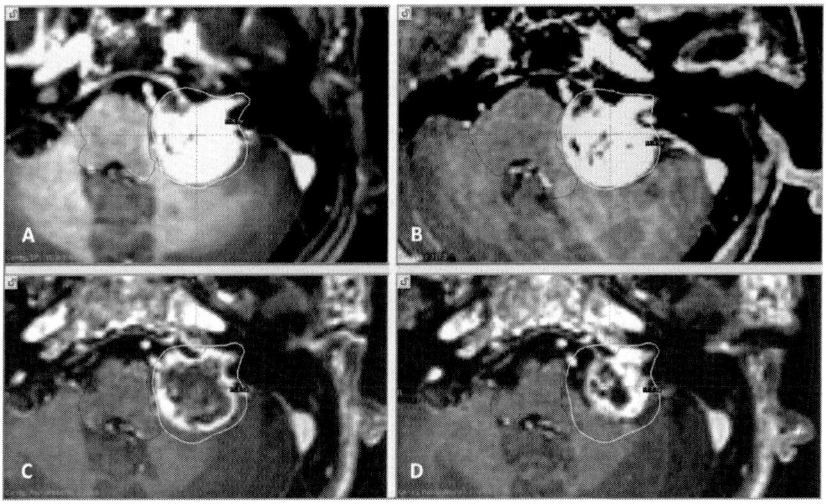

Figure 2. A. Shows images of a 70-year-old patient with left side vestibular schwannoma treated with radiosurgery, B, C and D shows subsequent scans done at 6 months intervals showing initial internal necrosis and later reduction in size of lesion.

Majority of meningiomas are WHO Gr. I tumours hence preservation of quality of life and avoidance of neurological morbidity are major treatment goals. The prescription dose for meningiomas is variable depending on the size of the lesion (Chin, Szerlip, and Regine 2003). Tumour control rate ranges from 84% (Seo et al. 2018) to 100% (Lee et al. 2016) (D. Kondziolka et al. 2016).

Proactive GKRS for asymptomatic meningiomas versus observation was assessed by Kim et al., showing radiological tumour control rate of 94.1% in GKRS group and progression was noted in 70.1% of observational group. Five year and 10-year survival rate in GKRS group (n = 153) was 98.7%, and 92.9% vs in observation groups (n = 201) was 64.6% and 42.7%, respectively in their study. (K. H. Kim et al. 2019) (Gupta et al. 2019)

Skull base meningiomas has shown PFS of 99% at three years to 97.2% at ten years. (Kreil et al. 2005) Tumours in petroclival or cavernous sinus regions develop considerable morbidity after microsurgical resection due to close proximity to critical neurovascular structures. Here GKRS can be a primary treatment modality with 5 year and 10 year PFS of 91% and 86%, respectively (Flannery et al. 2010) Systematic review of GKRS for posterior fossa meningiomas shows control rate of over 90%. (Jumah et al. 2020) Success rate for higher grade meningiomas is poor compared to grade I meningiomas with high local recurrence (C. K. Park et al. 2019) or progression in size (Kaprealian et al. 2016). Similarly, re-radiosurgery is viable option for gr. I meningiomas (M. Kim et al. 2017). Non-sporadic meningiomas associated with NF2 presenting with multiple lesions can be well controlled (90.7%) with GKRS; higher grade tumour, >2 lesions, peritumoral oedema, >1 GKRS in past are poor prognostic factors (Chen et al. 2019).

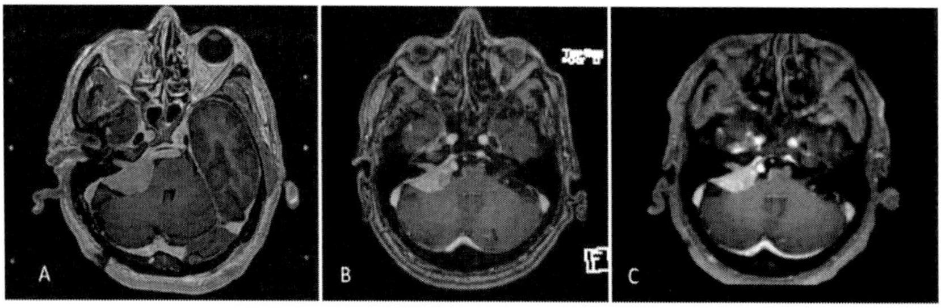

Figure 3. A shows a post-contrast axial MRI image of 60-year-old female with right petrous meningioma which was treated with gamma knife radiosurgery. B and C show subsequent images done yearly showing gradual decline in volume.

For large volume meningiomas in patients with multiple comorbidities who are at high risk for microsurgical resection, fractionated or single session GKRS provides an alternative form of treatment for tumour control. The 5-year tumour control rate in fractionated GKRS of 92.9% vs single session GKRS of 88.1% was noted (Bledsoe et al. 2010).

Pituitary Adenomas

Pituitary tumours are benign tumours, which are either hormone secreting (functioning), or non-functioning tumours which can cause mass effect on optic chiasm. The goal of treatment is different in both. In functioning tumours, it is biochemical cure, while in non-functioning tumour, reduction of mass effect by reducing tumour volume is attempted. Trans-sphenoidal surgery is presently a standard of care except in prolactinoma where medical management is the preferred first line of treatment. Other than surgery, medical management has a limited but definitive role in functioning tumours but not so much in non-functioning ones.

Radiotherapy plays an important role in recurrent or residual tumours which are not resectable due to their extent in critical areas like cavernous sinus. Conventional RT has its limitation in these tumours due to close proximity to chiasm and normal pituitary and post-RT delayed neuropathy or hypopituitarism are common complications in long-term (Casanueva et al. 2006)(Sholmo Melmed 2006).

In general, single session radiosurgical margin dose varies form 12-18 Gy for non-functioning and 15 to 30 Gy for functioning adenomas (Jagannathan et al. 2008)(Jagannathan et al. 2007)(J. P. Sheehan et al. 2013)(J. P. Sheehan et al. 2011)(J. M. Sheehan et al. 2000). Dose restriction of <8Gy to optic apparatus with minimum distance of 1 to 2mm from top of the adenoma to chiasm is desirable (Lim et al. 1998)(J. P. Sheehan et al. 2006)(Witt 2003).

Functioning tumours except prolactinomas require surgical excision and residual tumours in critical locations or recurrent lesions and surgically unfit candidates can be considered for GKRS. The major limitation of GKRS in functioning tumours is delayed response which averages to around 24 to 36 months, requiring effective medical treatment during this period.

Tumour control rate is excellent varying from 93% (J. P. Sheehan et al. 2011) (Mingione et al. 2006) to 100% (Castro, Cecílio, and Canteras 2010) (Hayashi et al. 2010) (Wilson et al. 2012) in non-functioning tumours. Cushing's disease demonstrates mean biochemical remission rate in 51% at an average time interval of 12 months (Jagannathan et al. 2007). Mean remission rate for acromegaly is 44.7%, with a median time to remission of 24 months (J. P. Sheehan et al. 2011). Hypothalamic-pituitary dysfunction is the commonest late complication of SRS seen in 30-50% developing new hormone deficiency 5 to 10 years after SRS (J. P. Sheehan et al. 2013)(J. P. Sheehan et al. 2011). Most SRS series report cranial neuropathy with neurological deficit in in <5%, with optic neuropathy being commonest (J. P.

Sheehan et al. 2013). Delayed recurrence after initial biochemical cure is rare but known (Jagannathan et al. 2007). Lifelong radiological and endocrinologic follow up is recommended after radiosurgery.

Glomus

Glomus jugulare and glomus Tympanicum are benign locally invasive tumours arising from the paraganglionic chemoreceptors. They can be sympathetic or parasympathetic with head and neck lesions being predominantly of the latter category. These are indolent locally destructive tumours. Treatment options available for them include microsurgical resection, embolization, fractioned RT or SRS and any combination of these. Surgical resection following embolization is a common strategy. Still, it is associated with significant morbidity with cranial nerve deficits. Hence, fractionated RT or SRS with primary aim to control tumor growth has become an attractive alternative. Marginal dose of 12-15 Gy for volume of less than 15cc is used depending on the volume location and cranial nerve function. Metanalysis published by Ivan et al. on tumour control rate in various treatment modalities of glomus included 869 patients from 46 publications. It showed tumour control rate of 86%, 71%, 95% following surgery, surgery f/b SRS and SRS alone, respectively with less cranial nerve deficits in SRS group (Ivan et al. 2011). Guss et al. reported 97% of tumour control and 95% of clinical control in another metanalysis of 335 patients (Zachary D. Guss, A.B., Sachin Batra, Charles J. Limb, Gordon Li, Michael E. Sughrue, Kristin Redmond, Daniele Rigamonti, Andrew T. Parsa, Steven Chang and Michael Lim 2011).

Hemangioblastomas

These are highly vascular solid cystic lesion in which primary treatment is microsurgery. 75-80% of them are sporadic and 20-25% of them are multiple and associated with syndromic transmission in the form of Von Hippel Lindau disease (VHL Syndrome). The role of SRS is mainly for deep seated lesion as a primary modality, or as salvage treatment in recurrent lesions.

Marginal dose of up to 18 Gy has been used with better long-term tumour control. A muticentre retrospective trial in American and Japanese GKRS centres showed PFS of 92% at three years, 89% at five years, and 79% at ten years. Factors associated with improved PFS included tumours associated with VHL syndrome, solid tumours, smaller volume, and higher marginal dose. (Kano et al. 2015) SRS is more effective on solid tumours or acts on mural nodule and cystic component may need drainage if symptomatic. (Moss et al. 2009) Tumour control rate varies from 69% to 100% (L. Pan et al. 1998)(Patrice et al. 1996)(Sayer et al. 2011).

Non-Vestibular Schwannomas

Schwannomas can arise from other cranial nerves, but trigeminal and jugular foramen are common. In these locations microsurgical resection needs complex skull base approaches. GKRS for residual lesions following microsurgery or upfront for small asymptomatic or minimally symptomatic lesions is a viable option. Dosages can be as high as 20Gy depending on the volume and location of the lesion and critical structures at risk. Tumour control rate ranges from 70-100%. (Sedney et al. 2013)(McRackan et al. 2012)(Fukuda et al. 2009)

Chordomas and Chondrosarcomas

These are slow growing indolent tumours of the skull base or spine. They are locally destructive and many are inaccessible for complete en-block resections at presentation. Conventional therapy consists of maximal surgical resection followed by fractionated RT. Recently, charged particle therapy like proton showed significant tumour control, but this is costly and not routinely available. SRS is useful as it can deliver a high dose of radiation in single fraction or sometimes in 2-5 fraction. This gives relative biological effectiveness, especially important in treatment of chordomas which are relatively radioresistant in nature. (Kano and Lunsford 2013) Tumour control rate of 40 to 67% is achieved with GKRS in chordomas (Cho et al. 2008) (Krishnan et al. 2005).

Chondrosarcomas are similar indolent tumours but with better clinical prognosis compared to chordomas. It is difficult to differentiate on routine imaging from chordomas. Surgical resection to reduce tumour burden is primary treatment. SRS is used as adjuvant therapy mainly for small residual tumours. Tumour control rate varies from 72% (Iyer et al. 2012) to 100%

(Krishnan et al. 2005) (Koga, Shin, and Saito 2010) at 5 years for marginal dose of minimum 15Gy.

Gliomas

Typically, gliomas are infiltrative tumours with ill-defined borders and variable size and are actually not ideal for GKRS. Only RCT, RTOG 93-05 investigated additional SRS to boost conventional therapy showed no survival advantage. Treatment protocol for gliomas is maximal safe surgical resection followed by concurrent chemo-radiotherapy with adjuvant chemotherapy. There is not much progress beyond this other than bevacizumab or few unconventional experimental therapies like vaccines and immune modulating therapies.

Pilocytic astrocytomas are circumscribed, Gr. I tumours which are ideal for surgical resection margins. Rarely, by virtue of their location in optic nerves, chiasm, or tectal plate, surgical resection especially in residual or recurrent settings is not an acceptable option. In such cases SRS can be an effective alternative. The dose can vary depending on the tolerability of the surrounding neurovascular structures.

In High grade astrocytomas (Gr. 3 and 4) post treatment recurrence usually occurs within 2 cm of the enhancing edge in 80% and within 1 cm in 50% (Wallner et al. 1989)(Fred H. Hochberg, M.D., and Amy Pruitt 1980). Consequently, use of WBRT for local control has limited benefit and higher dose used in SRS for focal region seems more logical. There are many small case series showing benefit of SRS boost in recurrent setting with improvement in OS by 9 months, with decrease in requirement of steroid dose, seizures and improvement in neurological deficits (M. van Kampen, R. Engenhart-Cabillic, J. Debus, M. FuB, B. Rhein 1998). Majority of these series are limited by selection bias and most cases eventually developed recurrence. At present SRS has limited but definite role in carefully selected cases with focal recurrence if other treatment resources have been exhausted. Extended field SRS enlarges a target tumour volume by an additional 0.5 to 1 cm beyond enhancing portion, trying to cover microscopic areas of infiltration (M. van Kampen, R. Engenhart-Cabillic, J. Debus, M. FuB, B. Rhein 1998).

In newly diagnosed GBM, SRS can be part of initial treatment contrary to the RTOG 93-05 study findings. There are some important criticisms of this study like use of carmustine (as it was before TMZ approval) and use of SRS before conventional therapy rather than as a boost to conventional RT

(Pouratian et al. 2009)(J. Sheehan 2012). Use of SRS in glioma is still debatable and needs further literature support for it to come into routine treatment protocols. The addition of bevacizumab to SRS may potentiate tumour control while lessening the risk of radiation necrosis.

In paediatric malignancies SRS can be used as an alternative to cranio-spinal radiation since long term side effects of radiation exposure on neuropsychological quotient and risk of secondary malignancy are known. The biggest hurdle in paediatric SRS is the application of rigid frame fixation and requirement of sedation or anaesthesia for treatment planning and precise delivery of high dose radiation. Frameless modalities for immobilisation are alternatives which can be tried with their own limitations.

Ependymomas

They are well circumscribed moderately cellular gliomas with sharp demarcation from surrounding brain. Also, they contain early responding tissue with no intervening normal brain tissue. Surgical resection is the most important prognostic factor in ependymoma with no effective chemo-therapeutic options, and postoperative EBRT is standard of care. SRS is a minimally invasive, localized treatment modality which may achieve local tumour control (>70% at 3 years). (Kano et al. 2010)(Stauder et al. 2012) Marginal and distant relapses can still occur. Post EBRT, in local recurrence which are not amenable to re-surgery by virtue of its location can be considered good candidates for SRS. Dose range varies from 9 to 22 Gy as a boost or as a salvage therapy.

Medulloblastoma

Role of radiotherapy with cranio-spinal radiation and posterior fossa boost is standard of care in medulloblastoma after surgery with chemotherapy. SRS can be used as an additional boost to deliver high dose to residual tumour or as a salvage therapy in recurrent tumours. Long-term side effects of cranio-spinal radiation in paediatric age group on memory, intellect and neuropsychological quotient are well established (Yeole et al. 2020) and attempts at reducing dosage of RT have been going along for decades. In such situations SRS can be useful but at a risk of distant failure, for which chemotherapy will be necessary. Presently literature support is scarce for use of SRS routinely and further evaluation with randomized trials is essential.

Metastasis

Whole brain Radiation Therapy (WBRT) was a gold standard treatment for brain metastasis for more than half a century. There are established early (impaired neurocognitive function) or delayed (radiation induced dementia or leukoencephalopathy) toxicities with WBRT (Chang et al. 2009). However, surgery may not be feasible either due to burden of disease or multiple metastasis or due to poor general condition of the patient. WBRT given following surgery for solitary metastasis decreases intracranial disease progression and the risk of neurological death while not impacting overall survival or performance status. (Patchell et al. 1998) (Kocher et al. 2011) Concerns with WBRT are due to neurotoxicity, cognitive impairment, and decline in quality of life (Chang et al. 2009) (Pulenzas et al. 2014).

SRS precisely delivers high-dose radiation to <3cm diameter target in a single session with steep dose falloff. It is minimally invasive compared to surgical excision with excellent local tumour control. Multiple lesions can be tackled in the same sitting and tumour shrinkage and oedema reduction both ameliorate neurological signs and symptoms, usually within few weeks of SRS treatment. It avoids leukoencephalopathy seen with WBRT (Pulenzas et al. 2014) and is effective on radioresistant tumours like melanoma, RCC and sarcoma. SRS is recommended for small multiple deep lesions or in patients not suitable for surgery.

In randomized trials, when compared to WBRT, WBRT+ SRS showed advantage of better local control, improved KPS and decreased dependency on steroids. (D. S. Kondziolka et al. 1999)(Andrews et al. 2004) Although there was no OS advantage, there was a favourable trend towards improved survival (M. Tsao, Xu, and Sahgal 2012). On the other hand, the use of SRS alone versus use of SRS+WBRT showed improved local control and distant control with addition of WBRT but with no added OS advantage (Aoyama et al. 2006). There is memory impairment at 4 months post WBRT when it was combined with SRS (Chang et al. 2009). Hence recommendation is to ideally combine both or use SRS alone if neurocognitive issues are high and use WBRT alone if patient is cognizant of radiation induced neurocognitive deficits.

Dose prescription is size dependent with 20Gy for lesions <2cm lesion, 18Gy for 2-3cm lesions and 15Gy for lesions 3-4 cm in size (Shaw et al. 2000)(Shehata et al. 2004). Isodose line above 70 is recommended for 1-3 brain metastasis to reduce treatment time without increase in local failure or radiation necrosis (Shiue et al. 2014).

Complications associated with SRS include radiation necrosis which is symptomatic and can be treated with steroids or bevacizumab and in case of significant mass effect with surgery. It is difficult to differentiate necrosis from recurrence completely without histopathological confirmation. MR spectroscopy, perfusion imaging and amino acid PET scan can help to a certain extent. Neurocognitive decline is another problem seen with combination of SRS with WBRT (Soffietti et al. 2013) and especially with WBRT (Chang et al. 2009).

For multiple intracranial metastases (>5), usual consensus guidelines from NCCN and American Society of Radiation Oncology (M. N. Tsao et al. 2012) say that WBRT is the preferred modality of treatment as SRS is unable to cover micro metastases in remaining brain. On the contrary, in the well-designed, sufficiently powered prospective JLGK 0901 trial, patients with 5 to 10 brain metastases with total volume < 15 mL fared no worse than patients with 2 to 4 in all end points analysed, including OS, intracranial tumour control, neurologic deterioration, and salvage therapy (Yamamoto et al. 2014). For recurrent metastases, local or new second SRS median survival time increases with actuarial survival rate of 58% and 35% at 6 and 12 months seen with maintenance of neurological status (Koiso et al. 2016).

Due to recent advances in systemic anti-cancer agent treatments, i.e., chemotherapeutic agents, tyrosine kinase inhibitors, immune check-point inhibitors, vascular endothelial growth factor inhibitors, and so on, increasing numbers of patients have been surviving longer. This makes it imperative for us to consider radiosurgery for brain metastasis as soon as they are detected. It is becoming increasingly evident that the mortality in cases of cancer is not dictated by brain metastasis, thanks to radiosurgery.

Conclusion

Gamma knife Radiosurgery is a valuable management strategy for a wide variety of neurosurgical patients. For lesions from benign tumours to malignant ones, for functional disorders from trigeminal neuralgia to obsessive compulsive disorder, radiosurgery has found its place as a management option. It is imperative for a neurosurgeon to have a basic knowledge of case selection as well as outcomes of gamma knife radiosurgery.

References

A.R., Prabhuraj, Ujwal Yeole, Arivazhagan Arimappamagan, K.V.L. Narasinga Rao, Dhananjaya I. Bhat, Srinivas Dwarakanath, Bhanumathi Govindswamy, and Sampath Somanna. 2019. "Effect of Gamma Knife Radiosurgery on Vestibular Schwannoma with Serviceable Hearing: A Single-Center Indian Study." *World Neurosurgery*, 127 (July): e114–23. https://doi.org/10.1016/j.wneu.2019.02.169.

Andrews, David W, Charles B Scott, Paul W Sperduto, Adam E Flanders, Laurie E Gaspar, Michael C Schell, Maria Werner-Wasik, et al. 2004. "Whole Brain Radiation Therapy with or without Stereotactic Radiosurgery Boost for Patients with One to Three Brain Metastases: Phase III Results of the RTOG 9508 Randomised Trial." *Lancet*, 363: 1665–72. http://www.ncbi.nlm.nih.gov/pubmed/15158627.

Aoyama, Hidefumi, Hiroki Shirato, Masao Tago, Keiichi Nakagawa, Tatsuya Toyoda, Kazuo Hatano, Masahiro Kenjyo, et al. 2006. "Stereotactic Radiosurgery plus Whole-Brain Radiation Therapy vs Stereotactic Radiosurgery Alone for Treatment of Brain Metastases: A Randomized Controlled Trial." *Journal of the American Medical Association*, 295 (21): 2483–91. https://doi.org/10.1001/jama.295.21.2483.

Bailo, Michele, Nicola Boari, Filippo Gagliardi, Alberto Franzin, Martina Piloni, Alfio Spina, Marco Gemma, Antonella Del Vecchio, Angelo Bolognesi, and Pietro Mortini. 2017. "Gamma Knife Radiosurgery for Residual and Recurrent Vestibular Schwannomas After Previous Surgery: Clinical Results in a Series of 90 Patients and Review of the Literature." *World Neurosurgery*, 98 (February): 60–72. https://doi.org/10.1016/j.wneu.2016.10.066.

Baschnagel, Andrew M., Peter Y. Chen, Dennis Bojrab, Daniel Pieper, Jack Kartush, Oksana Didyuk, Ilka C. Naumann, Ann Maitz, and Inga S. Grills. 2013. "Hearing Preservation in Patients with Vestibular Schwannoma Treated with Gamma Knife Surgery." *Journal of Neurosurgery*, 118 (3): 571–78. https://doi.org/10.3171/2012.10.JNS12880.

Bledsoe, Jonathan M., Michael J. Link, Scott L. Stafford, Paul J. Park, and Bruce E. Pollock. 2010. "Radiosurgery for Large-Volume (> 10 Cm3) Benign Meningiomas." *Journal of Neurosurgery*, 112 (5): 951–56. https://doi.org/10.3171/2009.8.JNS09703.

Boari, Nicola, Michele Bailo, Filippo Gagliardi, Alberto Franzin, Marco Gemma, Antonella Del Vecchio, Angelo Bolognesi, Piero Picozzi, and Pietro Mortini. 2014. "Gamma Knife Radiosurgery for Vestibular Schwannoma: Clinical Results at Long-Term Follow-up in a Series of 379 Patients." *Journal of Neurosurgery*, 121 (Suppl_2): 123–42. https://doi.org/10.3171/2014.8.GKS141506.

Casanueva, Felipe F., Mark E. Molitch, Janet A. Schlechte, Roger Abs, Vivien Bonert, Marcello D. Bronstein, Thierry Brue, et al. 2006. "Guidelines of the Pituitary Society for the Diagnosis and Management of Prolactinomas." *Clinical Endocrinology*, 65 (2): 265–73. https://doi.org/10.1111/j.1365-2265.2006.02562.x.

Castro, Douglas G., Soraya A.J. Cecílio, and Miguel M. Canteras. 2010. "Radiosurgery for Pituitary Adenomas: Evaluation of Its Efficacy and Safety." *Radiation Oncology*, 5 (1): 1–6. https://doi.org/10.1186/1748-717X-5-109.

Chang, Eric L., Jeffrey S. Wefel, Kenneth R. Hess, Pamela K. Allen, Frederick F. Lang, David G. Kornguth, Rebecca B. Arbuckle, et al. 2009. "Neurocognition in Patients with Brain Metastases Treated with Radiosurgery or Radiosurgery plus Whole-Brain Irradiation: A Randomised Controlled Trial." *The Lancet Oncology*, 10 (11): 1037–44. https://doi.org/10.1016/S1470-2045(09)70263-3.

Chen, Wei, Xiaoyu Wang, F. Liu, and Jing Chen. 2019. "Gamma Knife Radiosurgery for Patients with Multiple Intracranial Meningiomas." *World Neurosurgery*, 128: e495–500. https://doi.org/10.1016/j.wneu.2019.04.184.

Chin, Lawrence S., Nicholas J. Szerlip, and William F. Regine. 2003. "Stereotactic Radiosurgery for Meningiomas." *Neurosurgical Focus*, 14 (5): 1–6. https://doi.org/10.3171/foc.2003.14.5.7.

Cho, Young Hyun, Jeong Hoon Kim, Shin Kwang Khang, Jung Kyo Lee, and Chang Jin Kim. 2008. "Chordomas and Chondrosarcomas of the Skull Base: Comparative Analysis of Clinical Results in 30 Patients." *Neurosurgical Review*, 31 (1): 35–43. https://doi.org/10.1007/s10143-007-0099-z.

Flannery, Thomas J., Hideyuki Kano, L. Dade Lunsford, Sait Sirin, Matthew Tormenti, Ajay Niranjan, John C. Flickinger, and Douglas Kondziolka. 2010. "Long-Term Control of Petroclival Meningiomas through Radiosurgery: Clinical Article." *Journal of Neurosurgery*, 112 (5): 957–64. https://doi.org/10.3171/2009.8.JNS09695.

Flickinger, J. C., D. Kondziolka, A. Niranjan, and L. D. Lunsford. 2001. "Results of Acoustic Neuroma Radiosurgery: An Analysis of 5 Years' Experience Using Current Methods." *Journal of Neurosurgery*, 94 (1): 1–6. https://doi.org/10.3171/jns.2001.94.1.0001.

Flickinger, John C., Douglas Kondziolka, Ajay Niranjan, Ann Maitz, George Voynov, and L. Dade Lunsford. 2004. "Acoustic Neuroma Radiosurgery with Marginal Tumor Doses of 12 to 13 Gy." *International Journal of Radiation Oncology Biology Physics*, 60 (1): 225–30. https://doi.org/10.1016/j.ijrobp.2004.02.019.

Fred H. Hochberg, M.D., and Amy Pruitt, M.D. 1980. "Assumptions in the Radiotherapy of Glioblastoma." *Neurology*, 30 (9): 907–11. https://doi.org/10.1212/wnl.30.9.907.

Frischer, Josa M., Elise Gruber, Verena Schöffmann, Adolf Ertl, Romana Höftberger, Ammar Mallouhi, Stefan Wolfsberger, et al. 2018. "Long-Term Outcome after Gamma Knife Radiosurgery for Acoustic Neuroma of All Koos Grades: A Single-Center Study." *Journal of Neurosurgery*. https://doi.org/10.3171/2017.8.JNS171281.

Fukuda, Masafumi, Makoto Oishi, Akihiko Saito, and Yukihiko Fujii. 2009. "Long-Term Outcomes after Surgical Treatment of Jugular Foramen Schwannoma." *Skull Base*, 19 (6): 401–8. https://doi.org/10.1055/s-0029-1220197.

Gupta, Amitabh, Zhiyuan Xu, Or Cohen-Inbar, M. Harrison Snyder, Landon K. Hobbs, Chelsea Li, Quoc Tuan Nguyen, and Jason P. Sheehan. 2019. "Treatment of Asymptomatic Meningioma with Gamma Knife Radiosurgery: Long-Term Follow-up with Volumetric Assessment and Clinical Outcome." *Clinical Neurosurgery*, 85 (5): E889–99. https://doi.org/10.1093/neuros/nyz126.

Hasegawa, Toshinori, Yoshihisa Kida, Takenori Kato, Hiroshi Iizuka, and Takashi Yamamoto. 2011. "Factors Associated with Hearing Preservation after Gamma Knife Surgery for Vestibular Schwannomas in Patients Who Retain Serviceable Hearing." *Journal of Neurosurgery*, 115 (6): 1078–86. https://doi.org/10.3171/2011.7.JNS 11749.

Hayashi, Motohiro, Mikhail Chernov, Noriko Tamura, Mariko Nagai, Shoji Yomo, Taku Ochiai, Kosaku Amano, et al. 2010. "Gamma Knife Robotic Microradiosurgery of Pituitary Adenomas Invading the Cavernous Sinus: Treatment Concept and Results in 89 Cases." *Journal of Neuro-Oncology*, 98 (2): 185–94. https://doi.org/10.1007/s11060-010-0172-2.

Huang, Cheng-wei, Hsien-tang Tu, Chun-yi Chuang, Cheng-siu Chang, Hsi-hsien Chou, Ming-tsung Lee, and Chuan-fu Huang. 2018. "Gamma Knife Radiosurgery for Large Vestibular Schwannomas Greater than 3 Cm in Diameter." *Journal of Neurosurgery*, 128 (May): 1380–87. https://doi.org/10.3171/2016.12.JNS161530.J.

Huang, Marshall J, Hideyuki Kano, Seyed H Mousavi, Ajay Niranjan, Edward A 3rd Monaco, Yoshio Arai, John C Flickinger, and L Dade Lunsford. 2017. "Stereotactic Radiosurgery for Recurrent Vestibular Schwannoma after Previous Resection." *Journal of Neurosurgery*, 126 (5): 1506–13. https://doi.org/10.3171/2016.5.JNS1645.

Ivan, Michael E., Michael E. Sughrue, Aaron J. Clark, Ari J. Kane, Derick Aranda, Igor J. Barani, and Andrew T. Parsa. 2011. "A Meta-Analysis of Tumor Control Rates and Treatment-Related Morbidity for Patients with Glomus Jugulare Tumors." *Journal of Neurosurgery*, 114 (5): 1299–1305. https://doi.org/10.3171/2010.9.JNS10699.

Iwai, Yoshiyasu, Kazuhiro Yamanaka, and Tomoya Ishiguro. 2003. "Surgery Combined with Radiosurgery of Large Acoustic Neuromas." *Surgical Neurology*, 59 (4): 283–89. https://doi.org/10.1016/S0090-3019(03)00025-9.

Iyer, Aditya, Hideyuki Kano, Douglas Kondziolka, Xiaomin Liu, Ajay Niranjan, John C. Flickinger, and L. Dade Lunsford. 2012. "Stereotactic Radiosurgery for Intracranial Chondrosarcoma." *Journal of Neuro-Oncology*, 108 (3): 535–42. https://doi.org/10.1007/s11060-012-0858-8.

Jagannathan, Jay, Jason P. Sheehan, Nader Pouratian, Edward R. Laws, Ladislau Steiner, and Mary Lee Vance. 2007. "Gamma Knife Surgery for Cushing's Disease." *Journal of Neurosurgery*, 106: 980–87. https://doi.org/10.3171/JNS-07/07/0007.

———. 2008. "Gamma Knife Radiosurgery for Acromegaly: Outcomes after Failed Transsphenoidal Surgery: Commentary." *Neurosurgery*, 62 (6): 1270. https://doi.org/10.1227/01.NEU.0000316818.41382.A1.

Jain, Deepali, Mehar Chand Sharma, Chitra Sarkar, Deepak Gupta, Manmohan Singh, and A. K. Mahapatra. 2006. "Comparative Analysis of Diagnostic Accuracy of Different Brain Biopsy Procedures." *Neurology India*, 54 (4): 394–98. https://doi.org/10.4103/0028-3886.28113.

Jumah, Fareed, Vinayak Narayan, Amjad Samara, Travis R. Quinoa, Rimal Hanif Dossani, Gaurav Gupta, and Anil Nanda. 2020. "Efficacy and Safety of Gamma Knife Radiosurgery for Posterior Cranial Fossa Meningioma: A Systematic Review." *Neurosurgical Review*, 43 (4): 1089–99. https://doi.org/10.1007/s10143-019-01144-x.

Kano, Hideyuki, Douglas Kondziolka, Aftab Khan, John C Flickinger, and L Dade Lunsford. 2013. "Predictors of Hearing Preservation after Stereotactic Radiosurgery for Acoustic Neuroma: Clinical Article." *Journal of Neurosurgery*. https://doi.org/10.3171/2008.12.JNS08611.

Kano, Hideyuki, and L. Dade Lunsford. 2013. "Stereotactic Radiosurgery of Intracranial Chordomas, Chondrosarcomas, and Glomus Tumors." *Neurosurgery Clinics of North America*, 24 (4): 553–60. https://doi.org/10.1016/j.nec.2013.05.009.

Kano, Hideyuki, Takashi Shuto, Yoshiyasu Iwai, Jason Sheehan, Masaaki Yamamoto, Heyoung L. McBride, Mitsuya Sato, et al. 2015. "Stereotactic Radiosurgery for Intracranial Hemangioblastomas: A Retrospective International Outcome Study." *Journal of Neurosurgery*, 122 (6): 1469–78. https://doi.org/10.3171/ 2014.10.JNS 131602.

Kano, Hideyuki, Huai Che Yang, Douglas Kondziolka, Ajay Niranjan, Yoshio Arai, John C. Flickinger, and L. Dade Lunsford. 2010. "Stereotactic Radiosurgery for Pediatric Recurrent Intracranial Ependymomas: Clinical Article." *Journal of Neurosurgery: Pediatrics*, 6 (5): 417–23. https://doi.org/10.3171/2010.8.PEDS10252.

Kaprealian, Tania, David R. Raleigh, Penny K. Sneed, Nima Nabavizadeh, Jean L. Nakamura, and Michael W. McDermott. 2016. "Parameters Influencing Local Control of Meningiomas Treated with Radiosurgery." *Journal of Neuro-Oncology*, 128 (2): 357–64. https://doi.org/10.1007/s11060-016-2121-1.

Kim, Kyung Hwan, So Jeong Kang, Jung Won Choi, Doo Sik Kong, Ho Jun Seol, Do Hyun Nam, and Jung Il Lee. 2019. "Clinical and Radiological Outcomes of Proactive Gamma Knife Surgery for Asymptomatic Meningiomas Compared with the Natural Course without Intervention." *Journal of Neurosurgery*, 130 (5): 1740–49. https://doi.org/10.3171/2017.12.JNS171943.

Kim, Moinay, Do Hee Lee, Hyun Jung Kim RN, Young Hyun Cho, Jeong Hoon Kim, and Do Hoon Kwon. 2017. "Analysis of the Results of Recurrent Intracranial Meningiomas Treated with Re-Radiosurgery." *Clinical Neurology and Neurosurgery*, 153: 93–101. https://doi.org/10.1016/j.clineuro.2016.12.014.

Kocher, Martin, Riccardo Soffietti, Ufuk Abacioglu, Salvador Villà, Francois Fauchon, Brigitta G. Baumert, Laura Fariselli, et al. 2011. "Adjuvant Whole-Brain Radiotherapy versus Observation after Radiosurgery or Surgical Resection of One to Three Cerebral Metastases: Results of the EORTC 22952-26001 Study." *Journal of Clinical Oncology*, 29 (2): 134–41. https://doi.org/10.1200/JCO.2010.30.1655.

Koga, Tomoyuki, Masahiro Shin, and Nobuhito Saito. 2010. "Treatment with High Marginal Dose Is Mandatory to Achieve Long-Term Control of Skull Base Chordomas and Chondrosarcomas by Means of Stereotactic Radiosurgery." *Journal of Neuro-Oncology*, 98 (2): 233–38. https://doi.org/10.1007/s11060-010-0184-y.

Koiso, Takao, Masaaki Yamamoto, Takuya Kawabe, Shinya Watanabe, Yasunori Sato, Yoshinori Higuchi, Tetsuya Yamamoto, Akira Matsumura, and Hidetoshi Kasuya. 2016. "Follow-up Results of Brain Metastasis Patients Undergoing Repeat Gamma Knife Radiosurgery." *Journal of Neurosurgery*, 125 (December): 2–10. https://doi.org/10.3171/2016.6.gks161404.

Kondziolka, Douglas, Agam D. Patel, Hideyuki Kano, John C. Flickinger, and L. Dade Lunsford. 2016. "Long-Term Outcomes after Gamma Knife Radiosurgery for

Meningiomas." *American Journal of Clinical Oncology: Cancer Clinical Trials*, 39 (5): 453–57. https://doi.org/10.1097/COC.0000000000000080.

Kondziolka, Douglas S., Atul Patel, L. Dade Lunsford, Kassam Amin, and John C. Flickinger. 1999. "Stereotactic Radiosurgery plus Whole Brain Radiotherapy Alone for Patients with Multiple Brain Metastases." *International Journal of Radiation Oncology, Biology, Physics*, 45 (2): 427–34. https://doi.org/10.1016/s0360-3016(00) 00498-3.

Kreil, W., J. Luggin, I. Fuchs, V. Weigl, S. Eustacchio, and G. Papaefthymiou. 2005. "Long Term Experience of Gamma Knife Radiosurgery for Benign Skull Base Meningiomas." *Journal of Neurology, Neurosurgery and Psychiatry*, 76 (10): 1425–30. https://doi.org/10.1136/jnnp.2004.049213.

Krishnan, Sunil, Robert L. Foote, Paul D. Brown, Bruce E. Pollock, Michael J. Link, and Yolanda I. Garces. 2005. "Radiosurgery for Cranial Base Chordomas and Chondrosarcomas." *Neurosurgery*, 56 (4): 777–83. https://doi.org/10.1227/ 01. NEU.0000156789.10394.F5.

Lee, Seungjoo, Do Hoon Kwon, Chang Jin Kim, and Jeong Hoon Kim. 2016. "Long-Term Outcomes Following Gamma Knife Radiosurgery for Small, Newly Diagnosed Meningiomas." *Clinical Neurology and Neurosurgery*, 142: 1–7. https://doi.org/ 10.1016/j.clineuro.2016.01.009.

Lim, Y. J., W. Leem, T. S. Kim, B. A. Rhee, and G. K. Kim. 1998. "Four Years' Experiences in the Treatment of Pituitary Adenomas with Gamma Knife Radiosurgery." *Stereotactic and Functional Neurosurgery*, 70 (SUPPL. 1): 95–109. https://doi.org/10.1159/000056412.

Lobato-Polo, Javier, Douglas Kondziolka, Oscar Zorro, Hideyuki Kano, John C. Flickinger, and L. Dade Lunsford. 2009. "Gamma Knife Radiosurgery in Younger Patients with Vestibular Schwannomas." *Neurosurgery*, 65 (2): 294–300. https://doi.org/10.1227/01.NEU.0000345944.14065.35.

M. van Kampen, R. Engenhart-Cabillic, J. Debus, M. FuB, B. Rhein, M. Wannenmacher. 1998. "Originalarbeit Radiochirurgie Des Glioblastoma Multiforme." *Strahlentherapie Und Onkologi*, 174 (1): 19–24.

Ma, Lijun, Paula Petti, Brian Wang, Martina Descovich, Cynthia Chuang, Igor J. Barani, Sandeep Kunwar, Dennis C. Shrieve, Arjun Sahgal, and David A. Larson. 2011. "Apparatus Dependence of Normal Brain Tissue Dose in Stereotactic Radiosurgery for Multiple Brain Metastases: Technical Note." *Journal of Neurosurgery*, 114 (6): 1580–84. https://doi.org/10.3171/2011.1.JNS101056.

Marston, Alexander P., Jeffrey T. Jacob, Matthew L. Carlson, Bruce E. Pollock, Colin L.W. Driscoll, and Michael J. Link. 2017. "Pretreatment Growth Rate as a Predictor of Tumor Control Following Gamma Knife Radiosurgery for Sporadic Vestibular Schwannoma." *Journal of Neurosurgery*, 127 (2): 380–87. https://doi.org/10.3171/ 2016.5.JNS153013.

McRackan, Theodore R., Alejandro Rivas, George B. Wanna, Mi Jin Yoo, Marc L. Bennett, Mary S. Deitrich, Michael E. Glasscock, and David S. Haynes. 2012. "Facial Nerve Outcomes in Facial Nerve Schwannomas." *Otology and Neurotology*, 33 (1): 78–82. https://doi.org/10.1097/MAO.0b013e31823c8ef1.

Mezey, Geza, Julian Cahill, Jeremy G. Rowe, John Yianni, Debapriya Bhattacharyya, Lee Walton, Joanne Rodgers, and Matthias W.R. Radatz. 2020. "A Retrospective Analysis of the Role of Single-Session Gamma Knife Stereotactic Radiosurgery in Sporadic Vestibular Schwannomas with Tumor Volumes Greater Than 10 Cm^3: Is It Worth Stretching the Boundaries?" *Stereotactic and Functional Neurosurgery*, 98 (2): 85–94. https://doi.org/10.1159/000504857.

Mindermann, Thomas, and Ines Schlegel. 2014. "How to Distinguish Tumor Growth from Transient Expansion of Vestibular Schwannomas Following Gamma Knife Radiosurgery." *Acta Neurochirurgica*, 156 (6): 1121–23. https://doi.org/10.1007/s00701-014-2063-3.

Mingione, Vincenzo, Po Yen Chun, Mary Lee Vance, Melita Steiner, Jason Sheehan, Edward R. Laws, and Ladislau Steiner. 2006. "Gamma Surgery in the Treatment of Nonsecretory Pituitary Macroadenoma." *Journal of Neurosurgery*, 104 (6): 876–83. https://doi.org/10.3171/jns.2006.104.6.876.

Moss, Jason M., Clara Y.H. Choi, John R. Adler, Scott G. Soltys, Iris C. Gibbs, and Steven D. Chang. 2009. "Stereotactic Radiosurgical Treatment of Cranial and Spinal Hemangioblastomas." *Neurosurgery*, 65 (1): 79–85. https://doi.org/10.1227/01.NEU.0000348015.51685.D2.

Nagano, Osamu, Yoshinori Higuchi, Toru Serizawa, Junichi Ono, Shinji Matsuda, Iwao Yamakami, and Naokatsu Saeki. 2008. "Transient Expansion of Vestibular Schwannoma Following Stereotactic Radiosurgery: Clinical Article." *Journal of Neurosurgery*, 109 (5): 811–16. https://doi.org/10.3171/JNS/2008/109/11/0811.

Nagano, Osamu, Toru Serizawa, Yoshinori Higuchi, Shinji Matsuda, Makoto Sato, Iwao Yamakami, Koichi Okiyama, Junichi Ono, and Naokatsu Saeki. 2010. "Tumor Shrinkage of Vestibular Schwannomas after Gamma Knife Surgery: Results after More than 5 Years of Follow-Up." *Journal of Neurosurgery*, 113 Suppl (December): 122–27.

Pan, Hung-Chuan, Jason Sheehan, Meei-Ling Sheu, Wen-Ta Chiu, and Dar-Yu Yang. 2012. "Intracapsular Decompression or Radical Resection Followed by Gamma Knife Surgery for Patients Harboring a Large Vestibular Schwannoma." *Journal of Neurosurgery*, 117 Suppl (December): 69–77. https://doi.org/10.3171/ 2012.6.GKS 12697.

Pan, L., E. M. Wang, B. J. Wang, L. F. Zhou, N. Zhang, P. W. Cai, and J. Z. Da. 1998. "Gamma Knife Radiosurgery for Hemangioblastomas." *Stereotactic and Functional Neurosurgery*, 70 (SUPPL. 1): 179–86. https://doi.org/10.1159/000056420.

Park, Chang Kyu, Na Young Jung, Won Seok Chang, Hyun Ho Jung, and Jin Woo Chang. 2019. "Gamma Knife Radiosurgery for Postoperative Remnant Meningioma: Analysis of Recurrence Factors According to World Health Organization Grade." *World Neurosurgery*, 132: e399–402. https://doi.org/10.1016/j.wneu.2019.08.136.

Park, Chul-Kee, Hee-Won Jung, Jeong Eun Kim, Young-Je Son, Sun Ha Paek, and Dong Gyu Kim. 2006. "Therapeutic Strategy for Large Vestibular Schwannomas." *Journal of Neuro-Oncology*, 77 (2): 167–71. https://doi.org/10.1007/s11060-005-9015-y.

Patchell, Roy A., Phillip A. Tibbs, William F. Regine, Robert J. Dempsey, Mohammed Mohiuddin, Richard J. Kryscio, William R. Markesbery, Kenneth A. Foon, and Byron Young. 1998. "Postoperative Radiotherapy in the Treatment of Single Metastases to the Brain: A Randomized Trial." *Journal of the American Medical Association*, 280 (17): 1485–89. https://doi.org/10.1001/jama.280.17.1485.

Patrice, Stephen J., Penny K. Sneed, John C. Flickinger, Dennis C. Shrieve, Bruce E. Pollock, Eben Alexander, David A. Larson, et al. 1996. "Radiosurgery for Hemangioblastoma: Results of a Multiinstitutional Experience." *International Journal of Radiation Oncology Biology Physics*, 35 (3): 493–99. https://doi.org/10.1016/S0360-3016(96)80011-3.

Pollock, Bruce E. 2006. "Management of Vestibular Schwannomas That Enlarge after Stereotactic Radiosurgery: Treatment Recommendations Based on a 15 Year Experience." *Neurosurgery*, 58 (2): 241–46. https://doi.org/10.1227/01.NEU.0000194833.66593.8B.

Pollock, Bruce E, and Michael J Link. 2008. "Vestibular Schwannoma Radiosurgery after Previous Surgical Resection or Stereotactic Radiosurgery." *Progress in Neurological Surgery*, 21: 163–68. https://doi.org/10.1159/000156904.

Pouratian, Nader, R. Webster Crowley, Jonathan H. Sherman, Jay Jagannathan, and Jason P. Sheehan. 2009. "Gamma Knife Radiosurgery after Radiation Therapy as an Adjunctive Treatment for Glioblastoma." *Journal of Neuro-Oncology*, 94 (3): 409–18. https://doi.org/10.1007/s11060-009-9873-9.

Pulenzas, Natalie, Luluel Khan, May Tsao, Liying Zhang, Breanne Lechner, Nemica Thavarajah, Elizabeth Barnes, et al. 2014. "Fatigue Scores in Patients with Brain Metastases Receiving Whole Brain Radiotherapy." *Supportive Care in Cancer*, 22 (7): 1757–63. https://doi.org/10.1007/s00520-014-2140-4.

Régis, Jean, William Pellet, Christine Delsanti, Henry Dufour, Pierre Hughes Roche, Jean Marc Thomassin, Michel Zanaret, and Jean Claude Peragut. 2002. "Functional Outcome after Gamma Knife Surgery or Microsurgery for Vestibular Schwannomas." *Journal of Neurosurgery*, 97 (5): 1091–1100. https://doi.org/10.3171/jns.2002.97.5.1091.

Rueß, Daniel, Lea Pöhlmann, Alexandra Hellerbach, Christina Hamisch, Mauritius Hoevels, Harald Treuer, Stefan Grau, Karolina Jablonska, Martin Kocher, and Maximilian I. Ruge. 2018. "Acoustic Neuroma Treated with Stereotactic Radiosurgery: Follow-up of 335 Patients." *World Neurosurgery*, 116 (August): e194–202. https://doi.org/10.1016/j.wneu.2018.04.149.

Sahgal, Arjun, Lijun Ma, Eric Chang, Almon Shiu, David A. Larson, Normand Laperriere, Fang Fang Yin, et al. 2009. "Advances in Technology for Intracranial Stereotactic Radiosurgery." *Technology in Cancer Research and Treatment*, 8 (4): 271–80. https://doi.org/10.1177/153303460900800404.

Sayer, Faisal T., James Nguyen, Robert M. Starke, Chun Po Yen, and Jason P. Sheehan. 2011. "Gamma Knife Radiosurgery for Intracranial Hemangioblastomas-Outcome at 3 Years." *World Neurosurgery*, 75 (1): 99–105. https://doi.org/10.1016/j.wneu.2010.09.032.

Sedney, Cara L., Yoichi Nonaka, Ketan R. Bulsara, and Takanori Fukushima. 2013. "Microsurgical Management of Jugular Foramen Schwannomas." *Neurosurgery*, 72 (1): 42–46. https://doi.org/10.1227/NEU.0b013e3182770e74.

Seo, Youngbeom, Dong Gyu Kim, Jin Wook Kim, Jung Ho Han, Hyun Tai Chung, and Sun Ha Paek. 2018. "Long-Term Outcomes after Gamma Knife Radiosurgery for

Benign Meningioma: A Single Institution's Experience with 424 Patients." *Clinical Neurosurgery*, 83 (5): 1040–49. https://doi.org/10.1093/neuros/nyx585.

Sharma, Manish Singh, Rakesh Singh, Shashank S. Kale, Deepak Agrawal, Bhawani Shankar Sharma, and Ashok Kumar Mahapatra. 2010. "Tumor Control and Hearing Preservation after Gamma Knife Radiosurgery for Vestibular Schwannomas in Neurofibromatosis Type 2." *Journal of Neuro-Oncology*, 98 (2): 265–70. https://doi.org/10.1007/s11060-010-0181-1.

Shaw, Edward, Charles Scott, Luis Souhami, Robert Dinapoli, Robert Kline, Jay Loeffler, and Nancy Farnan. 2000. "Single Dose Radiosurgical Treatment of Recurrent Previously Irradiated Primary Brain Tumors and Brain Metastases: Final Report of RTOG Protocol 90- 05." *International Journal of Radiation Oncology Biology Physics*, 47 (2): 291–98. https://doi.org/10.1016/S0360-3016(99)00507-6.

Sheehan, J. M., M. L. Vance, J. P. Sheehan, D. B. Ellegala, and Jr Laws. 2000. "Radiosurgery for Cushing's Disease after Failed Transsphenoidal Surgery." *Journal of Neurosurgery*, 93 (5): 738–42. https://doi.org/10.3171/jns.2000.93.5.0738.

Sheehan, Jason. 2012. "Stereotactic Radiosurgery for Glioblastoma - Time to Revisit This Approach." *World Neurosurgery*, 78 (6): 592–93. https://doi.org/10.1016/j.wneu.2012.05.023.

Sheehan, Jason P., Jay Jagannathan, Nader Pouratian, and Ladislau Steiner. 2006. "Stereotactic Radiosurgery for Pituitary Adenomas: A Review of the Literature and Our Experience." *Frontiers of Hormone Research*, 34: 185–205. https://doi.org/10.1159/000091581.

Sheehan, Jason P., Nader Pouratian, Ladislau Steiner, Edward R. Laws, and Mary Lee Vance. 2011. "Gamma Knife Surgery for Pituitary Adenomas: Factors Related to Radiological and Endocrine Outcomes: Clinical Article." *Journal of Neurosurgery*, 114 (2): 303–9. https://doi.org/10.3171/2010.5.JNS091635.

Sheehan, Jason P., Robert M. Starke, David Mathieu, Byron Young, Penny K. Sneed, Veronica L. Chiang, John Y.K. Lee, et al. 2013. "Gamma Knife Radiosurgery for the Management of Nonfunctioning Pituitary Adenomas: A Multicenter Study." *Journal of Neurosurgery*, 119 (2): 446–56. https://doi.org/10.3171/2013.3.JNS12766.

Shehata, Michael K., Byron Young, Brady Reid, Roy A. Patchell, William St. Clair, Jackie Sims, Michael Sanders, Ali Meigooni, Mohammed Mohiuddin, and William F. Regine. 2004. "Stereotatic Radiosurgery of 468 Brain Metastases ≤2 Cm: Implications for SRS Dose and Whole Brain Radiation Therapy." *International Journal of Radiation Oncology Biology Physics*, 59 (1): 87–93. https://doi.org/10.1016/j.ijrobp.2003.10.009.

Shiue, Kevin, Gene H. Barnett, John H. Suh, Michael A. Vogelbaum, Chandana A. Reddy, Robert J. Weil, Lilyana Angelov, Gennady Neyman, and Samuel T. Chao. 2014. "Using Higher Isodose Lines for Gamma Knife Treatment of 1 to 3 Brain Metastases Is Safe and Effective." *Neurosurgery*, 74 (4): 360–64. https://doi.org/10.1227/NEU.0000000000000289.

Sholmo Melmed. 2006. "Review Article: Medical Progress Acromegaly." *The New England Journal of Medicine*, 355 (24): 2558–73. https://doi.org/10.1177/ 1461444810365020.

Soffietti, Riccardo, Martin Kocher, Ufuk M. Abacioglu, Salvador Villa, François Fauchon, Brigitta G. Baumert, Laura Fariselli, et al. 2013. "A European Organisation for Research and Treatment of Cancer Phase III Trial of Adjuvant Whole-Brain Radiotherapy versus Observation in Patients with One to Three Brain Metastases from Solid Tumors after Surgical Resection or Radiosurgery: Quality-of-Life." *Journal of Clinical Oncology*, 31 (1): 65–72. https://doi.org/10.1200/ JCO.2011.41.0639.

Stauder, Michael C., Nadia Ni Laack, Kamran A. Ahmed, Michael J. Link, Paula J. Schomberg, and Bruce E. Pollock. 2012. "Stereotactic Radiosurgery for Patients with Recurrent Intracranial Ependymomas." *Journal of Neuro-Oncology*, 108 (3): 507–12. https://doi.org/10.1007/s11060-012-0851-2.

Tsao, May N., Dirk Rades, Andrew Wirth, Simon S. Lo, Brita L. Danielson, Laurie E. Gaspar, Paul W. Sperduto, et al. 2012. "Radiotherapeutic and Surgical Management for Newly Diagnosed Brain Metastasis(Es): An American Society for Radiation Oncology Evidence-Based Guideline." *Practical Radiation Oncology*, 2 (3): 210–25. https://doi.org/10.1016/j.prro.2011.12.004.

Tsao, May, Wei Xu, and Arjun Sahgal. 2012. "A Meta-Analysis Evaluating Stereotactic Radiosurgery, Whole-Brain Radiotherapy, or Both for Patients Presenting with a Limited Number of Brain Metastases." *Cancer*, 118 (9): 2486–93. https://doi.org/ 10.1002/cncr.26515.

Wackym, P Ashley, Christina L Runge-Samuelson, John J Nash, David M Poetker, Katherine Albano, Joseph Bovi, Michelle A Michel, David R Friedland, Yong-ran Zhu, and Maureen T Hannley. 2010. "Gamma Knife Surgery of Vestibular Schwannomas: Volumetric Dosimetry Correlations to Hearing Loss Suggest Stria Vascularis Devascularization as the Mechanism of Early Hearing Loss." *Otology & Neurotology: Official Publication of the American Otological Society, American Neurotology Society [and] European Academy of Otology and Neurotology*, 31 (9): 1480—1487. https://doi.org/10.1097/mao.0b013e3181f7d7d4.

Wallner, Kent E., Joseph H. Galicich, George Krol, Ehud Arbit, and Mark G. Malkin. 1989. "Patterns of Failure Following Treatment for Glioblastoma Multiforme and Anaplastic Astrocytoma." *International Journal of Radiation Oncology, Biology, Physics*, 16 (6): 1405–9. https://doi.org/10.1016/0360-3016(89)90941-3.

Wilson, P. J., K. J. De-Loyde, J. R. Williams, and R. I. Smee. 2012. "A Single Centre's Experience of Stereotactic Radiosurgery and Radiotherapy for Non-Functioning Pituitary Adenomas with the Linear Accelerator (Linac)." *Journal of Clinical Neuroscience*, 19 (3): 370–74. https://doi.org/10.1016/j.jocn.2011.07.025.

Witt, Thomas C. 2003. "Stereotactic Radiosurgery for Pituitary Tumors." *Neurosurgical Focus*, 14 (5). https://doi.org/10.3171/foc.2003.14.5.11.

Yamamoto, Masaaki, Toru Serizawa, Takashi Shuto, Atsuya Akabane, Yoshinori Higuchi, Jun Kawagishi, Kazuhiro Yamanaka, et al. 2014. "Stereotactic Radiosurgery for Patients with Multiple Brain Metastases (JLGK0901): A Multi-Institutional Prospective Observational Study." *The Lancet Oncology*, 15 (4): 387–95. https://doi.org/10.1016/S1470-2045(14)70061-0.

Yang, Isaac, Michael E. Sughrue, Seunggu J. Han, Shanna Fang, Derick Aranda, Steven W. Cheung, Lawrence H. Pitts, and Andrew T. Parsa. 2009. "Facial Nerve

Preservation after Vestibular Schwannoma Gamma Knife Radiosurgery." *Journal of Neuro-Oncology*, 93 (1): 41–48. https://doi.org/10.1007/s11060-009-9842-3.

Yeole, Ujwal, Shantala Hegde, Mohit Gothwal, Prabhuraj AR, K Thennarasu, and Arimappamagan Arivazhagan. 2020. ""What Happens after Therapy? Quality of Life and Neurocognitive Functions of Children with Malignant Posterior Fossa Tumors after Adjuvant Therapy."" *Neurology India*.

Yeole, Ujwal, A. R. Prabhuraj, Arimappamagan Arivazhagan, Vazhayil Narasingarao, K. V. L. Vikas, Govindswamy Dhananjaya, Bhat Dwarakanath, Srinivas Bhanumathi, and Somanna. Sampath. 2021. "Gamma Knife Radiosurgery for Large Vestibular Schwannoma More Than 10 Cm 3 : A Single-Center Indian Tudy." *J Neurol Surg B Skull Base*. https://doi.org/https://doi.org/ 10.1055/s-0041-1729977.

Zachary D. Guss, A.B., Sachin Batra, Charles J. Limb, Gordon Li, Michael E. Sughrue, Kristin Redmond, Daniele Rigamonti, Andrew T. Parsa, Steven Chang, Lawrence Kleinberg, and Michael Lim. 2011. "Radiosurgery of Glomus Jugulare Tumors: A Meta- Analysis." *Int J Radiat Oncol Biol Phys*, 81 (4): e497–502. https://doi.org/ 10.1016/j.ijrobp.2011.05.006.

Chapter 16

Guidelines on the Management of Cerebral Metastasis

Maruti Nandan, Priyadarshi Dikshit, Ved Prakash Maurya, Kamlesh Rangari, Pawan Kumar Verma and Anant Mehrotra

Department of Neurosurgery, Sanjay Gandhi Postgraduate Institute of Medical Sciences, Lucknow, India

Abstract

Cerebral metastases are the most common brain malignancies, and these are four times more common than the primary tumor of the brain. Over the last few decades, there has been a significant surge in these metastatic deposits because of the increased life expectancy of the ageing population, improved diagnostic modalities, and better therapeutic measures.

Lung, breast, skin, colorectal, and renal malignancies are the maximum contributors to cerebral metastases. In about 15% of brain metastases, occult primary remains unknown and manifests only as a space-occupying lesion in the brain.

The presence of brain metastasis carries a significant impact on the quality of life (QOL) of an individual because of primary pathology and the cerebral deposit. The symptomatology is akin to any other space-occupying lesions in the brain and is often ignored in their initial stages. The presence of metastatic brain lesions carries diagnostic and therapeutic challenges to the treating physicians and are universally fatal over a few months if left untreated.

The treatment algorithm needs to be tailored according to the nature of the individual lesion, location, and other systemic manifestations. In

In: Advances in Neurosurgery Research
Editors: Amit Agrawal, Pradeep Chouksey, Adesh Shrivastava et al.
ISBN: 978-1-68507-859-1

this chapter, we will briefly focus on the available modalities of management for metastatic brain lesions, which extends from conventional options and the targeted therapy.

Introduction

Brain metastases (BM) are the most common intracranial neoplasm of the central nervous system (Arnold and Patchell, 2001). The incidence of BM is four times higher than the primary malignant brain tumor (Owonikoko et al., 2014). The most frequently encountered tumor presenting in the emergency or outpatient department is due to intratumoral haemorrhage, raised intracranial pressure (ICP), seizure, and neurological deficit. It is one of the leading causes of morbidity and mortality in a patient afflicted with malignant pathology. The incidence of metastatic brain tumors is increasing day by day owing to advancements in neuroimaging and development in targeted and immunotherapy with subsequent prolonged survival in cancer patients. The incidence of brain metastasis in cancer patients is approximately 8.5-9.6%, with a true annual incidence of >100,000 per year (Barnholtz-Sloan et al., 2004). Incidence of BM also depends upon the type of primary tumor as it has been observed that the risk of metastasis is more in cancer of lung, breast, and melanoma. Non-melanoma skin cancer, head and neck malignancy rarely metastasize to the brain (Cagney et al., 2017; Sperduto et al., 2017). Mainly cerebral metastasis occurs via hematogenous spread and may also affect leptomeninges, dura, and the overlying skull bone (Pekmezci and Perry, 2013a). Cerebral blood flow is an essential determinant of localization and proportion of BM, and therefore 80% of BM occurs in the cerebral hemisphere, 15% in the cerebellum, and 3% in basal ganglia (Fink and Fink, 2013). These metastatic tumors are most commonly found in the gray-white junction and watershed areas of arterial territory in cerebral circulation (Pekmezci and Perry, 2013b). Five primary tumors comprising lung cancer, renal cell carcinoma, breast cancer, melanoma, and gastrointestinal (GI) tract adenocarcinoma account for approximately 80% of all BM (Robbins et al., 2010). Leptomeningeal spread is more familiar with SCLC (small cell lung cancer), melanoma, breast cancer, whereas posterior fossa metastasis mainly occurs with pelvic and gastrointestinal tumors. SCLC and melanoma mostly have solitary metastasis, whereas breast, renal and colorectal carcinoma are more commonly associated with multiple lesions (Pekmezci and Perry 2013a).

Management of Brain Metastasis

Metastatic brain space-occupying lesion (SOL), once diagnosed, represents a diagnostic and management dilemma.

These include uncertainty in the diagnosis of the primary focus of the metastasis as well their optimal management. The management of the primary lesion may include surgical resection and chemo/ radiotherapy depending upon the morphology and histopathology of the lesions. Nowadays, advancements in radiosurgery and systemic therapy and targeted immunotherapy have expanded the available treatment paradigm spectrum. Brain metastasis, when diagnosed, must be tackled with a multidisciplinary approach with various combinations of surgery, radiotherapy, and targeted immunotherapy (Franchino, Rudà, and Soffietti, 2018; Cairncross, Kim, and Posner, 1980).

Surgical Resection

Surgical resection is the most invasive option amongst the treatment options available. However, it helps decrease the mass effect, brain edema, and associated symptoms immediately in large tumor refractory with corticosteroid therapy. Also, the tissue obtained helps in the histological diagnostic confirmation (Soffietti et al., 2017; Han and Brastianos, 2017). Genomic analysis of BM, primary tumor, and extracranial metastasis revealed that these tumors harbour potentially actionable driver mutations unique to them. Hence, targeted therapy against these tumors drastically improves the overall survival and neurologic outcome (Han and Brastianos, 2017).

Patchell et al. in their landmark paper described that surgical resection in combination with radiotherapy in a single metastatic lesion improves overall survival, decreases recurrence rate, and improves the quality of life compared to the patient treated with radiotherapy alone (Patchell et al., 1990). Binda et al., in their study, concluded that in cases of multiple metastatic lesions, surgical intervention might be beneficial in patients who have < 4 metastasis where all the lesions can be resected (Bindal et al., 1993). Factors influencing survival in recurrent BM are:

1. Time of recurrence >200 days
2. Number of the lesion (Single Vs Multiple)
3. Completeness of resection
4. Recursive partitioning analysis (RPA)- classification

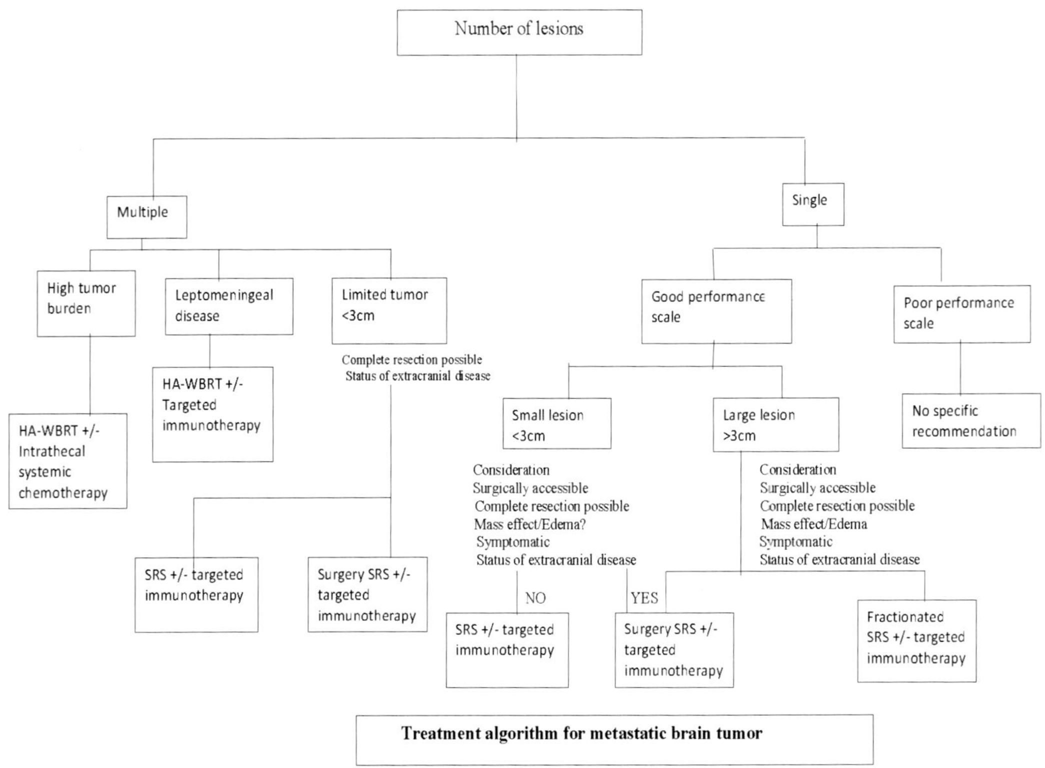

Figure 1. Represents a treatment algorithm that suggests the management of the cerebral metastatic lesion.

Surgical technique is also essential to minimize the risk of recurrence and leptomeningeal dissemination. En bloc resection without violation of tumor capsule along the brain tumor interface is preferred over piecemeal resection for prevention of recurrence and dissemination. Gross total resection has a better outcome and survival benefit than subtotal resection. However, the risk of permanent neurological deficit is there if the tumor is located in eloquent areas of the brain. With the help of advanced surgical techniques and modern advancements, i.e., neuronavigation, intraoperative ultrasound, cortical and subcortical mapping, laser interstitial thermal therapy significantly improved the rate of GTR with no or minimal neurological deficit. Several studies conducted over the years support surgical resection in a patient with an excellent functional score. Those patients who underwent complete surgical resection of all the possible lesions were absent or controlled extracranial tumour activity.

Stereotactic Radiosurgery (SRS)

SRS consists of delivering a hefty dose of radiation in a single session by using multiple nonparallel radiation beams converging on a precisely defined target lesion. By delivering radiation through a nonparallel converging radiation beam, the entire dose is delivered only where all the beams overlap, thus reducing the radiation dose to normal surrounding tissue significantly (Halperin et al., 2013). SRS can be used either as a single treatment modality or as adjuvant or neoadjuvant therapy, depending on the size, the number of the lesion, and its location in eloquent and non-eloquent areas of the brain. It is a viable option for the BM not amenable to surgical resection due to the high risk of neurological injury in deep-seated and lesion in eloquent areas of the brain. Historically, a maximum of four lesions was considered the cut-off for SRS treatment. However, studies have nowadays revealed that SRS can be used in patients with >4 lesions (Ehrlich et al., 2019; Yamamoto et al., 2014). SRS is suitable for smaller well-circumscribed lesions regardless of tumor cell radiosensitivity. As the tumor size increases, the risk of radiation toxicity to the surrounding normal brain tissue also increases. RTOG (Radiation treatment oncology group) previously concluded that the use of SRS could not achieve adequate tumour control when the tumor was >4cm in diameter and therefore determined the maximum tolerable dose for non-brainstem BM with diameters <2cm, >2-3cm, and >3-4cm to be 24 Gy, 18Gy and 12 Gy respectively (Shaw et al., 2000; 1996). Alternatively, if a large lesion (>4cm) is present, SRS can be split into 2 to 5 fractions named fractionated SRS or hypo fractionated SRS. Another method of reducing the radiation toxicity in the large tumor is volume staged SRS. A specific portion of the large lesion is targeted over time and achieve superior tumor control in patients with large BM (Angelov et al., 2017; Dohm et al., 2018). Apart from number and size, the location of the BM is also an essential factor while SRS is being employed as a treatment strategy. Lesions located in areas with the lowest risk of post-SRS neurological sequelae (Frontal/temporal lobe) are treated with higher radiation doses than lesions in high-risk areas such as the thalamus, basal ganglia, and brainstem. Lower radiation dose is also considered when BM is located in the eloquent areas of the brain. These eloquent areas are the primary motor cortex, primary somatosensory cortex, primary visual cortex, primary auditory cortex, Broca's area (Posterior inferior frontal gyrus), and Wernicke's areas (Halperin et al., 2013; Hsu et al., 2015). The CN II and CN VIII are most sensitive to radiation injury in the cranium, which is why SRS is contraindicated for any lesion within or adjacent to the optic apparatus that requires more than 10 Gy of radiation (Ito et al., 1997; Stafford et al., 2003). However, it has been observed that when SRS was used alone as an adjuvant therapy without WBRT, it had a poor local control rate and increased risk of recurrence (Brown et al., 2016; Chang et al., 2009). The following factors can be used to predict recurrence in patients treated with SRS alone:

1. Number of brain metastasis
2. Patient age
3. Cancer type (HER-2 breast cancer, colorectal cancer, melanoma)
4. Progressive systemic disease/ increasing extracranial disease burden.

It is essential to follow up on the patient with a serial scan due to the higher recurrence rate when SRS is used alone postoperatively. SRS use is also linked to radiation necrosis (RN) and leptomeningeal dissemination (LMD). RN is the most significant complication of SRS, which develops between six months to several years. The risk of RN is more in a single-fraction SRS, and it depends on radiation dose and prior SRS or WBRT received for the same lesion. Treatment option for RNs includes corticosteroid therapy, vascular endothelial growth factor (VEGF) inhibitor (Bevacizumab), hyperbaric oxygen therapy, surgical resection, and interstitial thermotherapy (Bodensohn et al., 2020; Mehta, Shah, and Jung, 2017; Ahluwalia et al., 2018) 29-31. Postop SRS is associated with leptomeningeal dissemination (LMD), more so in the case of breast cancer, infratentorial lesion, multiple BM, and distant intracranial failure.

Whole-Brain Radiation Therapy (WBRT)

Historically, WBRT has long been the standard modality of treatment for multiple BM and continues to be one of the critical treatment modalities despite SRS development. It can be used after radiosurgery or after surgical resection for tumor control. Studies have also shown that adjuvant WBRT can reduce the risk of recurrence of BM in the adjacent area and help control local tumor growth (Aoyama et al., 2006). However, adjuvant WBRT was associated with poor quality of life and learning and memory functions deterioration. There may also be an extracranial factor contributing to these patients' lack of survival benefit. Adjuvant WBRT, either post-SRS or surgery, is beneficial in local tumor control and reduces the risk of distant metastases. However, it has no survival benefit when administered after surgical resection. Therefore, SRS may be more beneficial in limited intracranial tumor burden (< 4 lesions that are <3cm in diameter) (Andrews et al., 2004). To minimize the adverse neurocognitive effect of WBRT, memantine or hippocampal avoidance intensity-modulated radiation therapy (IMRT) should be used. Helical tomotherapy and linear accelerator-IMRT (LINAC-IMRT) effectively spare the hippocampus and reduce the total dose delivered to it. In helical tomotherapy, the median and the maximum dose for the hippocampus are 5.5Gy and 12.8Gy, respectively, while in LINAC-based IMRT, it is 7.8Gy and 15.3Gy (Gondi et al., 2014).

Systemic Therapy

The treatment of BM with systemic chemotherapy agents has been relatively limited for decades due to poor blood-brain barrier penetration, the presence of efflux pumps, and uneven distribution caused by blood tumor barriers. The efficacy of chemotherapy depends upon the sensitivity of the primary tumor to chemotherapeutic agents. The highest rate of extracranial response is seen in small cell lung carcinoma (30-80%) and the lowest in melanoma (10-15%) (Soffietti et al., 2017). Because of the new mutations acquired by metastatic lesions, the intracranial response does not always correlate with the systemic response. Therefore, chemotherapeutic agents have a limited role in treating the metastatic tumor. However, it plays a critical role in controlling the extracranial disease. Certain patients may benefit from targeted and immunotherapy treatments. Patients with the primary tumor from non-small-cell lung carcinomas (NSCLC), human epidermal growth factor receptor 2 (HER 2) positive breast cancers, and melanoma harboring the BRAF mutation have benefited from targeted therapy.(Peters et al., 2017; Bachelot et al., 2013; Long et al., 2012). The use of first-generation EGFR inhibitors such as Gefitinib and Erlotinib has been shown to improve response rate and progression-free survival in EGFR mutant BM patients and overall survival. Now 2nd and 3rd generation EGFR inhibitors (Aftinib and Osimeritinib, respectively) are also available, targeting EGFR mutation more effectively (Kim et al., 2009; Porta et al., 2011).

Similarly, For patients with ALK-rearranged NSCLC with brain metastases, Alectinib, Ceritinib, Brigatinib, and Lorlatinib should be considered (Venur and Ahluwalia, 2016). HER 2 positive breast cancer not amenable to surgery, WBRT, and SRS may be treated with systemic therapy. HER2 inhibitor Lapatinib, Neratinib, Tuvatinib, Tesevatinib have shown promising results in HER2-positive breast cancer. Combination therapy with Tucatinib, Capecitabine, and Trastuzumab has also demonstrated improved progression-free survival (PFS) and overall survival (OS) (Lin et al., 2008; 2009). Dabrafenib and vemurafenib are beneficial for patients who have previously been treated with disease progression and those who have never been treated before (Long et al., 2012). In patients without prior treatment, a combination of the BRAF and MEK inhibitors Dabrafenib and Trametinib demonstrated a response rate of 58% (Davies et al., 2017).

Immunotherapy

Immunotherapy has developed significantly in the last few decades, with immune checkpoint inhibitors providing hope for a more efficacious therapeutic approach to intracranial neoplasms. Combining CLTA4 inhibitors (Ipilimumab) and PD-1 inhibitors (Nivolumab) demonstrated better response rates (46-56%) in BM compared to nivolumab alone (20%) (H. A. Tawbi et al., 2018). It is advisable to take precautions while taking steroids in immunotherapy since they alter the response to the therapy (25% vs 10%). Also, concomitant SRS and immunotherapy improve both survival and intracranial response (H. A.-H. Tawbi et al., 2017). Nivolumab and

Ipilimumab, and SRS improve overall survival in patients with melanoma BM. Studies have revealed superior benefits when SRS and immunotherapy are used concurrently (Schoenfeld et al., 2015).

Hopefully, more studies will help treat the BM patient more effectively with immunotherapeutic agents.

Recurrence of Metastatic Brain Lesion

Resection of recurrent BM lesions is not beneficial in the following situations:

1. KPS score <70
2. Time to recurrence <4 months
3. Age > 40 years
4. Primary lung cancer
5. Primary breast cancer or melanoma (Arbit et al., 1995).

In their study, Binda et al. determined that patients who meet 1 criterion have a 5-year survival rate of 57%, whereas those meeting >2 criteria have an 11% 5-year survival rate (Bindal et al., 1995). Repeat SRS can also be considered in recurrent metastatic brain tumors.

Conclusion

The management strategy of brain metastases requires a multidisciplinary approach in close collaboration with general medicine, medical and radiation oncology, one anaesthesiologist, and a neurosurgeon. Even though there is a significant variation in the opinion between treating physicians, an evidence-based treatment protocol is needed for better management.

References

Ahluwalia Manmeet, Barnett Gene H, Di Deng, Tatter Stephen B, Laxton Adrian W, Mohammadi Alireza M, Leuthardt Eric, Chamoun Roukoz, Judy Kevin and Asher Anthony. 2018. "Laser Ablation after Stereotactic Radiosurgery: A Multicenter Prospective Study in Patients with Metastatic Brain Tumors and Radiation Necrosis". *Journal of Neurosurgery*, 130 (3): 804–11.

Andrews David W, Scott Charles B, Sperduto Paul W, Flanders Adam E, Gaspar Laurie E, Schell Michael C, Werner-Wasik Maria, Demas William, Ryu Janice and Bahary Jean-Paul. 2004. "Whole Brain Radiation Therapy with or without Stereotactic Radiosurgery Boost for Patients with One to Three Brain Metastases: Phase III Results of the RTOG 9508 Randomised Trial". *The Lancet,* 363 (9422): 1665–72.

Angelov Lilyana, Mohammadi Alireza M, Bennett Elizabeth E, Abbassy Mahmoud, Elson Paul, Chao Samuel T, Montgomery Joshua S, Habboub Ghaith, Vogelbaum Michael A and Suh John H. 2017. "Impact of 2-Staged Stereotactic Radiosurgery for Treatment of Brain Metastases ≥2 Cm". *Journal of Neurosurgery,* 129 (2): 366–82.

Aoyama Hidefumi, Hiroki Shirato, Masao Tago, Keiichi Nakagawa, Tatsuya Toyoda, Kazuo Hatano, Masahiro Kenjyo, Natsuo Oya, Saeko Hirota and Hiroki Shioura. 2006. "Stereotactic Radiosurgery plus Whole-Brain Radiation Therapy vs Stereotactic Radiosurgery Alone for Treatment of Brain Metastases: A Randomized Controlled Trial". *JAMA,* 295 (21): 2483–91.

Arbit Ehud, Wroński Marek, Burt Michael and Galicich Joseph H. 1995. "The Treatment of Patients with Recurrent Brain Metastases. A Retrospective Analysis of 109 Patients with Nonsmall Cell Lung Cancer". *Cancer,* 76 (5): 765–73.

Arnold Susanne M and Patchell Roy A, 2001. "Diagnosis and Management of Brain Metastases". *Hematology/Oncology Clinics,* 15 (6): 1085–1108.

Bachelot Thomas, Romieu Gilles, Campone Mario, Diéras Véronique, Cropet Claire, Dalenc Florence, Jimenez Marta, Le Rhun Emilie, Pierga Jean-Yves and Gonçalves Anthony. 2013. "Lapatinib plus Capecitabine in Patients with Previously Untreated Brain Metastases from HER2-Positive Metastatic Breast Cancer (LANDSCAPE): A Single-Group Phase 2 Study". *The Lancet Oncology,* 14 (1): 64–71.

Barnholtz-Sloan Jill S, Sloan Andrew E, Davis Faith G, Vigneau Fawn D, Lai Ping and Sawaya Raymond E. 2004. "Incidence Proportions of Brain Metastases in Patients Diagnosed (1973 to 2001) in the Metropolitan Detroit Cancer Surveillance System". *Journal of Clinical Oncology,* 22 (14): 2865–72.

Bindal Rajesh K, Sawaya Raymond, Leavens Milam E, Hess Kenneth R and Taylor Sarah H. 1995. "Reoperation for Recurrent Metastatic Brain Tumors". *Journal of Neurosurgery,* 83 (4): 600–604.

Bindal Rajesh K, Sawaya Raymond, Leavens Milam E and Jack Lee J. 1993. "Surgical Treatment of Multiple Brain Metastases". *Journal of Neurosurgery,* 79 (2): 210–16.

Bodensohn Raphael, Indrawati Hadi, Daniel Felix Fleischmann, Corradini Stefanie, Thon N, Rauch J, Belka C and Niyazi M. 2020. "Bevacizumab as a Treatment Option for Radiation Necrosis after Cranial Radiation Therapy: A Retrospective Monocentric Analysis". *Strahlentherapie und Onkologie,* 196 (1): 70–76.

Brown Paul D, Jaeckle Kurt, Ballman Karla V, Farace Elana, Cerhan Jane H, Keith Anderson S, Carrero Xiomara W, Barker Fred G, Deming Richard and Burri Stuart H. 2016. "Effect of Radiosurgery Alone vs Radiosurgery with Whole Brain Radiation Therapy on Cognitive Function in Patients with 1 to 3 Brain Metastases: A Randomized Clinical Trial". *JAMA,* 316 (4): 401–9.

Cagney Daniel N, Martin Allison M, Catalano Paul J, Redig Amanda J, Lin Nancy U, Lee Eudocia Q, Wen Patrick Y, Dunn Ian F, Wenya Linda Bi and Weiss Stephanie E. 2017. "Incidence and Prognosis of Patients with Brain Metastases at Diagnosis of

Systemic Malignancy: A Population-Based Study". *Neuro-Oncology,* 19 (11): 1511–21.

Cairncross J Gregory, Jae-Ho Kim and Posner Jerome B. 1980. "Radiation Therapy for Brain Metastases". *Annals of Neurology: Official Journal of the American Neurological Association and the Child Neurology Society,* 7 (6): 529–41.

Chang Eric L, Wefel Jeffrey S, Hess Kenneth R, Allen Pamela K, Lang Frederick F, Kornguth David G, Arbuckle Rebecca B, Swint J Michael, Shiu Almon S and Maor Moshe H. 2009. "Neurocognition in Patients with Brain Metastases Treated with Radiosurgery or Radiosurgery plus Whole-Brain Irradiation: A Randomised Controlled Trial". *The Lancet Oncology,* 10 (11): 1037–44.

Davies Michael A, Saiag Philippe, Robert Caroline, Grob Jean-Jacques, Flaherty Keith T, Arance Ana, Chiarion-Sileni Vanna, Thomas Luc, Lesimple Thierry and Mortier Laurent. 2017. "Dabrafenib plus Trametinib in Patients with BRAFV600-Mutant Melanoma Brain Metastases (COMBI-MB): A Multicentre, Multicohort, Open-Label, Phase 2 Trial". *The Lancet Oncology,* 18 (7): 863–73.

Dohm Ammoren, McTyre Emory R, Okoukoni Catherine, Henson Adrianna, Cramer Christina K, LeCompte Michael C, Ruiz Jimmy, Munley Michael T, Qasem Shadi and Hui-Wen Lo. 2018. "Staged Stereotactic Radiosurgery for Large Brain Metastases: Local Control and Clinical Outcomes of a One-Two Punch Technique". *Neurosurgery,* 83 (1): 114–21.

Ehrlich Matthew I, Schiff Elliot, Knisely Jonathan PS, Jenghwa Chang, Xin Qian, Anuj Goenka and Michael Schulder. 2019. "Tumor Control and Survival in Patients with Ten or More Brain Metastases Treated with Stereotactic Radiosurgery: A Retrospective Analysis". *Journal of Neuro-Oncology,* 143 (1): 167–74.

Fink Kathleen R and Fink James R. 2013. "Imaging of Brain Metastases". *Surgical Neurology International,* 4 (Suppl 4): S209.

Franchino Federica, Rudà Roberta and Soffietti Riccardo. 2018. "Mechanisms and Therapy for Cancer Metastasis to the Brain". *Frontiers in Oncology,* 8: 161.

Gondi Vinai, Pugh Stephanie L, Tome Wolfgang A, Caine Chip, Corn Ben, Kanner Andrew, Rowley Howard, Kundapur Vijayananda, DeNittis Albert and Greenspoon Jeffrey N. 2014. "Preservation of Memory with Conformal Avoidance of the Hippocampal Neural Stem-Cell Compartment during Whole-Brain Radiotherapy for Brain Metastases (RTOG 0933): A Phase II Multi-Institutional Trial". *Journal of Clinical Oncology,* 32 (34): 3810.

Halperin Edward C, Brady Luther W, Wazer David E and Perez Carlos A. 2013. *Perez & Brady's Principles and Practice of Radiation Oncology*. Lippincott Williams & Wilkins.

Han Catherine H and Brastianos Priscilla K. 2017. "Genetic Characterization of Brain Metastases in the Era of Targeted Therapy". *Frontiers in Oncology,* 7: 230.

Hsu Fred, Nichol Alan, Ma Roy, Kouhestani Para, Toyota Brian and McKenzie Michael. 2015. "Stereotactic Radiosurgery for Metastases in Eloquent Central Brain Locations". *Canadian Journal of Neurological Sciences,* 42 (5): 333–37.

Ito Ken, Hiroki Kurita, Keiko Sugasawa, Masahiro Mizuno and Tomio Sasaki. 1997. "Analyses of Neuro-Otological Complications after Radiosurgery for Acoustic

Neurinomas". *International Journal of Radiation Oncology, Biology, Physics,* 39 (5): 983–88.

Kim Jeong-Eun, Dae Ho Lee, Yunsuk Choi, Dok Hyun Yoon, Sang-We Kim, Cheolwon Suh and Jung-Shin Lee. 2009. "Epidermal Growth Factor Receptor Tyrosine Kinase Inhibitors as a First-Line Therapy for Never-Smokers with Adenocarcinoma of the Lung Having Asymptomatic Synchronous Brain Metastasis". *Lung Cancer,* 65 (3): 351–54.

Lin Nancy U, Carey Lisa A, Liu Minetta C, Younger Jerry, Come Steven E, Ewend Matthew, Harris Gordon J, Bullitt Elizabeth, Van den Abbeele Annick D and Henson John W. 2008. "Phase II Trial of Lapatinib for Brain Metastases in Patients with Human Epidermal Growth Factor Receptor 2–Positive Breast Cancer". *Journal of Clinical Oncology: Official Journal of the American Society of Clinical Oncology,* 26 (12): 1993.

Lin Nancy U, Diéras Véronique, Devchand Paul, Lossignol Dominique, Christodoulou Christos, Stemmler Hans-Joachim, Roché Henri, Liu Minetta C, Greil Richard and Ciruelos Eva. 2009. "Multicenter Phase II Study of Lapatinib in Patients with Brain Metastases from HER2-Positive Breast Cancer". *Clinical Cancer Research,* 15 (4): 1452–59.

Long Georgina V, Trefzer Uwe, Davies Michael A, Kefford Richard F, Ascierto Paolo A, Chapman Paul B, Puzanov Igor, Hauschild Axel, Robert Caroline and Algazi Alain. 2012. "Dabrafenib in Patients with Val600Glu or Val600Lys BRAF-Mutant Melanoma Metastatic to the Brain (BREAK-MB): A Multicentre, Open-Label, Phase 2 Trial." *The Lancet Oncology,* 13 (11): 1087–95.

Mehta Swapnil, Aatman Shah and Jung Henry. 2017. "Diagnosis and Treatment Options for Sequelae Following Radiation Treatment of Brain Tumors". *Clinical Neurology and Neurosurgery,* 163: 1–8.

Owonikoko Taofeek K, Arbiser Jack, Zelnak Amelia, Hui-Kuo G Shu, Hyunsuk Shim, Robin Adam M, Kalkanis Steven N, Whitsett Timothy G, Salhia Bodour and Tran Nhan L. 2014. "Current Approaches to the Treatment of Metastatic Brain Tumours". *Nature Reviews Clinical Oncology,* 11 (4): 203–22.

Patchell Roy A, Tibbs Phillip A, Walsh John W, Dempsey Robert J, Maruyama Yosh, Kryscio Richard J, Markesbery William R, Macdonald John S and Byron Young. 1990. "A Randomized Trial of Surgery in the Treatment of Single Metastases to the Brain". *New England Journal of Medicine,* 322 (8): 494–500.

Pekmezci Melike and Perry Arie. 2013a. "Neuropathology of Brain Metastases". *Surgical Neurology International,* 4 (Suppl 4): S245.

Pekmezci Melike and Perry Arie. 2013b. "Neuropathology of Brain Metastases". *Surgical Neurology International,* 4 (Suppl 4): S245.

Peters Solange, Ross Camidge D, Shaw Alice T, Gadgeel Shirish, Ahn Jin S, Dong-Wan Kim, Sai-Hong I. Ou, Maurice Pérol, Dziadziuszko Rafal and Rosell Rafael. 2017. "Alectinib versus Crizotinib in Untreated ALK-Positive Non–Small-Cell Lung Cancer". *New England Journal of Medicine,* 377 (9): 829–38.

Porta R, Sanchez-Torres JM, Paz-Ares L, Massuti B, Reguart N, Mayo C, Lianes P, Queralt C, Guillem V and Salinas P. 2011. "Brain Metastases from Lung Cancer Responding to Erlotinib: The Importance of EGFR Mutation". *European Respiratory Journal,* 37 (3): 624–31.

Robbins Stanley L, Ramzi S. Cotran, Vinay Kumar, Abul K. Abbas, Nelson Fausto and Aster Jon C. 2010. "Robbins and Cotran Pathologic Basis of Disease". In *Robbins and Cotran Pathologic Basis of Disease*, 1450–1450.

Schoenfeld Jonathan D, Mahadevan Anand, Floyd Scott R, Dyer Michael A, Catalano Paul J, Alexander Brian M, McDermott David F and Kaplan Irving D. 2015. "Ipilmumab and Cranial Radiation in Metastatic Melanoma Patients: A Case Series and Review". *Journal for Immunotherapy of Cancer,* 3 (1): 1–6.

Shaw Edward, Scott Charles, Souhami Luis, Dinapoli Robert, Bahary Jean-Paul, Kline Robert, Wharam Moody, Schultz Christopher, Davey Phillip and Loeffler Jay. 1996. "Radiosurgery for the Treatment of Previously Irradiated Recurrent Primary Brain Tumors and Brain Metastases: Initial Report of Radiation Therapy Oncology Group Protocol 90-05". *International Journal of Radiation Oncology* Biology* Physics,* 34 (3): 647–54.

Shaw Edward, Scott Charles, Souhami Luis, Dinapoli Robert, Kline Robert, Loeffler Jay and Farnan Nancy. 2000. "Single Dose Radiosurgical Treatment of Recurrent Previously Irradiated Primary Brain Tumors and Brain Metastases: Final Report of RTOG Protocol 90-05". *International Journal of Radiation Oncology* Biology* Physics,* 47 (2): 291–98.

Soffietti Riccardo, Ufuk Abacioglu, Baumert Brigitta, Combs Stephanie E, Kinhult Sara, Kros Johan M, Marosi Christine, Metellus Philippe, Radbruch Alexander and Villa Freixa Salvador S. 2017. "Diagnosis and Treatment of Brain Metastases from Solid Tumors: Guidelines from the European Association of Neuro-Oncology (EANO)". *Neuro-Oncology,* 19 (2): 162–74.

Sperduto Paul W, Yang T Jonathan, Beal Kathryn, Pan Hubert, Brown Paul D, Bangdiwala Ananta, Shanley Ryan, Yeh Norman, Gaspar Laurie E and Braunstein Steve. 2017. "Estimating Survival in Patients with Lung Cancer and Brain Metastases: An Update of the Graded Prognostic Assessment for Lung Cancer Using Molecular Markers (Lung-MolGPA)". *JAMA Oncology,* 3 (6): 827–31.

Stafford Scott L, Pollock Bruce E, Leavitt Jacqueline A, Foote Robert L, Brown Paul D, Link Michael J, Gorman Deborah A and Schomberg Paula J. 2003. "A Study on the Radiation Tolerance of the Optic Nerves and Chiasm after Stereotactic Radiosurgery". *International Journal of Radiation Oncology* Biology* Physics,* 55 (5): 1177–81.

Tawbi Hussein A, Forsyth Peter A, Algazi Alain, Hamid Omid, Hodi F Stephen, Moschos Stergios J, Khushalani Nikhil I, Lewis Karl, Lao Christopher D and Postow Michael A. 2018. "Combined Nivolumab and Ipilimumab in Melanoma Metastatic to the Brain". *New England Journal of Medicine,* 379 (8): 722–30.

Tawbi Hussein Abdul-Hassan, Forsyth Peter AJ, Patrick Algazi Alain, Hamid Omid, Hodi F Stephen, Moschos Stergios J, Khushalani Nikhil I, Gonzalez Rene, Lao Christopher D and Andrew Postow Michael. 2017. "Efficacy and Safety of Nivolumab (NIVO) plus Ipilimumab (IPI) in Patients with Melanoma (MEL) Metastatic to the Brain: Results of the Phase II Study CheckMate 204". *American Society of Clinical Oncology.*

Venur Vyshak A and Ahluwalia Manmeet S. 2016. "Targeted Therapy in Brain Metastases: Ready for Primetime?" *American Society of Clinical Oncology,* Educational Book, 36: e123–30.

Yamamoto Masaaki, Toru Serizawa, Takashi Shuto, Atsuya Akabane, Yoshinori Higuchi, Jun Kawagishi, Kazuhiro Yamanaka, Yasunori Sato, Hidefumi Jokura and Shoji Yomo. 2014. "Stereotactic Radiosurgery for Patients with Multiple Brain Metastases (JLGK0901): A Multi-Institutional Prospective Observational Study". *The Lancet Oncology,* 15 (4): 387–95.

Chapter 17

The Role of Sex Steroid Receptors in Glioblastoma Biology

Helga Fariña-Jerónimo and Julio Plata-Bello
Neurosurgery Department, Hospital Universitario de Canarias, Tenerife, Spain

Abstract

Glioblastoma is the most common primary tumor of the brain and is associated with an awful prognosis despite the use of different therapeutic modalities. In this regard, the identification of new therapeutic targets or strategies for glioblastoma patient management is considered a priority.

The expression and functionality of sex steroid receptors in glioblastoma have been studied in recent decades, but this new foundation of knowledge has not been translated into new therapeutic options for this tumor.

The present chapter critically reviews the evidence reported in the literature regarding the expression of sex steroid receptors (progesterone, estrogenic and androgen receptors) and their putative roles in glioblastoma development, growth and recurrence.

Introduction

Glioblastoma is the most common primary brain tumor in adults, with an incidence of approximately 4 cases/100,000 inhabitants/year (Ostrom et al. 2019), (Lapointe, Perry, and Butowski 2018). In the central nervous system, it is the tumor with the worst prognosis (mean overall survival of 12-15 months) (Ostrom et al. 2019)-(Gately et al. 2017). Glioblastoma presents a higher

In: Advances in Neurosurgery Research
Editors: Amit Agrawal, Pradeep Chouksey, Adesh Shrivastava et al.
ISBN: 978-1-68507-859-1

incidence in men than in women (3: 2) (Lapointe, Perry, and Butowski 2018). Most of these tumors arise without any prior clinical or histological evidence of a lower grade precursor (primary glioblastoma); however, a small percentage results from the progression of an astrocytoma of lower histological grade (secondary glioblastoma). The standard treatment of glioblastoma consists of surgical resection (trying to achieve the highest degree of resection without compromising brain function), followed by adjuvant treatment consisting of radiochemotherapy (Stupp Scheme) that comprises a total dose of 60 Gy (approximately 2 Gy/day, 5 days per week) and temozolomide concomitant and after radiotherapy (at least 6 cycles) (Stupp et al. 2009). However, despite this treatment, only 5% of patients with GB survive 5 years after diagnosis (Lapointe, Perry, and Butowski 2018). Since the integration of the Stupp scheme for the treatment of these tumors in 2005, only a few therapeutic alternatives have demonstrated an improvement in prognosis, but with a poor impact on overall survival (Stupp et al. 2015), (Stupp et al. 2017). Therefore, the study of new possible therapeutic targets in glioblastoma is an essential task.

Bearing this in mind, sex steroid receptors could be a suitable target in glioblastoma patients. First, they are expressed in glioblastoma tissues; second, it has been demonstrated, in preclinical studies, that they may play a role in glioblastoma biology by modulating cell growth, migration, invasion and chemo-/radioresistance. Finally, significant clinical experience exists in other tumors for the use of drugs that modulate sex steroid receptors (e.g., breast or prostate cancer); thus, the period of time between basic/preclinical research and the possibility of initiating clinical trials should be shorter.

In the present chapter, we review and discuss the role of sex steroid receptors (progesterone, estrogen and androgen receptors) in glioblastoma biology. We first describe the expression of each receptor in glioblastoma tissue and, afterward, the effects of their activation related to tumor behavior.

The Role of Progesterone in Glioblastoma

Progesterone Receptor(s)

Progesterone receptor (PR) is a ligand-induced transcription factor that regulates the expression of several genes by interacting with specific DNA sequences called hormone responsive elements (Gronemeyer 1991), (Mangelsdorf et al. 1995). PR has a DNA binding domain (DBD) between an upstream N-terminal region, which contains activation and inhibitory functions, and a C-terminal ligand binding domain (LBD) (Jacobsen and Horwitz 2011), (Hovland et al. 1998). Two PR isoforms have been described in humans (PRA and PRB) (McDonnell 1995). The PRB isoform (114 kD) contains an additional 164 amino acids compared to the PRA isoform (94 kD), which can be considered an N-terminally truncated form of PRB (G González-Agüero et al. 2001). Both isoforms are encoded by the same gene and are generated from either alternative transcriptional or translational start sites (Conneely et al. 1987), (Kastner et al. 1990), but they have distinctive transcriptional activities (Jacobsen and Horwitz 2011).

The process of gene transcription mediated by PR activation does not differ from other steroid hormone receptors. The receptor is mainly located in the cytoplasm when it is not active. Once its ligand binds to the receptor, this complex is translocated to the nucleus and links with other hormone-receptor complexes to undergo dimerization, and this new complex binds to specific DNA sequences. Nevertheless, in some contexts, PR differs from other steroid receptors in certain aspects. First, PR may be largely located in the nucleus, even in the absence of its ligand (progesterone [P]); second, dimerization may not be required for PR-mediated transcription; and finally, PR also signals through the cell membrane and cytoplasmic pathways (Jacobsen and Horwitz 2011). This last mechanism is mediated by membrane progesterone receptors, which consist of two groups of nonclassical progesterone signaling molecules. On the one hand, the members of the Class II progestin and adipQ receptor (PAQR) family, called membrane progestin receptors (mPRs), include PAQR7, PAQR8, PAQR5, PAQR6 and PAQR9. On the other hand, other members of the nonclassical progesterone signaling molecules are some receptors of the b5-like heme/steroid-binding protein family: PGRMC1, PGRMC2, neudesin and neuferricin (Valadez-Cosmes et al. 2016), (Petersen et al. 2013). These membrane receptors mediate a variety of rapid, cell surface-initiated progesterone actions involving activation of intracellular signaling pathways (Thomas and Pang 2012). Most of them are constitutively expressed in the brain (Pang, Dong, and Thomas 2013), (Tang et al. 2005) and they are involved in neuroprotective mechanisms (Pang, Dong, and Thomas 2013).

Expression of Progesterone Receptor(s) in Glioblastoma

The expression of PR in glioma tissues has already been studied. In 1997, Khalid H et al. reported PR immunoreactivity in 73% of astrocytic tumors.

Regarding only glioblastoma cases (primary or recurrent cases), this percentage rose up to 94%. Thus, high-grade gliomas presented higher PR expression than lower grades (Khalid et al. 1997). Furthermore, these authors described that positivity was observed in most tumors, solely in the nucleus or solely in the cytoplasm. The presence of PR in the nucleus is considered a sign of a functionally active receptor, which has translocated from the cytoplasm after progestin binding. However, these authors did not find any correlation between PR expression and prognostic variables (recurrence and survival) (Khalid et al. 1997).

Gonzalez-Agüero et al. (2001) studied the differential expression of PR isoforms in biopsies of 6 grade III and 7 grade IV gliomas. They described a higher expression of PR in grade IV vs. grade III gliomas and that the most highly expressed PR isoform was PRB at both the mRNA and protein level (G González-Agüero et al. 2001). Furthermore, PRB was mainly localized in the nucleus, and interestingly, biopsies that presented the highest number of immunoreactive cells also presented intense immunostaining (G González-Agüero et al. 2001), suggesting a possible association between PR expression and activation of the antitumor immune response. Nevertheless, other studies (see below) showed that the activation of PR is associated with a suppression of antitumor immunity.

The importance of investigating the expression of PR isoforms in glioblastoma is justified because each isoform can regulate different genes in the same tissue (Mulac-Jericevic et al. 2000). In this regard, in different cell contexts, PRB may function as a transcriptional progesterone-responsive gene activator, and PRA may act as a transcriptional repressor of various steroid receptors, including PRB (Giangrande and McDonnell 1999), (Vegeto et al. 1993). This differential regulation has been associated with different affinities between PRA and PRB with some corepresors and coactivators (Giangrande et al. 2000).

Progesterone membrane receptors may also play a role in glioblastoma biology. Many of these receptors are downregulated in glioblastoma, but the upregulation of PAQR9 (mPRε) seems to be associated with a worse prognosis (Del Moral-Morales et al. 2020), and the activation of PAQR7 (mPRα) has been associated with higher aggressiveness of glioblastoma cells (González-Orozco et al. 2018). Interestingly, the expression of membrane progesterone receptors is superior to PR in glioma stem cells (GSCs), which seem to be the cells responsible for resistance to therapy and recurrence (Hlavaty et al. 2016).

Effects of Progesterone Receptor(s) Activity in Glioblastoma

The effects of progesterone on glioblastoma have also been studied. Not only this hormone but also its metabolites seem to have an influence on glioblastoma cell biology. For instance, the effects of progesterone during pregnancy (a period where progesterone levels rise up to 200-fold) have been analyzed. In a multi-institutional retrospective study with 50 pregnant women diagnosed with glioma, 87% of the cases diagnosed with this tumor before pregnancy (24 patients) showed an increase in the growth rate of the tumor. The other 28 women were diagnosed with glioma during pregnancy (29% during the second and 54% during the third trimesters). These authors concluded that pregnancy may unfavorably impact glioma progression, not only in their growth rate but also in its associated symptoms, with an improvement after delivery in some cases (Peeters et al. 2018).

However, the effects of progesterone on glioblastoma may be different depending on the hormone concentration. Some authors have described an increase in cell proliferation and viability when glioblastoma cell line cultures are exposed to physiological concentrations of progesterone (Gabriela González-Agüero et al. 2007), (Marquina-Sánchez et al. 2017). Furthermore, these effects seem to be mediated by PR activation because they are blocked when RU486 (an antagonist of PR) is used (Gabriela González-Agüero et al. 2007), (Marquina-Sánchez et al. 2017). The stimulation of proliferation by progesterone seems to be mediated by the increase in EGFR and Cyclin D1 expression, as well as the recruitment of steroid receptor coactivator-1 (SRC-1) (Hernández-Hernández, González-García, and Camacho-Arroyo 2012). Moreover, the interplay between PR and protein kinase C seems to play a pivotal role in these effects of progesterone on glioblastoma cells (Marquina-Sánchez et al. 2017).

In contrast, other authors have reported a decrease in cell viability when glioblastoma cell line cultures are exposed to high concentrations of progesterone (or derivatives) (Atif, Yousuf, and Stein 2015), (Altinoz et al. 2020), (Altinoz et al. 2018). In this regard, the antitumoral effect of high progesterone concentrations has been associated with the reduction of glycolytic metabolism and the induction of cell senescence by decreasing Glut1 expression and attenuating the PI3K/Akt/mTOR signaling pathway (Atif et al. 2019). Furthermore, high progresterone concentrations seem to induce changes in detoxification mechanisms, stress and immune response (Altinoz et al. 2020), enhance the cytotoxic effect of temozolamide and reduce its toxic side effects in healthy primary cells (Atif et al. 2015). In line with this, an experimental rat model of glioblastoma showed that progesterone was more effective than dexamethasone in prolonging overall survival and preserving neurologic function (Cheng et al. 2019).

Progesterone also promotes the migration and invasion of glioblastoma-derived cell lines, and these actions seem to be mediated by PR activation because they are blocked by RU-486 (Piña-Medina et al. 2016). These actions seem to be associated with a modulatory effect of progesterone on the phosphorylation state of some molecules involved in cytoskeletal remodeling (Piña-Medina et al. 2016). Moreover, another *in vivo* experiment showed the same effects of progesterone in the rat brain (Germán-Castelán et al. 2014).

Furthermore, another mechanism associated with the development of glioblastoma mediated by progesterone is the expression of progesterone-induced blocking factor (PIBF). This protein has been associated with the proliferative and immunologic effects of progesterone (Gutiérrez-Rodríguez, Hansberg-Pastor, and Camacho-Arroyo 2017), (Bello-Alvarez and Camacho-Arroyo 2021) and the expression of PIBF has been reported in glioblastoma cells (Kyurkchiev et al. 2014). PIBF suppresses antitumor immunity in a similar way as the embryo experiences during pregnancy (Check et al. 2001). The increase in PIBF induced by progesterone leads to an increase in glioblastoma cell proliferation by activating the IL-4 receptor/JAK1/STAT6 signaling pathway.

In conclusion, there is some evidence for the role of progesterone in glioblastoma biology. First, both classic cytoplasmic-nuclear and membrane progesterone receptors are expressed in glioblastoma cells. Second, the activation of these receptors by progesterone or its analogs is associated with changes in the proliferation, migration and invasiveness capacity of glioblastoma cells. Third, those changes are hormone dose-dependent, i.e., physiological doses seem to increase cell viability, proliferation and migration capacity, while high progesterone doses seem to be associated with an antitumoral effect. However, all these data are mainly based on *in vitro* or *in vivo* studies. Only a few retrospective clinical studies have been performed, and because of this, there is a lack of clinical evidence for the role of this hormone in glioblastoma behavior. In this regard, new prospective clinical studies (focusing on prognosis and quality of life) should be performed to test the effect of progesterone pathway modulation in glioblastoma patients.

The Role of Estrogens in Glioblastoma

Estrogen Receptor(s)

There are three main types of estrogens: estrone (E1), estradiol (E2) and estriol (E3), with estradiol being the one with the most powerful estrogenic activity. Estrogens play a neuroprotective role and display neuroproliferative and anti-inflammatory activity in the brain. They modulate neuronal excitability, synaptic plasticity, and neuronal development. This activity is mediated by estrogen receptors, which can be nuclear or membrane receptors (Haas et al. 2012), (Hirtz et al. 2020).

On the one hand, the nuclear receptors ERα and ERβ are encoded by the ESR1 and ESR2 genes, respectively. The ESR1 gene encodes four isoforms (ERα 66, ERα 46, ERα 36, ERα 30), while the ESR2 gene encodes five isoforms (Erβ-1, Erβ-2, Erβ-3, Erβ-4 and Erβ-5). These receptors act as transcription factors; that is, once they are activated, they translocate to the nucleus and modify the expression of target genes (TORAN-ALLERAND 2005). In the brain, both ERα and ERβ are widely distributed and expressed in both neuronal and nonneuronal cell types but with different distribution patterns. For example, ERα is expressed primarily in the hypothalamus and amygdala (autonomic nervous system regulation, reproductive and neuroendocrine response and emotional reactions) (Shughrue, Lane, and Merchenthaler 1997), (Österlund et al. 2000), while ERβ has a higher expression in the cerebral cortex and hippocampus (cognitive functions and mood) (Walf, Koonce, and Frye 2008).

On the other hand, GPER (G-protein associated estrogen receptor) is a nonspecific estrogen membrane receptor capable of activating a rapid, nongenomic and ERα/ERβ-independent estrogen signaling pathway (Cui, Shen, and Li 2013) and is expressed mainly in the hippocampus, cortex, hypothalamus, midbrain nuclei and the Purkinje layer of the cerebellum (Revankar et al. 2005).

Estrogen Signaling Pathways

The estrogen signaling pathways are usually ER-dependent, but in a minority of cases, they are ER-independent; that is, instead of binding to the ER, estrogens interact with other nuclear receptors and regulate enzymatic activities without associating with the ER (Cui, Shen, and Li 2013).

Transcriptional estrogen activity begins when ERα and ERβ receptors interact with estrogens, form homodimers (ERα/ERα, ERβ/ERβ) or heterodimers (ERα/ERβ) and move from the cytoplasm to the nucleus to regulate the expression of genes that contain specific target sequences called EREs (estrogen response elements) (Hewitt et al. 2010).

Another ER-dependent signaling pathway, more rapid than the one previously discussed, is the pathway initiated from the cellular membrane (ERα, ERβ and GPER). Although ERα and ERβ are considered classical nuclear receptors, the existence of these receptors on the cellular membrane has been demonstrated in brain tissue samples, including IGF-1 (insulin-like growth factor 1) and Trk (receptor tyrosine kinase), among others (Milner et al. 2001). At this point, we highlight the role of GPER, which can mediate the rapid activation of signaling cascades such as PI3K/AKT. In addition, a ligand-independent ER pathway activated by other neurotransmitters (dopamine, EGF and IGF-1) instead of estrogens exists (Hayashi and Yamaguchi 2008), (Ignar-Trowbridge et al. 1992), (Klotz et al. 2002).

Expression of Estrogen Receptor(s) in Glioblastoma

Regardless of age and ethnic origin, there is a higher incidence of glioblastoma in men than in women; in addition, the difference between the two decreases when women reach menopause, which suggests a role of sex hormones in glioma pathogenesis. In this regard, female sex hormones may have a protective effect on the development of glioblastoma (Kabat, Etgen, and Rohan 2010).

A few studies have demonstrated the presence of ER expression (ERα and ERβ) in low-grade and high-grade gliomas, showing lower expression in high-grade gliomas. Thus, ER expression seems to play a role in the pathological aggressiveness of gliomas (Tavares et al. 2018), (Fujimoto et al. 1984), (C. Liu et al. 2014). Furthermore, Hönikl et al. (2020) reported a relationship between the expression of ER (α and β) and the prognosis of glioblastoma patients. In this sense, higher ERα and ERβ expression was associated with longer overall survival (Batistatou et al. 2006).

Effects of Estrogen Receptor(s) Activity in Glioblastoma

In the last twenty years, several studies have investigated the role of estrogens in glioblastoma biology. The effect of estrogens on glioblastoma seems to depend on the dose. For example, Altiok N et al. (2011) described an inhibition of cell growth (T98G and C6 cell lines) and a promotion of apoptosis via JNK-c-jun signaling when these cell lines were exposed to higher 17β-estradiol concentrations (Altiok, Ersoz, and Koyuturk 2011). Bearing this in mind, a recent study described not only a lower viability of glioblastoma cells that received higher 17β-estradiol doses but also a greater sensitivity to temozolamide (Hönikl et al. 2020). Nevertheless, low estrogen doses have been associated with an increase in cell proliferation and migration (Bishop and Simpkins 1994), (Castracani et al. 2020). The dose-dependent effect in glioblastoma cells may be related to a complex interaction of different ER isoforms with different signaling pathways. In this regard, the expression of different ERβ isoforms seems to have a differential effect. For example, ERβ1 plays a putative tumor suppressor role, while ERβ5 has oncogenic properties and is overexpressed in high-grade gliomas (J. Liu et al. 2018). Regarding ERβ1, Liu et al. (2018) reported that the expression and activation of ERβ1 decreased the viability of glioblastoma cells *in vitro* through the downregulation of NF-kB, the JAK/STAT and mTor/S6 kinase signaling pathways, and the migratory and invasive potential by decreasing the activity of MMP2. This finding was also confirmed in an *in vivo* model (J. Liu et al. 2018). Subsequently, Zhou M et al. described that the overexpression of ERβ1 was associated with a downregulation of DNA repair genes in glioblastoma cells, enhancing the temozolamide effect by promoting apoptosis and cell cycle arrest both *in vitro* and *in vivo* (Zhou et al. 2019). Alternatively, the expression and activation of another ERβ isoform (i.e., ERβ5) has been associated with the promotion of tumor migration and invasion through the Akt/mTOR pathway (J. Liu et al. 2018).

On the other hand, the expression of ERα has been more commonly reported in low-grade gliomas than in high-grade gliomas, and its expression in high-grade tumors has been associated with a better prognosis. However, the activation of ERα *in vitro* has been associated with tumor cell growth (González-Arenas et al. 2012), and specific ERα isoforms (ERα-36) seem to be associated with the development of tamoxifen (a modulator of ER) resistance in glioblastoma cells (Qu et al. 2019).

Nevertheless, the balance between ERα/ERβ expression seems to be more important than the expression of each receptor individually. For example, cells with higher expression of ERα (i.e., ERα > ERβ) showed a downregulation of Conexin43, a tumor suppressor gene. If the expression of ERα decreased (without changes in the expression of ERβ), there was an increase in Conexin43 expression (Moinfar et al. 2016). The expression of Conexin43 has been observed in normal brain tissue and low-grade gliomas, with very weak or undetectable expression in glioblastoma (Huang et al. 1999). Therefore, glioblastoma cells respond to estrogens depending on the expression balance between ERα and ERβ. Furthermore, when the net modulatory effect of each receptor is considered, one must bear in mind the expression of the specific ERα and ERβ isoforms.

In conclusion, there is consistent evidence that estrogens play a relevant role in the pathogenesis of glioblastoma. The expression of nuclear ER in glioblastoma has been demonstrated, confirming that its activation modulates the proliferation and migration of tumor cells in glioblastoma in a dose-dependent manner.

However, the evidence is based mainly on *in vitro* and *in vivo* studies, and it is necessary to more precisely characterize the role of each isoform and the crosstalk between hormone responses to provide a better understanding. This would allow the development of clinical trials to create new therapeutic strategies in glioblastoma treatment.

The Role of Androgens in Glioblastoma

Androgen Receptor(s)

The androgen receptor (AR) is a type of nuclear receptor that is mainly activated by the binding of androgens, mainly testosterone and dihydrotestosterone. There are two prominent isoforms of the androgen receptors AR-A (87 kDa) and AR-B (110 kDa), with three major functional domains: the N-terminal domain, DNA-binding domain, and androgen-binding domain (Wilson and McPhaul 1994). When AR is not activated, it is located in the cytoplasm and associated with heat shock proteins. The union of an androgen molecule produces a conformational change in the receptor and a dissociation to heat shock proteins. Activated AR translocates to the nucleus, dimerizes and binds to specific gene sequences (called hormone response elements) of specific genes, termed androgen responsive genes (ARGs), whose expression is modulated by the activity of AR. This is the so-called genomic mechanism of action.

Nevertheless, AR may also have other actions that are independent of an interaction with DNA, i.e., the nongenomic mechanism of action. This mechanism consists of an interaction between AR and signal transduction proteins of some pathways in the cytoplasm. These interactions may produce changes in ion transport or regulate the cytoplasmic phosphorylation of other signal transduction pathway proteins (Heinlein and Chang 2002), (Fix et al. 2004). Some of these nongenomic actions modulated by androgens may be associated with the activation of membrane androgen receptors. Three distinct proteins have been proposed as membrane androgen receptors and meet the traditional criterion for their designation. These proteins are TRMP8, GPRC6A and ZIP9 (Thomas 2019). However, these receptors have not been extensively studied, and more information about their specific functions is needed.

Androgens are important for the maintenance of homeostasis in the central nervous system. In this regard, androgens regulate important functions in the central nervous system: neural differentiation and brain masculinization (Di Donato et al. 2015); learning and memory processes; and emotional states, impulsivity and aggressive behaviors (Almeida et al. 2004), (Welk et al. 2017). In addition, androgen levels are essential for the modulation of synaptic plasticity mechanisms (Soma et al. 2018). Thus, androgens, especially testosterone and dihydrotestosterone, are considered neuroprotective factors with actions generally mediated by the AR (Yao et al. 2017).

Expression of the Androgen Receptor in Glioblastoma

The activation of AR seems to have a pathogenic role in glioblastoma. Indeed, higher AR expression has been demonstrated in glioblastoma biopsies than in healthy brains (Yu et al. 2015), (Zalcman et al. 2018). This difference was confirmed in various databases included in the Oncomine™ repository (Bredel Brain and Sun Brain). The level of AR expression seems to be associated with the histological grade of glial tumors, in such a way that the highest expression is found in the highest-grade glial tumors. Furthermore, overexpression of AR has also been described in some glioblastoma cell lines (Bao et al. 2017).

On the other hand, it should be noted that testosterone levels appear to be higher in patients with gliomas than in patients with other neurosurgical diseases, such as benign tumors or patients with craniocerebral trauma (Bao et al. 2017). In addition, from an epidemiological point of view, the incidence of glioblastoma is higher in men than in women (3: 2) (Lapointe, Perry, and Butowski 2018). However, the relationship between blood androgen levels, the expression of the androgen receptor and the prognosis of patients with glioblastoma has not yet been determined.

Effects of Androgen Receptor Activity on Glioblastoma

The effects of AR activity on glioblastoma cells have been tested in cell line cultures and in a few *in vivo* and in silico studies. Rodríguez-Lozano DC et al. (2019) described an increase in the proliferative rates of tumor cells and a greater capacity for migration and invasiveness by the addition of testosterone *in vitro* (Rodríguez-Lozano et al. 2019). In fact, silencing the AR gene or its pharmacological blockade leads to cell death in *in vitro* and *in vivo* studies (Zalcman et al. 2018), (Bao et al. 2017). Furthermore, an *in vitro* study demonstrated that the activation of AR in glioblastoma is associated with radiation resistance by regulating transcriptional programs needed to repair radiation-induced DNA damage (Werner et al. 2020). All these findings suggest that, in terms of prognosis, the most important factor is not AR expression but its activity. This hypothesis was tested by our group in a study performed with data from The Cancer Genome Atlas (TCGA). We calculated a score of AR activity (AR score) by considering the expression of a specific set of ARGs (provided by previous functional *in vitro* experiments in prostate cancer cell lines), and we found that this score was negatively associated with overall survival (Submitted, June 2021). However, evidence for the putative influence of AR in the biology of glioblastoma is mainly based on glioblastoma cell lines. No study has been conducted on the expression and functionality of AR using primary glioblastoma cell cultures. Furthermore, the activity of AR has been evaluated by using some ARGs that are induced by AR activation in prostate cancer. Whether they are the most significant ARGs in glioblastoma is a question that has not yet been addressed.

Therefore, there is enough evidence in the literature to justify the link between androgens and glioblastoma, although there are many questions that need to be answered. Likewise, for the other sex steroid receptors, the main interest lies in the possible use of the androgenic pathway as a therapeutic target for the management of glioblastoma.

Conclusion

Sex steroid receptors are expressed in glioblastoma tissues and have been demonstrated to play a role in glioblastoma pathogenesis, modulating cell growth, migration and invasion. However, most of the studies are preclinical and use glioblastoma cell lines, which do not reflect the heterogeneity of glioblastoma. For this reason, it would be necessary to promote studies in primary cultures, which would provide more evidence for the role of sex steroid receptors in glioblastoma.

Thus, bearing in mind that sex steroid receptors may play a role in the pathogenesis of one of the worst prognostic tumors and that there is wide clinical experience in the use of sex steroid receptor modulating drugs in other tumors (e.g., breast cancer), it is appropriate to consider this strategy in new prospective clinical studies in glioblastoma patients, with the aim of improving the survival and quality of life of glioblastoma patients.

References

Almeida, Osvaldo P, Anna Waterreus, Nigel Spry, Leon Flicker, and Ralph N Martins. 2004. "One Year Follow-up Study of the Association between Chemical Castration, Sex Hormones, Beta-Amyloid, Memory and Depression in Men." *Psychoneuroendocrinology* 29 (8): 1071–81. doi:10.1016/j.psyneuen.2003.11.002.

Altinoz, Meric A, Josephine Nalbantoglu, Aysel Ozpinar, M Emin Ozcan, Rolando F Del Maestro, and Ilhan Elmaci. 2018. "From Epidemiology and Neurodevelopment to Antineoplasticity. Medroxyprogesterone Reduces Human Glial Tumor Growth *in Vitro* and C6 Glioma in Rat Brain *in Vivo*." *Clinical Neurology and Neurosurgery* 173. Neuroacademy Research Group, Istanbul, Turkey; Department of Psychiatry, Maastricht University, Holland, Netherlands. Electronic address: maltinoz@gmail.com.: 20–30. doi:10.1016/j.clineuro.2018.07.012.

Altinoz, Meric A, Yasemin Ucal, Muazzez C Yilmaz, İrem Kiris, Ozan Ozisik, Ugur Sezerman, Aysel Ozpinar, and İlhan Elmaci. 2020. "Progesterone at High Doses Reduces the Growth of U87 and A172 Glioblastoma Cells: Proteomic Changes Regarding Metabolism and Immunity." *Cancer Medicine* 9 (16). John Wiley and Sons Inc.: 5767–80. doi:10.1002/cam4.3223.

Altiok, Nedret, Melike Ersoz, and Meral Koyuturk. 2011. "Estradiol Induces JNK-Dependent Apoptosis in Glioblastoma Cells." *Oncol Lett* 2 (6). Yeni Yuzyil University School of Medicine, Department of Pharmacology, Cevizlibag-Topkapi, Istanbul, Turkey Institute of Medical Sciences, Istanbul Science/Bilim University, Istanbul, Turkey Department of Histology and Embryology of Istanbul Science/Bilim: 1281–85. doi:10.3892/ol.2011.385.

Atif, Fahim, Neil R Patel, Seema Yousuf, and Donald G Stein. 2015. "The Synergistic Effect of Combination Progesterone and Temozolomide on Human Glioblastoma Cells." *PloS One* 10 (6). Public Library of Science: e0131441–e0131441. doi:10.1371/journal.pone.0131441.

Atif, Fahim, Seema Yousuf, Claudia Espinosa-Garcia, Elena Sergeeva, and Donald G Stein. 2019. "Progesterone Treatment Attenuates Glycolytic Metabolism and Induces Senescence in Glioblastoma." *Scientific Reports*. Brain Research Laboratory, Department of Emergency Medicine, School of Medicine, Emory University, Atlanta, GA, 30322, USA. fatif@emory.edu. doi:10.1038/s41598-018-37399-5.

Atif, Fahim, Seema Yousuf, and Donald G Stein. 2015. "Anti-Tumor Effects of Progesterone in Human Glioblastoma Multiforme: Role of PI3K/Akt/mTOR Signaling." *The Journal of Steroid Biochemistry and Molecular Biology* 146. Department of Emergency Medicine, Brain Research Laboratory, Emory University, Atlanta, GA 30322, USA. Electronic address: fatif@emory.edu.: 62–73. doi:10.1016/j.jsbmb.2014.04.007.

Bao, Dejun, Chuandong Cheng, Xiaoqiang Lan, Rong Xing, Zhuo Chen, Hua Zhao, Junyan Sun, et al. 2017. "Regulation of p53wt Glioma Cell Proliferation by Androgen Receptor-Mediated Inhibition of Small VCP/p97-Interacting Protein Expression." *Oncotarget* 8 (14): 23142–54. doi:10.18632/oncotarget.15509.

Batistatou, Anna, Panayiotis A Kyzas, Ann Goussia, Evdokia Arkoumani, Spyridon Voulgaris, Konstantinos Polyzoidis, Niki J Agnantis, and Dimitrios Stefanou. 2006. "Estrogen Receptor Beta (ERβ) Protein Expression Correlates with BAG-1 and Prognosis in Brain Glial Tumours." *Journal of Neuro-Oncology* 77 (1): 17–23. doi:10.1007/s11060-005-9005-0.

Bello-Alvarez, Claudia, and Ignacio Camacho-Arroyo. 2021. "Impact of Sex in the Prevalence and Progression of Glioblastomas: The Role of Gonadal Steroid Hormones." *Biology of Sex Differences* 12 (1). BioMed Central: 28. doi:10.1186/s13293-021-00372-5.

Bishop, Jean, and James W Simpkins. 1994. "Estradiol Treatment Increases Viability of Glioma and Neuroblastoma Cells *in Vitro*." *Molecular and Cellular Neuroscience* 5 (4): 303–8. doi:https://doi.org/10.1006/mcne.1994.1036.

Castracani, Carlo Castruccio, Lucia Longhitano, Alfio Distefano, Daniela Anfuso, Stavroula Kalampoka, Enrico La Spina, Marinella Astuto, et al. 2020. "Role of 17*β*-Estradiol on Cell Proliferation and Mitochondrial Fitness in Glioblastoma Cells." *Journal of Oncology* 2020. Hindawi: 2314693. doi:10.1155/2020/2314693.

Check, J H, P Nazari, J Goldberg, W Yuen, and D Angotti. 2001. "A Model for Potential Tumor Immunotherapy Based on Knowledge of Immune Mechanisms Responsible for Spontaneous Abortion." *Medical Hypotheses* 57 (3): 337–43. doi:https://doi.org/10.1054/mehy.2001.1333.

Cheng, Yin, Wan Lung Yeung, Ping De Zhang, Ning Li, Mei Yee Kiang, and Gilberto K K Leung. 2019. "Progesterone Is More Effective Than Dexamethasone in Prolonging Overall Survival and Preserving Neurologic Function in Experimental Animals with Orthotopic Glioblastoma Allografts." *World Neurosurgery* 125 (May). United States: e497–507. doi:10.1016/j.wneu.2019.01.113.

Conneely, Orla M, Beth Lynn Maxwell, David O Toft, William T Schrader, and Bert W O'Malley. 1987. "The A and B Forms of the Chicken Progesterone Receptor Arise by Alternate Initiation of Translation of a Unique mRNA." *Biochemical and Biophysical Research Communications* 149 (2): 493–501. doi:https://doi.org/10.1016/0006-291X(87)90395-0.

Cui, Jie, Yong Shen, and Rena Li. 2013. "Estrogen Synthesis and Signaling Pathways during Aging: From Periphery to Brain." *Trends in Molecular Medicine* 19 (3). Center for Hormone Advanced Science and Education (CHASE), Roskamp Institute, Sarasota, FL 34243, USA.: 197–209. doi:10.1016/j.molmed.2012.12.007.

Del Moral-Morales, Aylin, Juan Carlos González-Orozco, José Moisés Capetillo-Velázquez, Ana Gabriela Piña-Medina, and Ignacio Camacho-Arroyo. 2020. "The Role of mPRδ and mPRε in Human Glioblastoma Cells: Expression, Hormonal Regulation, and Possible Clinical Outcome." *Hormones & Cancer* 11 (2). United States: 117–27. doi:10.1007/s12672-020-00381-7.

Di Donato, Marzia, Antonio Bilancio, Loredana D'Amato, Pamela Claudiani, Maria Antonietta Oliviero, Maria Vittoria Barone, Alberto Auricchio, et al. 2015. "Cross-Talk between Androgen Receptor/filamin A and TrkA Regulates Neurite Outgrowth in PC12 Cells." *Molecular Biology of the Cell* 26 (15): 2858–72. doi:10.1091/mbc.E14-09-1352.

Fix, Charity, Cynthia Jordan, Patricia Cano, and William H Walker. 2004. "Testosterone Activates Mitogen-Activated Protein Kinase and the cAMP Response Element Binding Protein Transcription Factor in Sertoli Cells." *Proceedings of the National Academy of Sciences of the United States of America* 101 (30). Department of Cell Biology and Physiology, University of Pittsburgh, PA 15261, USA.: 10919–24. doi:10.1073/pnas.0404278101.

Fujimoto, M, E Yoshino, K Hirakawa, J Fujimoto, and T Tamaya. 1984. "Estrogen Receptors in Brain Tumors." *Clinical Neuropharmacology* 7 (4): 357–62. doi:10.1097/00002826-198412000-00015.

Gately, L, S A McLachlan, A Dowling, and J Philip. 2017. "Life beyond a Diagnosis of Glioblastoma: A Systematic Review of the Literature." *Journal of Cancer Survivorship : Research and Practice* 11 (4): 447–52. doi:10.1007/s11764-017-0602-7.

Germán-Castelán, Liliana, Joaquín Manjarrez-Marmolejo, Aliesha González-Arenas, María Genoveva González-Morán, and Ignacio Camacho-Arroyo. 2014. "Progesterone Induces the Growth and Infiltration of Human Astrocytoma Cells Implanted in the Cerebral Cortex of the Rat." *BioMed Research International* 2014. Hindawi Publishing Corporation: 393174. doi:10.1155/2014/393174.

Giangrande, P H, E A Kimbrel, D P Edwards, and D P McDonnell. 2000. "The Opposing Transcriptional Activities of the Two Isoforms of the Human Progesterone Receptor Are due to Differential Cofactor Binding." *Molecular and Cellular Biology* 20 (9). Department of Pharmacology, Duke University Medical Center, Durham, North Carolina 27710, USA.: 3102–15. doi:10.1128/mcb.20.9.3102-3115.2000.

Giangrande, P H, and D P McDonnell. 1999. "The A and B Isoforms of the Human Progesterone Receptor: Two Functionally Different Transcription Factors Encoded by a Single Gene." *Recent Progress in Hormone Research* 54. United States: 291–94.

González-Agüero, Gabriela, Andrés A Gutiérrez, Diana González-Espinosa, José D Solano, Rocío Morales, Aliesha González-Arenas, Edith Cabrera-Muñoz, and Ignacio Camacho-Arroyo. 2007. "Progesterone Effects on Cell Growth of U373 and D54 Human Astrocytoma Cell Lines." *Endocrine* 32 (2). Facultad de Química, Departamento de Biología, Universidad Nacional Autónoma de México, Mexico DF, 04510, Mexico.: 129–35. doi:10.1007/s12020-007-9023-0.

González-Agüero, G, R Ondarza, A Gamboa-Domínguez, M A Cerbón, and I Camacho-Arroyo. 2001. "Progesterone Receptor Isoforms Expression Pattern in Human Astrocytomas." *Brain Research Bulletin* 56 (1). Departamento de Biología, Facultad de Química, Universidad Nacional Autónoma de México, Coyoacán, México.: 43–48. doi:10.1016/s0361-9230(01)00590-1.

González-Arenas, Aliesha, Valeria Hansberg-Pastor, Olivia Tania Hernández-Hernández, Tania Karina González-García, Joshua Henderson-Villalpando, Diana Lemus-Hernández, Aglaé Cruz-Barrios, Mariana Rivas-Suárez, and Ignacio Camacho-Arroyo. 2012. "Estradiol Increases Cell Growth in Human Astrocytoma Cell Lines through ERα Activation and Its Interaction with SRC-1 and SRC-3 Coactivators." *Biochimica et Biophysica Acta* 1823 (2). Facultad de Química, Departamento de Biología, Universidad Nacional Autóma de México, Ciudad Universitaria, Coyoacán, Mexico.: 379–86. doi:10.1016/j.bbamcr.2011.11.004.

González-Orozco, Juan Carlos, Valeria Hansberg-Pastor, Paulina Valadez-Cosmes, Walter Nicolas-Ortega, Yenifer Bastida-Beristain, Marisol De La Fuente-Granada, Aliesha González-Arenas, and Ignacio Camacho-Arroyo. 2018. "Activation of Membrane Progesterone Receptor-Alpha Increases Proliferation, Migration, and Invasion of Human Glioblastoma Cells." *Molecular and Cellular Endocrinology* 477 (December). Ireland: 81–89. doi:10.1016/j.mce.2018.06.004.

Gronemeyer, H. 1991. "Transcription Activation by Estrogen and Progesterone Receptors." *Annual Review of Genetics* 25. Laboratoire de Génétique Moléculaire des Eucaryotes CNRS, Unité 184 de Biologie Moléculaire et de Génie Génétique de l'INSERM, Faculté de Médecine, Strasbourg, France.: 89–123. doi:10.1146/annurev.ge.25.120191.000513.

Gutiérrez-Rodríguez, Araceli, Valeria Hansberg-Pastor, and Ignacio Camacho-Arroyo. 2017. "Proliferative and Invasive Effects of Progesterone-Induced Blocking Factor in Human Glioblastoma Cells." *BioMed Research International* 2017. Hindawi Publishing Corporation: 1295087. doi:10.1155/2017/1295087.

Haas, Michael J, Prafull Raheja, Sarada Jaimungal, Mae Sheikh-Ali, and Arshag D Mooradian. 2012. "Estrogen-Dependent Inhibition of Dextrose-Induced Endoplasmic Reticulum Stress and Superoxide Generation in Endothelial Cells." *Free Radical Biology & Medicine* 52 (11–12). Division of Endocrinology, Diabetes and Metabolism, Department of Medicine, University of Florida College of Medicine, Jacksonville, FL 32209, USA.: 2161–67. doi:10.1016/j.freeradbiomed.2012.04.009.

Hayashi, Shin-ichi, and Yuri Yamaguchi. 2008. "Estrogen Signaling Pathway and Hormonal Therapy." *Breast Cancer (Tokyo, Japan)* 15 (4). Department of Molecular and Functional Dynamics, Laboratory Medicine and Sciences, Tohoku University Graduate School of Medicine, Aoba-ku, Sendai 980-8575, Japan. shayashi@mail.tains.tohoku.ac.jp: 256–61. doi:10.1007/s12282-008-0070-z.

Heinlein, Cynthia A, and Chawnshang Chang. 2002. "The Roles of Androgen Receptors and Androgen-Binding Proteins in Nongenomic Androgen Actions." *Molecular Endocrinology (Baltimore, Md.)* 16 (10). United States: 2181–87. doi:10.1210/me.2002-0070.

Hernández-Hernández, Olivia Tania, Tania Karina González-García, and Ignacio Camacho-Arroyo. 2012. "Progesterone Receptor and SRC-1 Participate in the Regulation of VEGF, EGFR and Cyclin D1 Expression in Human Astrocytoma Cell Lines." *The Journal of Steroid Biochemistry and Molecular Biology* 132 (1–2). Facultad de Química, Departamento de Biología, Universidad Nacional Autónoma de México, Mexico.: 127–34. doi:10.1016/j.jsbmb.2012.04.005.

Hewitt, Sylvia C, Yin Li, Leping Li, and Kenneth S Korach. 2010. "Estrogen-Mediated Regulation of Igf1 Transcription and Uterine Growth Involves Direct Binding of Estrogen Receptor Alpha to Estrogen-Responsive Elements." *The Journal of Biological Chemistry* 285 (4). Receptor Biology Section, Laboratory of Reproductive and Developmental Toxicology, NIEHS, National Institutes of Health, Research Triangle Park, North Carolina 27709, USA. curtiss@niehs.nih.gov: 2676–85. doi:10.1074/jbc.m109.043471.

Hirtz, Alex, Fabien Rech, Hélène Dubois-Pot-Schneider, and Hélène Dumond. 2020. "Astrocytoma: A Hormone-Sensitive Tumor?" *International Journal of Molecular Sciences* 21 (23). MDPI: 9114. doi:10.3390/ijms21239114.

Hlavaty, Juraj, Reinhard Ertl, Ingrid Miller, and Cordula Gabriel. 2016. "Expression of Progesterone Receptor Membrane Component 1 (PGRMC1), Progestin and AdipoQ Receptor 7 (PAQPR7), and Plasminogen Activator Inhibitor 1 RNA-Binding Protein (PAIRBP1) in Glioma Spheroids *In Vitro*." *BioMed Research International* 2016. Institute of Anatomy, Histology and Embryology, University of Veterinary Medicine, 1210 Vienna, Austria.: 8065830. doi:10.1155/2016/8065830.

Hönikl, Lisa Stefanie, Friederike Lämmer, Jens Gempt, Bernhard Meyer, Jürgen Schlegel, and Claire Delbridge. 2020. "High Expression of Estrogen Receptor Alpha and Aromatase in Glial Tumor Cells Is Associated with Gender-Independent Survival Benefits in Glioblastoma Patients." *Journal of Neuro-Oncology* 147 (3): 567–75. doi:10.1007/s11060-020-03467-y.

Hovland, A R, R L Powell, G S Takimoto, L Tung, and K B Horwitz. 1998. "An N-Terminal Inhibitory Function, IF, Suppresses Transcription by the A-Isoform but Not the B-Isoform of Human Progesterone Receptors." *The Journal of Biological Chemistry* 273 (10). Department of Medicine, University of Colorado Health Sciences Center, Denver, Colorado 80262, USA.: 5455–60. doi:10.1074/jbc.273.10.5455.

Huang, R P, M Z Hossain, A Sehgal, and A L Boynton. 1999. "Reduced connexin43 Expression in High-Grade Human Brain Glioma Cells." *Journal of Surgical Oncology* 70 (1). Molecular Medicine, Northwest Hospital, Seattle, Washington 98125, USA. rphuang@nwlink.com: 21–24. doi:10.1002/(sici)1096-9098(199901)70:1<21::aid-jso4>3.0.co;2-0.

Ignar-Trowbridge, D M, K G Nelson, M C Bidwell, S W Curtis, T F Washburn, J A McLachlan, and K S Korach. 1992. "Coupling of Dual Signaling Pathways: Epidermal Growth Factor Action Involves the Estrogen Receptor." *Proceedings of the National Academy of Sciences of the United States of America* 89 (10). Laboratory of

Reproductive and Developmental Toxicology, National Institute of Environmental Health Sciences, National Institutes of Health, Research Triangle Park, NC 27709.: 4658–62. doi:10.1073/pnas.89.10.4658.

Jacobsen, Britta, and Kathryn Horwitz. 2011. "Progesterone Receptors, Their Isoforms and Progesterone Regulated Transcription." *Molecular and Cellular Endocrinology* 357 (September): 18–29. doi:10.1016/j.mce.2011.09.016.

Kabat, Geoffrey C, Anne M Etgen, and Thomas E Rohan. 2010. "Do Steroid Hormones Play a Role in the Etiology of Glioma?" *Cancer Epidemiology Biomarkers & Prevention*, September, 658–1055. doi:10.1158/1055-9965.EPI-10-0658.

Kastner, P, A Krust, B Turcotte, U Stropp, L Tora, H Gronemeyer, and P Chambon. 1990. "Two Distinct Estrogen-Regulated Promoters Generate Transcripts Encoding the Two Functionally Different Human Progesterone Receptor Forms A and B." *The EMBO Journal* 9 (5). John Wiley & Sons, Ltd: 1603–14. doi:https://doi.org/10.1002/j.1460-2075.1990.tb08280.x.

Khalid, H, S Shibata, M Kishikawa, A Yasunaga, M Iseki, and T Hiura. 1997. "Immunohistochemical Analysis of Progesterone Receptor and Ki-67 Labeling Index in Astrocytic Tumors." *Cancer* 80 (11). Department of Neurosurgery, Nagasaki University School of Medicine, Japan.: 2133–40. doi:10.1002/(sici)1097-0142(19971201)80:11<2133::aid-cncr13>3.0.co;2-#.

Klotz, Diane M, Sylvia Curtis Hewitt, Paolo Ciana, Michele Raviscioni, Jonathan K Lindzey, Julie Foley, Adriana Maggi, Richard P DiAugustine, and Kenneth S Korach. 2002. "Requirement of Estrogen Receptor-Alpha in Insulin-like Growth Factor-1 (IGF-1)-Induced Uterine Responses and *in Vivo* Evidence for IGF-1/estrogen Receptor Cross-Talk." *The Journal of Biological Chemistry* 277 (10). United States: 8531–37. doi:10.1074/jbc.M109592200.

Kyurkchiev, Dobroslav, Emanuil Naydenov, Kalina Tumangelova-Yuzeir, Ekaterina Ivanova-Todorova, Kalina Belemezova, Ivan Bochev, Krasimir Minkin, et al. 2014. "Cells Isolated from Human Glioblastoma Multiforme Express Progesterone-Induced Blocking Factor (PIBF)." *Cellular and Molecular Neurobiology* 34 (4). United States: 479–89. doi:10.1007/s10571-014-0031-3.

Lapointe, Sarah, Arie Perry, and Nicholas A Butowski. 2018. "Primary Brain Tumours in Adults." *Lancet (London, England)* 392 (10145): 432–46. doi:10.1016/S0140-6736(18)30990-5.

Liu, Chang, Yanlei Zhang, Kaiyuan Zhang, Chen Bian, Yangang Zhao, and Jiqiang Zhang. 2014. "Expression of Estrogen Receptors, Androgen Receptor and Steroid Receptor Coactivator-3 Is Negatively Correlated to the Differentiation of Astrocytic Tumors." *Cancer Epidemiology* 38 (3). Netherlands: 291–97. doi:10.1016/j.canep.2014.03.001.

Liu, Jinyou, Gangadhara R Sareddy, Mei Zhou, Suryavathi Viswanadhapalli, Xiaonan Li, Zhao Lai, Rajeshwar R Tekmal, Andrew Brenner, and Ratna K Vadlamudi. 2018. "Differential Effects of Estrogen Receptor β Isoforms on Glioblastoma Progression." *Cancer Research* 78 (12): 3176–89. doi:10.1158/0008-5472.CAN-17-3470.

Mangelsdorf, D J, C Thummel, M Beato, P Herrlich, G Schütz, K Umesono, B Blumberg, et al. 1995. "The Nuclear Receptor Superfamily: The Second Decade." *Cell* 83 (6). Howard Hughes Medical Institute, University of Texas Southwestern Medical Center, Dallas 75235-9050, USA.: 835–39. doi:10.1016/0092-8674(95)90199-x.

Marquina-Sánchez, Brenda, Jesús González-Jorge, Valeria Hansberg-Pastor, Talia Wegman-Ostrosky, Noemi Baranda-Ávila, Sonia Mejía-Pérez, Ignacio Camacho-Arroyo, and Aliesha González-Arenas. 2017. "The Interplay between Intracellular Progesterone Receptor and PKC Plays a Key Role in Migration and Invasion of Human Glioblastoma Cells." *The Journal of Steroid Biochemistry and Molecular Biology* 172. Departamento de Medicina Genómica y Toxicología Ambiental, Programa de Investigación en Cancer de Mama, Instituto de Investigaciones Biomédicas, Universidad Nacional Autónoma de México, Ciudad de México, Mexico.: 198–206. doi:10.1016/j.jsbmb.2016.10.001.

McDonnell, Donald P. 1995. "Unraveling the Human Progesterone Receptor Signal Transduction Pathway: Insights into Antiprogestin Action." *Trends in Endocrinology & Metabolism* 6 (4): 133–38. doi:https://doi.org/10.1016/1043-2760(95)00065-P.

Milner, T A, B S McEwen, S Hayashi, C J Li, L P Reagan, and S E Alves. 2001. "Ultrastructural Evidence That Hippocampal Alpha Estrogen Receptors Are Located at Extranuclear Sites." *The Journal of Comparative Neurology* 429 (3). Division of Neurobiology, Department of Neurology and Neuroscience, Weill Medical College of Cornell University, New York, New York 10021, USA. tmilner@mail.med.cornell.edu: 355–71. doi:10.1002/1096-9861(20010115)429:3<355::aid-cne1>3.0.co;2-#.

Moinfar, Zahra, Hannes Dambach, Bodo Schoenebeck, Eckart Förster, Nora Prochnow, and Pedro Michael Faustmann. 2016. "Estradiol Receptors Regulate Differential Connexin 43 Expression in F98 and C6 Glioma Cell Lines." *PLOS ONE* 11 (2). Public Library of Science: e0150007.

Mulac-Jericevic, B, R A Mullinax, F J DeMayo, J P Lydon, and O M Conneely. 2000. "Subgroup of Reproductive Functions of Progesterone Mediated by Progesterone Receptor-B Isoform." *Science (New York, N.Y.)* 289 (5485). Department of Molecular and Cellular Biology, Baylor College of Medicine, One Baylor Plaza, Houston, TX 77030, USA.: 1751–54. doi:10.1126/science.289.5485.1751.

Österlund, Marie K, Jan-Åke Gustafsson, Eva Keller, and Yasmin L Hurd. 2000. "Estrogen Receptor β (ERβ) Messenger Ribonucleic Acid (mRNA) Expression within the Human Forebrain: Distinct Distribution Pattern to ERα mRNA1." *The Journal of Clinical Endocrinology & Metabolism* 85 (10): 3840–46. doi:10.1210/jcem.85.10.6913.

Ostrom, Quinn T, Haley Gittleman, Carol Kruchko, and Jill S Barnholtz-Sloan. 2019. "Primary Brain and Other Central Nervous System Tumors in Appalachia: Regional Differences in Incidence, Mortality, and Survival." *Journal of Neuro-Oncology* 142 (1): 27–38. doi:10.1007/s11060-018-03073-z.

Pang, Yefei, Jing Dong, and Peter Thomas. 2013. "Characterization, Neurosteroid Binding and Brain Distribution of Human Membrane Progesterone Receptors δ and {epsilon} (mPRδ and mPR{epsilon}) and mPRδ Involvement in Neurosteroid Inhibition of Apoptosis." *Endocrinology* 154 (1). Endocrine Society: 283–95. doi:10.1210/en.2012-1772.

Peeters, Sophie, Mélanie Pagès, Guillaume Gauchotte, Catherine Miquel, Stéphanie Cartalat-Carel, Jean-Sébastien Guillamo, Laurent Capelle, et al. 2018. "Interactions between Glioma and Pregnancy: Insight from a 52-Case Multicenter Series." *Journal of Neurosurgery* 128 (1). United States: 3–13. doi:10.3171/2016.10.JNS16710.

Petersen, Sandra L, Karlie A Intlekofer, Paula J Moura-Conlon, Daniel N Brewer, Javier Del Pino Sans, and Justin A Lopez. 2013. "Novel Progesterone Receptors: Neural Localization and Possible Functions." *Frontiers in Neuroscience* 7 (September). Frontiers Media S.A.: 164. doi:10.3389/fnins.2013.00164.

Piña-Medina, Ana Gabriela, Valeria Hansberg-Pastor, Aliesha González-Arenas, Marco Cerbón, and Ignacio Camacho-Arroyo. 2016. "Progesterone Promotes Cell Migration, Invasion and Cofilin Activation in Human Astrocytoma Cells." *Steroids* 105. Unidad de Investigación en Reproducción Humana, Instituto Nacional de Perinatología-Facultad de Química, Universidad Nacional Autónoma de México (UNAM), Ciudad Universitaria, Coyoacán 04510, México, D.F., Mexico.: 19–25. doi:10.1016/j.steroids.2015.11.008.

Qu, Chao, Jingyun Ma, Yejun Zhang, Chao Han, Liang Huang, Liming Shen, Hongyan Li, Xiaobo Wang, Jing Liu, and Wei Zou. 2019. "Estrogen Receptor Variant ER-α36 Promotes Tamoxifen Agonist Activity in Glioblastoma Cells." *Cancer Science* 110 (1): 221–34. doi:10.1111/cas.13868.

Revankar, Chetana M, Daniel F Cimino, Larry A Sklar, Jeffrey B Arterburn, and Eric R Prossnitz. 2005. "A Transmembrane Intracellular Estrogen Receptor Mediates Rapid Cell Signaling." *Science (New York, N.Y.)* 307 (5715). Department of Cell Biology and Physiology, University of New Mexico Health Sciences Center, Albuquerque, NM 87131, USA.: 1625–30. doi:10.1126/science.1106943.

Rodríguez-Lozano, Dulce Carolina, Ana Gabriela Piña-Medina, Valeria Hansberg-Pastor, Claudia Bello-Alvarez, and Ignacio Camacho-Arroyo. 2019. "Testosterone Promotes Glioblastoma Cell Proliferation, Migration, and Invasion Through Androgen Receptor Activation." *Frontiers in Endocrinology* 10: 16. doi:10.3389/fendo.2019.00016.

Shughrue, Paul J, Malcolm V Lane, and Istvan Merchenthaler. 1997. "Comparative Distribution of Estrogen Receptor-α and -β mRNA in the Rat Central Nervous System." *Journal of Comparative Neurology* 388 (4). John Wiley & Sons, Ltd: 507–25. doi:https://doi.org/10.1002/(SICI)1096-9861(19971201)388:4<507::AID-CNE1>3.0.CO;2-6.

Soma, Mika, Jonghyuk Kim, Asami Kato, and Suguru Kawato. 2018. "Src Kinase Dependent Rapid Non-Genomic Modulation of Hippocampal Spinogenesis Induced by Androgen and Estrogen." *Frontiers in Neuroscience* 12: 282. doi:10.3389/fnins.2018.00282.

Stupp, Roger, Monika E Hegi, Warren P Mason, Martin J van den Bent, Martin J B Taphoorn, Robert C Janzer, Samuel K Ludwin, et al. 2009. "Effects of Radiotherapy with Concomitant and Adjuvant Temozolomide versus Radiotherapy Alone on Survival in Glioblastoma in a Randomised Phase III Study: 5-Year Analysis of the EORTC-NCIC Trial." *The Lancet. Oncology* 10 (5): 459–66. doi:10.1016/S1470-2045(09)70025-7.

Stupp, Roger, Sophie Taillibert, Andrew A. Kanner, Santosh Kesari, David M. Steinberg, Steven A. Toms, Lynne P. Taylor, et al. 2015. "Maintenance Therapy With Tumor-Treating Fields Plus Temozolomide vs Temozolomide Alone for Glioblastoma." *JAMA* 314 (23): 2535. doi:10.1001/jama.2015.16669.

Stupp, Roger, Sophie Taillibert, Andrew Kanner, William Read, David M. Steinberg, Benoit Lhermitte, Steven Toms, et al. 2017. "Effect of Tumor-Treating Fields Plus Maintenance Temozolomide vs Maintenance Temozolomide Alone on Survival in Patients With Glioblastoma." *JAMA* 318 (23): 2306. doi:10.1001/jama.2017.18718.

Tang, Y Tom, Tianhua Hu, Matthew Arterburn, Bryan Boyle, Jessica M Bright, Peter C Emtage, and Walter D Funk. 2005. "PAQR Proteins: A Novel Membrane Receptor Family Defined by an Ancient7-Transmembrane Pass Motif." *Journal of Molecular Evolution* 61 (3): 372–80. doi:10.1007/s00239-004-0375-2.

Tavares, Cléciton Braga, Francisca das Chagas Sheyla Gomes-Braga, Emerson Brandão Sousa, Umbelina Soares Borges, Carla Solange Escórcio-Dourado, João Paulo da Silva-Sampaio, and Benedito Borges da Silva. 2018. "Evaluation of Estrogen Receptor Expression in Low-Grade and High-Grade Astrocytomas." *Revista Da Associacao Medica Brasileira (1992)* 64 (12). Brazil: 1129–33. doi:10.1590/1806-9282.64.12.1129.

Thomas, Peter. 2019. "Membrane Androgen Receptors Unrelated to Nuclear Steroid Receptors." *Endocrinology* 160 (4). United States: 772–81. doi:10.1210/en.2018-00987.

Thomas, Peter, and Yefei Pang. 2012. "Membrane Progesterone Receptors: Evidence for Neuroprotective, Neurosteroid Signaling and Neuroendocrine Functions in Neuronal Cells." *Neuroendocrinology* 96 (2): 162–71. doi:10.1159/000339822.

TORAN-ALLERAND, C.DOMINIQUE. 2005. "Estrogen and the Brain: Beyond ER-A, ER-B, and 17β-Estradiol." *Annals of the New York Academy of Sciences* 1052 (1). John Wiley & Sons, Ltd: 136–44. doi:https://doi.org/10.1196/annals.1347.009.

Valadez-Cosmes, Paulina, Edgar Ricardo Vázquez-Martínez, Marco Cerbón, and Ignacio Camacho-Arroyo. 2016. "Membrane Progesterone Receptors in Reproduction and Cancer." *Molecular and Cellular Endocrinology* 434: 166–75. doi:https://doi.org/10.1016/j.mce.2016.06.027.

Vegeto, E, M M Shahbaz, D X Wen, M E Goldman, B W O'Malley, and D P McDonnell. 1993. "Human Progesterone Receptor A Form Is a Cell- and Promoter-Specific Repressor of Human Progesterone Receptor B Function." *Molecular Endocrinology (Baltimore, Md.)* 7 (10). United States: 1244–55. doi:10.1210/mend.7.10.8264658.

Walf, Alicia A, Carolyn J Koonce, and Cheryl A Frye. 2008. "Estradiol or Diarylpropionitrile Administration to Wild Type, but Not Estrogen Receptor Beta Knockout, Mice Enhances Performance in the Object Recognition and Object Placement Tasks." *Neurobiology of Learning and Memory* 89 (4): 513–21. doi:10.1016/j.nlm.2008.01.008.

Welk, Blayne, Eric McArthur, Michael Ordon, Sarah A Morrow, Jade Hayward, and Stephanie Dixon. 2017. "The Risk of Dementia with the Use of 5 Alpha Reductase Inhibitors." *Journal of the Neurological Sciences* 379 (August): 109–11. doi:10.1016/j.jns.2017.05.064.

Werner, Christian K, Uchechi J Nna, Hanshi Sun, Kari Wilder-Romans, Joseph Dresser, Ayesha U Kothari, Weihua Zhou, et al. 2020. "Expression of the Androgen Receptor Governs Radiation Resistance in a Subset of Glioblastomas Vulnerable to Antiandrogen Therapy." *Molecular Cancer Therapeutics* 19 (10): 2163–74. doi:10.1158/1535-7163.MCT-20-0095.

Wilson, C M, and M J McPhaul. 1994. "A and B Forms of the Androgen Receptor Are Present in Human Genital Skin Fibroblasts." *Proceedings of the National Academy of Sciences of the United States of America* 91 (4): 1234–38. doi:10.1073/pnas.91.4.1234.

Yao, Peng-Le, Shu Zhuo, Hong Mei, Xiao-Fang Chen, Na Li, Teng-Fei Zhu, Shi-Ting Chen, Ji-Ming Wang, Rui-Xing Hou, and Ying-Ying Le. 2017. "Androgen Alleviates Neurotoxicity of β-Amyloid Peptide (Aβ) by Promoting Microglial Clearance of Aβ and Inhibiting Microglial Inflammatory Response to Aβ." *CNS Neuroscience & Therapeutics* 23 (11): 855–65. doi:10.1111/cns.12757.

Yu, Xiaoming, Yuhua Jiang, Wei Wei, Ping Cong, Yinlu Ding, Lei Xiang, and Kang Wu. 2015. "Androgen Receptor Signaling Regulates Growth of Glioblastoma Multiforme in Men." *Tumour Biology: The Journal of the International Society for Oncodevelopmental Biology and Medicine* 36 (2): 967–72. doi:10.1007/s13277-014-2709-z.

Zalcman, Nomi, Tamar Canello, Haim Ovadia, Hanna Charbit, Bracha Zelikovitch, Anat Mordechai, Yakov Fellig, et al. 2018. "Androgen Receptor: A Potential Therapeutic Target for Glioblastoma." *Oncotarget* 9 (28): 19980–93. doi:10.18632/oncotarget.25007.

Zhou, Mei, Gangadhara R Sareddy, Mengxing Li, Jinyou Liu, Yiliao Luo, Prabhakar Pitta Venkata, Suryavathi Viswanadhapalli, Rajeshwar R Tekmal, Andrew Brenner, and Ratna K Vadlamudi. 2019. "Estrogen Receptor Beta Enhances Chemotherapy Response of GBM Cells by down Regulating DNA Damage Response Pathways." *Scientific Reports* 9 (1): 6124. doi:10.1038/s41598-019-42313-8.

Chapter 18

Creating and Developing a Pediatric Comprehensive Spasticity Program: An Eight-Year Experience

Hector E. James[1], MD, Louise Z. Spierre[2], MD and Nathan J. Ranalli[3], MD, FAANS, FAAP

[1]Department of Neurosurgery, University of Florida College of Medicine and Pediatric Neurosurgery Consultant, Wolfson Children's Hospital/Baptist Health of Northeast Florida, Jacksonville, FL, USA

[2]Department of Pediatrics, University of Florida College of Medicine Jacksonville, and Department of Rehabilitation, Wolfson Children's Hospital, Jacksonville, FL, USA

[3]Department of Neurosurgery and Department of Oral and Maxillofacial Surgery, University of Florida College of Medicine Jacksonville, Jacksonville, FL, USA

Abstract

We describe the eight-year experience of a comprehensive multidisciplinary and multi-institutional program for the evaluation and management of youth with spasticity. The University of Florida Division of Pediatric Neurosurgery completed a staged process to develop a multidisciplinary multi-institutional working group. Physicians and allied health personnel volunteered to participate in monthly meetings for care coordination. The administrative matrix for development, structuring and care sequence is delineated. This report covers the period of June 2009 through July 2019. Following recruitment of a pediatric physical medicine (PPM) physician, a spasticity clinic was established. The PPM physician, advanced practice registered nurse (APRN), and pediatric physical therapist (PPT) evaluate patients in the clinic, and diagnosis and management decisions are made. Patients what may require surgical interventions are presented in the monthly

In: Advances in Neurosurgery Research
Editors: Amit Agrawal, Pradeep Chouksey, Adesh Shrivastava et al.
ISBN: 978-1-68507-859-1

multidisciplinary multi-institutional care conference. Following team management decisions, patients are referred to surgical specialists. Medical care is coordinated by the APRN. Quality improvement aspects and outcomes, as well as pertinent scientific literature is presented in the monthly conferences. A multidisciplinary group can be created with interested and motivated physicians and allied health personnel, to provide comprehensive management of youth with spasticity.

Introduction

Spasticity and motor tone alterations are a common finding in youth with cerebral palsy [1]. These create a chronic limitation in day to day activities, competitiveness and independence [2]. Chronic pain may occur as a consequence of contractures and spasticity, and can be managed with pediatric physical therapy (PPT) and pediatric occupational therapy (POT), with or without medications. At times, a more invasive approach with botulinum toxin injections, surgical tendon releases, orthopedic interventions, baclofen pumps and/or rhizotomies is employed [3].

Children with chronic medical conditions receive better care in a comprehensive multidisciplinary setting [4]. Few medical centers provide multidisciplinary venues with a team approach for children with spasticity. Existing programs differ in their structure according to the background and training of the various members of the team and leadership, evaluation process, and management protocols [5].

We previously reported on the initiation of the comprehensive pediatric spasticity program at Wolfson Children's Hospital (WCH), with multispecialty and multi-institutional support, and involving specialties from University of Florida College of Medicine Jacksonville (UFCOMJ), the WCH Department of Rehabilitation, and Nemours Children's Specialty Care Jacksonville (NCSCJ) [6]. We wish to share the eight-year experience and the initiation of the clinical program.

Materials and Methods

The current material addresses development and establishment of a spasticity program from June 2009 through July 2019.

A partnership between the leadership of the UFCOMJ Division of Pediatric Neurosurgery and WCH/Baptist Health of Northeast Florida was established in 2003. At that time, no program was in place for the care of children with spasticity. Communication proceeded between the UFCOMJ Department of Pediatrics and Division of Pediatric Neurosurgery, the administrative leadership teams, the WCH Department of Rehabilitation, and the NCSCJ Division of Orthopedics. The recruitment process began for a pediatric physical medicine (PPM) physician in June 2009, and the Physical Medicine and Rehabilitation Program was subsequently initiated.

A detailed report on the initiation of the program was previously published and explained the administrative phase as well as phases one through three [6]. In this report we will now summarize the initiation steps.

An initial educational venue was established by the PPM physician with a core group of PPT and POT personnel. These core team members visited the spasticity program in place at Primary Children's Medical Center/University of Utah in Salt Lake City where they observed the sequence of the care of spasticity. A designated outpatient rehabilitation area was identified, and an inpatient progressive care unit was established.

Results

A spasticity clinic was initiated in December 2009, following establishment of an outpatient pediatric rehabilitation area. Using a team approach in this clinic, youth with spasticity and related conditions are evaluated by the PPM advanced practice registered nurse (APRN) and PPT, and decisions are made with the parent and care providers in attendance. The clinic meets three days each week. The patient's primary care provider will receive treatment updates and results. If therapy or procedure authorizations are required, documentation is submitted to the pertinent medical insurance for approval.

Spasticity and Related Services

Following initial evaluation by the clinic team members, management decisions are made, and follow-up visits are arranged for patient progress. For patients requiring PPT or POT, appointments are coordinated for the pertinent regional outreach rehabilitation clinics of WCH. For patients needing botulinum toxin injection, sessions are performed by the PPM physician in the office or in the hospital under minimal sedation or general anesthesia, as needed, in a monitored area. A PPM physician performs baclofen trials in a progressive care area. Lumbar puncture and intrathecal baclofen administration are performed by pediatric radiology, under fluoroscopy, with or without sedation. These patients are admitted in the early morning hours and evaluated by PPT and POT prior to baclofen administration. They are examined following the baclofen injection and discharged home in the late morning/afternoon. If the trial is successful, the baclofen pump is instituted at a later date. All patients with a baclofen pump are followed by the PPM physician in the Spasticity Clinic.

Dorsal rhizotomy patients are also managed in the Spasticity Clinic for assessment, PPT modifications or related care issues.

Multidisciplinary Team Conference and Surgical Patient Management

A monthly team conference is held with specialty resources. These include the PPM physician, pediatric neurosurgery, pediatric orthopedics (PORTH), PPT, POT, and social services. Patients who failed conservative management are discussed. An overview of medical history, physical findings, management issues, and pre- and post-baclofen trial videos are reviewed. Further treatment options are discussed, and management recommendations made by the team. The PPM physician or APRN communicates team decisions to the parents/caregivers and primary care provider. Patients previously treated with baclofen pumps, rhizotomies, and/or related procedures are also discussed. PORTH patients may have spasticity as a comorbidity and are referred to PPM for evaluation and recommendations. PORTH is an active participant in the care sequence of spasticity. Monthly conferences may raise questions as to patient needs, such as, but not limited to surgery for tendon release, tendon lengthening, foot deformities, scoliosis surgery, and others.

Baclofen Pump Care Sequence and Quality Improvement

Prior to baclofen pump placement, the PPM physician and APRN explain to the parents/caregivers the indications, potential complications and subsequent care of the child with a baclofen pump, including the importance of long-term follow-up. In addition, symptoms of pump malfunction and baclofen withdrawal are discussed, and a parent pamphlet providing written guidelines and instructions for the parents of a child with a baclofen pump is provided. A social services assessment, as part of the multidisciplinary team conference, is discussed. Amongst the issues is not only the authorization process with the healthcare insurance agency/venue, but the importance of a dedicated parent/caregiver who will follow-up the necessary post pump placement appointments. Referral to pediatric neurosurgery for preoperative visit is performed after the parents/caregivers express their understanding of the care sequence and need for follow-up. A pediatric neurosurgery clinic appointment is then made, and during the appointment the technical aspects of the operative procedure, need for general anesthesia, and postoperative hospital care sequence is detailed. If the consent for the procedure is obtained, authorization request to the healthcare insurance agency/venue follows, and upon approval the patient is scheduled for surgery.

A protocol for the patient suspected of having a malfunctioning baclofen pump was created in which a PPM team member is always available for the management of a suspected malfunction. Evaluation of the pump is observed using radio opaque dye injection into side port followed by a spiral computer tomography to examine the length of the catheter. A management plan was prepared with the collaboration of PPM physician, pediatric radiology, and pediatric neurosurgery, for patient's needing magnetic resonance imaging (MRI). The MRI technologist follows instructions for special study sequencing provided specifically for baclofen pump patients. Upon completion of the study, a PPM team member will examine and reprogram the pump.

During the period between January 2010 and July 2019, a total of 96 baclofen pump procedures were performed. This includes baclofen pump insertions, revisions, and procedures for wound breakdown and/or infection. Further details are discussed in the section on "Quality Improvement by Periodic Review of Scientific Literature" in this chapter.

Selective Lumbar Dorsal Rhizotomy Care Sequence and Quality Improvement

The PPM physician discusses with the parents/caregivers the decision by the multidisciplinary team care conference that their child is a candidate for a selective dorsal rhizotomy (SDR). The physician explains the potential complications and outpatient care sequence following the rhizotomy procedure, highlighting the importance of follow-up with PPM physician and PPT. A handout written for the parents of a child who needs a rhizotomy is provided. Patient referral for consultation by pediatric neurosurgery is initiated. The pediatric neurosurgeon explains the preoperative and technical aspects of the operative procedure, as well as inpatient care sequence. Following discharge from the hospital, a follow-up appointment is made for postoperative care sequence and wound check. The patient is then referred for ongoing longitudinal care to the spasticity clinic for team care. Rhizotomies are performed collaboratively by the pediatric neurosurgeon, who performs the operative intervention, and a PPM physician who evaluates the response to stimulation. This SDR sequence follows the model of Salt Lake City Primary Children's Hospital [7].

In the period between January 2010 and July 2019, 46 selective lumbar dorsal rhizotomies were performed. Further details are discussed in the section on "Quality Improvement by Periodic Review of Scientific Literature" in this chapter.

Healthcare Insurance: A Recurring Administrative Burden

Approximately 70% of families managed in the spasticity clinic are insured by Medicaid and/or Children's Medical Services of the States of Florida or Georgia, military health coverage (Tricare), or related organizations. The remainder have private insurance. Prior to clinic visits and/or interventions/procedures, authorizations from the pertinent healthcare insurance agency/venue is required. In many situations, repeated requests are necessary due to the lack of understanding that more than one healthcare provider will be seen in a clinic visit, as part of team care. At times, appointments and/or interventions require rescheduling due to lack of timely completion of pertinent documentation and authorization. The social services worker participates in assisting parents/caregivers in navigating the administrative medical process.

Quality Improvement by Periodic Review of Scientific Literature

Pertinent and current scientific literature related to spasticity is periodically reviewed and discussed in the monthly team conferences to maintain an ongoing educational sequence with updated subject matter. These ongoing learning experiences are an attempt to facilitate a cohesive approach for children with spasticity. As an example of the process, a change in the patient care sequence occurred following the discussion of the work performed by D'Aquino et al., on SDR in the patients classified with the Gross Motor Function Classification System (GMFCS) IV and V [8]. D'Aquino and colleagues demonstrated these patients, in the past, were not considered candidates for SDR, responded with efficacy and therapeutic durability to the procedure [8]. Following identification and selection by PPM of patients with grade IV-V, the patients were presented in the monthly team conference. Following the conference, PPM presented the option to the parents/caregivers of patients felt to be candidates for SDR, and if they consented to the procedure, they were then referred to pediatric neurosurgery. Similarly, following the presentation of the work of Ingale et al. on the choice of SDR as an alternative to baclofen pump replacement in grade IV-V patients, the treatment paradigm was changed [9]. At the time of baclofen pump replacement was needed in patients with grade IV-V, PPM informed the parents/caregivers about SDR as an alternative to pump replacement. If they consented to SDR they were then referred for preoperative consultation with pediatric neurosurgery.

In patients with functioning pumps, delivery of baclofen is reduced gradually and monitored by PPM prior to operation to ensure a smooth transition. PPM may prescribe oral medication such as baclofen and others, as felt necessary, according to the patient's progress.

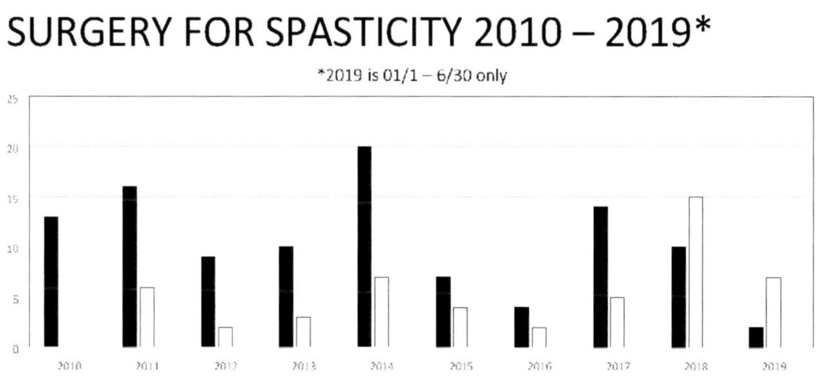

* Baclofen pumps include new, replacements and wound revisions.

Figure 1. Incidence and yearly distribution of baclofen pump procedures and selective dorsal rhizotomies.

Baclofen pumps have been traditionally employed over SDR when relief of spasticity of upper extremities was felt to be necessary. However, there are reports on a similar benefit from SDR [9-11]. Finding similar results in our patients, we have progressively modified our protocols and have selected more patients for SDR over intrathecal baclofen pump. In the period of January 2013 through December 2017, 76% of SDR were performed on patients with GMCS I-III, and 24% for GMFCS IV-V. Since January 2018, SDR was performed on GMFCS I-III in 43% of patients, and 57% with GMFCS IV-V. No *de novo* intrathecal baclofen pumps have been performed since December 2017.

These paradigm changes are reflected in Figure 1, which demonstrates an increase in the number of patients undergoing SDR, over baclofen pump.

Telemedicine Pilot Project

A pilot program is in the initial stages for telemedicine assessment and follow-up of youth with spasticity. The base site is the Spasticity Clinic PPM in Jacksonville, Florida and the remote site is the WCH Rehabilitation Clinic in Lake City, Florida with PPT and patient. Face to face interaction via telemedicine permits the PPM physician to evaluate the clinical scope with the PPT and the parents.

Current Developments

A database has been developed in collaboration with the Cerebral Palsy Research Network (CPRN) collecting data on the incidence, severity of spasticity, comparing botulinum toxin injections versus SDR, and other aspects. PPM is also exploring treatment paradigms that will incorporate gait analysis studies in youth with spasticity, where indicated.

A database on parent/caregiver satisfaction is in process. Healthcare costs, in reference to care coordination and outcome is being analyzed as part of the care sequence.

Discussion

The child with spasticity and their family require a variety of educational, developmental and necessary support services from many agencies and programs [12, 13]. Comprehensive healthcare models for children with chronic medical needs have been shown to lower healthcare and social costs, reduce hospitalizations, and lower the amount of lost work days for their parents/caregivers [4, 14-17]. The limited number of comprehensive multispecialty clinics is a result of many reasons that include restriction of full insurance reimbursement for care providers "outside of the network," lack of reimbursement for chronic healthcare coordination for individual patients or for services provided by non-medical staff members, and limitations to the number of services billed during a single visit or day [13, 14].

Cerebral palsy (CP) has been documented to have increased from 1.5 per 1000 live births in the 1960's to the rate of 2.5 per 1000 live births reported in 2006 [18]. Spasticity as an ongoing chronic medical condition is found in approximately 80% of youth with CP [19]. This can lead to multiple secondary medical problems including restriction in movement, ambulation, muscle contractures, and chronic pain [20, 21]. As a result, each child with spasticity should be evaluated and treated with insight of the multiple modalities and management strategies available.

For patients that do not respond to medical and physical therapy measures, the benefit of surgery for spasticity has been documented [22-25]. The long-term effect of SDR in 95 patients who were followed for 20-28 years after SDR was reported by Park et al. [26]. They noted positive long-term effects on quality of life and ambulation. When comparing adults who had SDR performed as children to those that did not have surgery (group mean age 27 years), Daunter et al. found lower decline in gross motor function over time in those who underwent SDR as children, as well as six fewer hours of daily assistance, than in those who did not have the operative procedure [27].

There is no consistent overall approach to deciding as to whether intrathecal baclofen pumps or SDR is best for youth with spasticity. In a recent report by Davidson, et al. with a systematic review of evidence of both procedures for treatment of GMFCS level IV-V patients found a lack of evidence as to which procedure is best [28]. They recommended further standardized studies be performed [28].

There are established spasticity programs for care of spasticity in children [7, 22-25]. Limitation in the number of comprehensive programs for the management spasticity in youth is not only due to the previously discussed conditions, but also because of a limited number of trained medical and non-medical personnel in the same region and/or medical facility. Currently there is no uniform and systematic approach to youth with spasticity provided by health care agencies in the continental and overseas territories of the United States, as well as other countries.

Conclusion

A comprehensive multidisciplinary spasticity program with multiple institutions can be developed in the presence of interested and motivated professionals. This collaborative approach requires administrative support and solid lines of interdisciplinary communication. Ongoing learning and quality improvement are necessary to maintain and achieve comprehensive patient care.

We wish to encourage and assist those who desire a similar comprehensive model in their location.

Acknowledgments

We wish to acknowledge the support of the Lucy Gooding Charitable Foundation Trust and Baptist Health Foundation of Northeast Florida (both are not-for-profit entities). We would also like to thank Jennifer Santarone for article preparation and assistance with electronic submission.

References

[1] Mac Keith, R. C., Mackenzie, I. C. K., and Polani, P. E. (1959) The Little Club: Memorandum on terminology and classification of "cerebral palsy." *Cerebral Palsy Bulletin* 5:27-35 https://onlinelibrary.wiley.com/doi/pdf/10.1111/j.1469-8749.1959.tb08073.x.

[2] Lance, J. W. Symposium synopsis. (1980) In: Feldman, R. G., Young, R. R., Koella, W. P., eds. *Spasticity: Disordered Motor Control*. Miami, FL: Symposia Specialists; distributed by Chicago, IL: Yearbook Medical Publishers; 485-494.

[3] Albright, A. L. (1996) Spasticity and movement disorders in cerebral palsy. *J. Child Neurol.* 11 Suppl 1:S1-S4. doi: 10.1177/0883073896011001S01.

[4] American Academy of Pediatrics Council on Children with Disabilities (2005). Care coordination in the medical home: integrating health and related systems of care for

children with special health care needs. *Pediatrics* 116(5):1238-1244. doi: 10.1542/peds.2005-2070.

[5] Stempien, L., and Tsai, T. (2000) Intrathecal baclofen pump use for spasticity: a clinical survey. *Am. J. Phys. Med. Rehabil.* 79(6):536-541 doi:10.1097/00002060-200011000-00010.

[6] James, H. E., Hofrichter, P. B., Spierre, L. Z., and Aldana, P. R. (2013) Initiating a pediatric spasticity program with multispecialty and multi-institutional support: a preliminary report. *Pediatr. Neurosurg.* 49(1):11-15. doi: 10.1159/000355125.

[7] Kan, P., Gooch, J., Amini, A., Ploeger, D., Grams, B., Oberg, W., Simonsen, S., Walker, M., and Kestle, J. (2008) Surgical treatment of spasticity in children: comparison of selective dorsal rhizotomy and intrathecal baclofen pump implantation. *Childs Nerv. Syst.* 24(4):239-243. doi:10.1007/s00381-007-0457-8.

[8] D'Aquino, D., Moussa, A. A., Ammar, A., Ingale, H., and Vloeberghs, M. (2018) Selective dorsal rhizotomy for the treatment of severe spastic cerebral palsy: efficacy and therapeutic durability in GMFCS grade IV and V children. *Acta Neurochir. (Wien)* 160(4):811-821. doi: 10.1007/s00701-017-3349-z.

[9] Ingale, H., Ughratadar, I., Muquit, S., Moussa A. A., and Vloeberghs, M. H. (2016) Selective dorsal rhizotomy as an alternative to intrathecal baclofen pump replacement in GMFCS grades 4 and 5 children. *Childs Nerv. Syst.* 32(2):321-325. doi: 10.1007/s00381-015-2950-9.

[10] Albright, A. L., Barry, M. J., Fasick, M. P., and Janosky, J. (1995) Effect of continuous intrathecal baclofen infusion and selected posterior rhizotomy on upper extremity spasticity. *Pediatr. Neurosurg.* 23(2):82-85. doi: 10.1159/000120941.

[11] Gigante, P., McDowell, M. M., Bruce, S. S., Chirelstein, G., Chiriboga, C. A., Dutkowsky, J., Fontana, E., Hyman, J., Kim, H., Morgan, D., Pearson, T. S., Roye, B. D., Boye Jr., D. P., Ryan, P., Vitale, M., and Anderson, R. C. E. (2013) Reduction in upper-extremity tone after lumbar selective dorsal rhizotomy in children with spastic cerebral palsy. *J. Neurosurg. Pediatr.* 12(6):588-594. doi: 10.3171/2013.9.PEDS12591.

[12] Kraus, M. W., Wells, N., Gulley, S., and Anderson, B. (2001) Navigating systems of care: results from a national survey of families of children with special health care needs. *Child Serv. Soc. Policy Res. Pract.* 4(4):165-187. doi: 10.1207/S15326918CS0404_02.

[13] Telfair, J., Haque, A., Etienne, M., Tang, S., and Strasser, S. (2003) Rural/urban differences in access to and utilization of services among people in Alabama with sickle cell disease. *Public Health Rep.* 118(1):27-36. doi: 10.1093/phr/118.1.27.

[14] Bilenker, J. H., Weller, W. E., Shaffer, T. J., Dover, G. J., and Anderson, G. F. (1998) The costs of children with sickle cell anemia; preparing for managed care. *J. Pediatr. Hematol. Oncol.* 20(6):528-533. doi: 10.1097/00043426-199811000-00003.

[15] Farmer, J. E., Clark, M. J., Sherman, A., Marien, W. E., and Selva, T. J. (2005) Comprehensive primary care for children with special health care needs in rural areas. *Pediatrics* 116(3):649-656. doi: 10.1542/peds.2004-0647.

[16] Hussey, P. S., Eibner, C., Ridgely, M. S., and McGlynn, E. A. (2009) Controlling U. S. health care spending-separating promising from unpromising approaches. *N. Engl. J. Med.* 361(22):2109-2111. doi: 10.1056/NEJMp0910315.

[17] Palfrey, J. S., Sofis, L. A., Davidson, E. J., Liu, J., Freeman, L., and Ganz, M. L. (2004) The Pediatric Alliance for Coordinated Care: evaluation of a medical home model. *Pediatrics* 113(5 Suppl):1507-1516.

[18] Odding, E., Roebroeck, M. E., and Stam, H. J. (2006) The epidemiology of cerebral palsy: incidence, impairments and risk factors. *Disabil. Rehabil.* 28(4):183-191. doi: 10.1080/09638280500158422.

[19] Stanley, F., Blair, E., and Alberman, E., eds. How common are the cerebral palsies? (2000) In: *Cerebral Palsies: Epidemiology and Causal Pathways.* Clinics in Developmental Medicine. London, England: MacKeith Press, 14-21.

[20] Aiona, M. D. and Sussman, M. D. (2004) Treatment of spastic diplegia in patients with cerebral palsy: Part II. *J. Pediatr. Orthrop. B* 13(3):S13-S38. doi: 10.1097/00009957-200405000-00016.

[21] Gage, J. R., ed. (2004) An overview of treatment. In: *The Treatment of Gait Problems in Cerebral Palsy.* Clinics in Developmental Medicine. London, England: MacKeith Press, 238-244.

[22] Park, T. S., Gaffney, P. T., Kaufman, B. A., and Molleston, M. C. (1993) Selective lumbosacral dorsal rhizotomy immediately caudal to the conus medullaris for cerebral palsy spasticity. *Neurosurgery* 33(5):929-933. doi: 10.1227/00006123-199311000-00026.

[23] Park, T. S. and Johnston, J. M. (2006) Surgical techniques of selective dorsal rhizotomy for spastic cerebral palsy. Technical note. *Neurosurg. Focus* 21(2):e7.

[24] Abbott, R., Forem, S. L., and Johann, M. (1989) Selective posterior rhizotomy for the treatment of spasticity: a review. *Childs Nerv. Syst.* 5(6):337-346. doi: 10.1007/BF00271889.

[25] Albright, A. L., Barron, W. B., Fasick, M. P., Polinko, P., and Janosky, J. (1993) Continuous intrathecal baclofen infusion for spasticity of cerebral origin. *JAMA* 270(20):2475-2477.

[26] Park, T. S., Liu, J. L., Edwards, C., Walter, D. M., and Dobbs, M. B. (2017) Functional outcomes of childhood selective dorsal rhizotomy 20 to 28 years later. *Cureus* 9(5):e1256. doi: 10.7759/cureus.1256.

[27] Daunter, A. K., Kratz, A. L., and Hurvitz, E. A. (2017) Long-term impact of childhood selective dorsal rhizotomy on pain, fatigue, and function: a case-control study. *Dev. Med. Child Neurol.* 59(10):1089-1095. doi: 10.1111/dmcn.13481.

[28] Davidson, B., Schoen, N., Sedighim, S., Haldenby, R., Dalziel, B., Breitbart, S., Fehlings, D., Milo-Manson, G., Narayanan, U. G., Drake, J. M., and Ibrahim, G. M. (2020) Intrathecal baclofen versus selective dorsal rhizotomy for children with cerebral palsy who are nonambulant: a systematic review. *J. Neurosurg. Pediatr.* 25:69-77. doi: 10.3171/2019.8.PEDS19282.

Chapter 19

Recent Advances in the Treatment of Parkinson's Disease and Dystonia

Ruchika Tandon[1], Pawan Kumar Verma[2,*] and Kuntal Kanti Das[2]
[1]Department of Neurology, SGPGI, Lucknow, Uttar Pradesh, India
[2]Department of Neurosurgery, SGPGI, Lucknow, Uttar Pradesh, India

Abstract

Parkinson's disease and dystonia are quite frequently encountered movement disorders in clinical practice. Though a number of treatment options are available for the management of both of these conditions, still the etiology and pathophysiology of these conditions is not fully understood. New insight into pathogenesis of these disorders draws us to explore new treatment options for these diseases, both medical and surgical. In this chapter, we aim to review the treatment options, both medical and surgical, which have come up and / or are coming up in the recent years.

Keywords: Parkinson's disease, dystonia, medical treatment, surgical treatment, neurostimulation, recent advances

Introduction

Parkinson's disease (PD) is the most common neurodegenerative movement disorder characterized by tremor, rigidity, bradykinesia/akinesia and postural

---

* Corresponding Author's Email: drkuntalkantidas@gmail.com.

In: Advances in Neurosurgery Research
Editors: Amit Agrawal, Pradeep Chouksey, Adesh Shrivastava et al.
ISBN: 978-1-68507-859-1

instability. Other motor and non-motor symptoms are also a part of Parkinson's disease [1]. In this section, we shall be dealing with the recent advances in the management of idiopathic Parkinson's disease.

Recent Advances in Drug Treatment

Medical cannabis may be effective in reducing levodopa-induced dyskinesias [2]. They may also respond to clozapine [3]. *Extended-release levodopa* has come up recently, which avoids off state. *AP09004 or accordion* pill, prolongs gastric retention and increases absorption of levodopa/carbidopa [3]. A trial evaluating *exenatide* in PD patients showed positive results, while others evaluating adenosine A_{2A} antagonist, preladenant and active control rasagiline in early Parkinson's disease patients were not effective. *Safinamide*, a mixed MAOB-I with glutamate release properties is already in market and it improves off-time dyskinesias. *Opicapone* is another new longer acting, once daily Caetchol-O-methyltransferase (COMT)-I that improves off time. For reducing off time in these patients, present options include injection of short-acting dopamine agonist *apomorphine* and a sublingual apomorphine. Intranasal levodopa (CVT-301) improved off time in clinical trial [4]. Gastroprokinetic motilin receptor agonist, *camicinal (GSK962040)* increases gastric emptying, thereby improving levodopa absorption in the small intestine. This molecule improved off time over 7–9 days, but did not improve peak levodopa levels. *Mucuna puriens,* a legume containing natural levodopa was noninferior to levodopa in a 16-week study. Caffeine tablets and mGluR5 antagonist, mavoglurant may not be effective. Long-acting, once a day *Amantadine* [ADS-5102 (Amantadine) extended-release capsules] has a US Food and Drug Administration (FDA) approval for levodopa induced dyskinesias [4]. For advanced PD patients, *levodopa-carbidopa intestinal gel (LCIG)* is FDA approved for infusion and it improves motor fluctuations, dyskinesias, sleep, mood and even cognition till at least 2 years. Intrajejunal levodopa pump is available commercially and can counter motor fluctuation and dyskinesias. However, dislocation, kinking and occlusion of catheter and infection of percutaneous gastrostomy site may limit its widespread use. For fluctuating PD, Japan has approved *Istradefylline*, a selective A2A antagonist [5]. Trials with another A2A antagonist, *Vipadenant* are undergoing [5]. *Pardoprunox* a 5-HT_{1A} agonist and partial dopamine D2/D3 agonist had lots of side effects and eltoprazine, a mixed $5\text{-HT}_{1A/1B}$ receptor agonist is on trial for levodopa induced dyskinesias [6]. *Methylphenidate* may improve gait and

Memantine may improve axial motor symptoms [6]. People nowadays, are doing drug repurposing or finding new uses for existing or abandoned drugs and also using prodrugs to enhance dopamine agonist and/or levodopa absorption for finding out novel treatment options for PD [7, 8]. Continuous subcutaneous infusion of apomorphine is another similar approach for patients with such an advanced disease [4]. Future may have in store many new strategies like targeting glucocerebrosidase (GBA), modulating calcium channels using *isradapine* and iron chelators like *deferiprone* [4].

For non-motor symptoms of PD, *atomoxetine*, a specific norepinephrine reuptake inhibitor, subjectively improved attention, working memory, processing speed and set-shifting [4]. *Oxycodone/naloxone* is under trial for chronic disabling pain in PD [9]. *Rotigotine* and *eszopiclone* may help in insomnia with PD and caffeine and may help in excessive day time sleepiness in PD [9]. Trials are evaluating rivastigmine, piribedil and donepezil for PD dementia, venlafaxine, S -Adenosyl-methionine and paroxetine for depression with psychosis, rasagiline for motor fluctuations, creatine to slow the progression of PD, amantadine for levodopa induced dyskinesia and freezing of gait and transdermal rotigotine, subcutaneous infusion of lisuride, transdermal ropinirole and tozadenant in PD [9].

A recent study of *Rivastigmine* in a dose of 3-12 mg/day over 32 weeks significantly reduced falls in PD [10] and another study of *Droxidopa* in a dose of 300-1800 mg/day over 10 weeks reduced falls in PD patients having orthostatic hypotension [10]. Cholinesterase inhibitors may work in PD dementia [11]. For psychosis with Parkinson's disease, FDA (United States Food and Drug Administration) has approved *Pimavanserin*, a highly selective 5-HT_{2A} inverse agonist [12]. It is also undergoing trials for treatment of levodopa induced dyskinesias [5]. *Metformin* may be neuroprotective in PD [13]. Glucagon-like peptide-1 may play a role in PD treatment [14].

For autonomic symptoms in advanced PD patients, sildenafil citrate (50 mg) may treat erectile dysfunction and apomorphine may help in erectile and anorectal dysfunction. More continuous drug delivery systems may improve sweating and polyethylene glycol may relieve constipation [3]. Melatonin agonists may help in sleep and so may sodium oxybate and imipramine, carbamazepine, levodopa, sodium oxybate, triazolam, zopiclone, quetiapine, clozapine and clonazepam may help in REM sleep behaviour disorder [3].

Using micro and nanotechnologies (like Cerium oxide nanoparticles), *pyrazole* scaffold synthesis and liposomes to deliver drugs which may reach their targets in the brain is another recent approach [15-17]. Computer-aided drug design might help in designing new drugs against PD [18].

Modulation of *neuromelanin* accumulation could be beneficial for PD patients and it could prevent PD or delay brain aging [19]. Among other possible neuroprotective agents, trials with *AVE8112, a phosphodiesterase type 4 inhibitor, rosiglitazone and pioglitazone* are undergoing [5]. Trials with many new molecules are going on and soon we shall get data on the efficacy of these drugs [20].

Newer imaging modalities like MR sequences sensitive to iron and nigral pigments (like neuromelanin imaging), meta-iodobenzylguanidine (MIBG) cardiac scintigraphy, dopamine transporter scintigraphy, ^{18}F-FDG PET, diffusion tensor imaging (DTI), Modified Driven Equilibrium Fourier Transform (MDEFT) MRI sequences, structural MRI advances like cholinergic basal forebrain nuclei atrophy for cognitive impairment in PD and so on, are paving way for development of new biomarkers and may help in newer treatment modalities in the future [21-23]. Similarly, other biomarkers are paving way for disease-modifying approach for patients with Parkinson's disease like α-synuclein immunotherapy, antioxidants, neurotrophic factors like cerebral dopamine neurotrophic factor, use of microRNAs, exosomes, gene therapy, protein injection therapy and cell transplantation therapy [24-27].

Several gene mutations of late, have come up in the picture of PD, thus gene therapy may assume greater significance in the future. New era is hopefully an era of personalized medicine. One step in this regard is the use of stem cells specific to a PD patient. The first human trial of induced pluripotent stem cells transplantation in patients suffering from Parkinson's disease began in Japan in 2018 [28]. Researchers are employing genome editing tools like CRISPR/Cas9 system for PD patients [29]. They are also studying active or passive vaccination against alpha synuclein using compounds like PRX002, an IgG monoclonal Ab against C terminus of alpha synuclein in trials [4]. People are studying an yeast model of α-synuclein toxicity to study PD and to test drugs [30]. However, cell based therapies have their own limitations and few people are close to drug development stage as of now.

Mammalian target of *rapamycin* (mTOR) signaling pathway regulates autophagy and inhibition of this pathway may be beneficial in the treatment of levodopa-induced dyskinesia [31]. People worldwide are also investigating the role of mitochondria and respiratory chain dysfunction in the pathogenesis of PD [32]. Glial cell line–derived neurotrophic factors, vaccines and anti-inflammatory and neuroprotective approaches are other therapies under evaluation [3].

Future may have in *store plants and plant products* like *Crocus sativus,* resveratrol, quercetin, catechins, lycopene, baicalein, Camellia sinensis, Gastrodia elata, Zingiber officinale, Magnolia obovata, ginseng, Curcuma longa, Bacopa monniera, Ginkgo biloba, Fallopia multiflora, Camellia sinensis, tyrosinase inhibitors and Vicia faba, for treating Parkinson's disease and its various complications [33-36].

Neurostimulation

We already know that DBS acts by stimulating axons in the subthalamic region causing change in motor cortical activity, thereby masking or desynchronizing pathologically enhanced beta-band oscillations in basal ganglia–thalamocortical circuit (Figure 1). We have to stimulate these neurons and avoid stimulating those in the surrounding areas (like corticospinal or corticobulbar fibres in the internal capsule causing walking or motor deficits) to avoid adverse effects. What is new in this field is the use of *directional leads*, current steering by dividing circle of ring-shaped electrode contact into three or four sectors, which allow separate activation, change in duration of current pulse, changing the shape of pulse waveform, computational models, optogenetics technique, future skull implantable miniature pacemakers, use of intraoperative MRI to guide lead placement, identifying symptom or disease specific physio markers and setting new stimulation patterns selectively suppressing disease specific brain activity [37, 38] (Figure 2).

New leads with segmented electrodes can improve the therapeutic window for programming at the cost of several permutations and combinations. Also, interleaving technique with two different alternating programs on one electrode with the same frequency may also be useful for optimum stimulation [39]. Closed loop DBS system delivers stimulus only when there is pathological physiological signal like an increase in oscillatory activity in patients with PD [4, 40]. In other words, it senses and records signals and delivers stimuli when needed, simultaneously. Proposed mechanisms of action are also changing from excitation and inhibition of neural circuits to long term neural and synaptic plasticity or so called disease modifying effects [40]. Newer advances in DBS may involve functional connectivity profiling which studies the relationship between multiple brain regions with respect to time and stimuli and structural connectivity profiling, which studies the physical connections between different brain regions by reconstructing the axons [41]. STN-DBS facilitates motor learning, according to a recent publication [42] (Figure 3). Recently a published study showed the effectiveness of patient-rated visual analogue scale (VAS) for real-time adjustment of DBS parameters in PD patients with STN-DBS [43]. Online remote programming technology is coming up. *Variable frequency stimulation (VFS)*, which applies alternating high and low frequency stimulation for freezing of gait in Parkinson's patients is another treatment approach [44]. *Adaptive DBS* for PD may take signals from basal ganglia local field potentials, cortical recordings (electrocorticography), wearable sensors, and eHealth and mHealth devices. These involve machine learning and take care of energy consumption as well [45]. An early DBS (EARLYSTIM) significantly reduces neuropsychiatric fluctuations and hyperdopaminergic behaviours compared to the best medical therapy alone, without aggravating hypodopaminergic behaviour and apathy [4]. STN-DBS improves bladder symptoms [4]. "Asleep" image guided and robot-assisted DBS may be as effective as an awake STN-DBS [46].

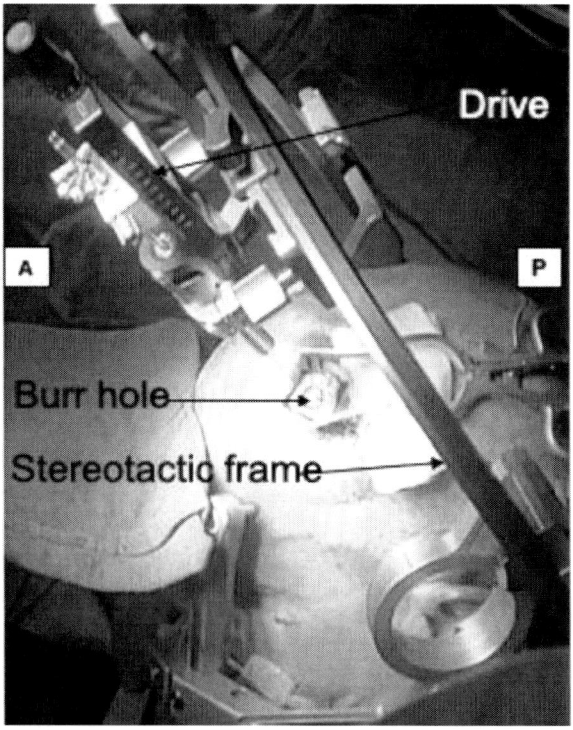

Figure 1. Showing the assembly of frame and drive targeted on left STN deep brain stimulation (DBS).

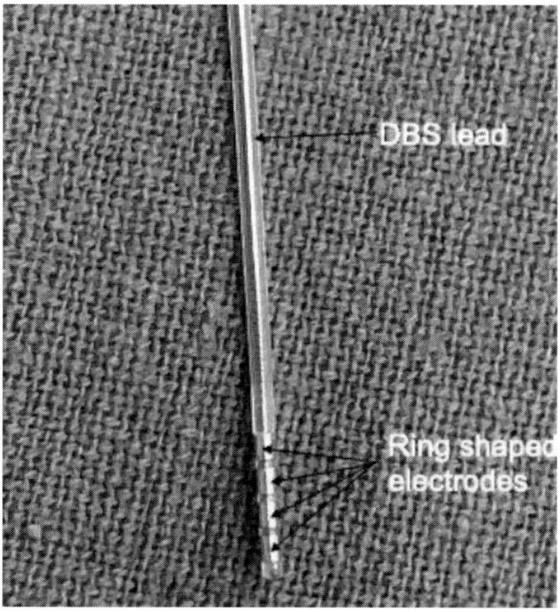

Figure 2. The recent '*directional lead*' showing circle of four ring-shaped electrode, which allow separate activation and changing the shape and site of site of stimulation.

Researchers are studying pedunculopontine nucleus (PPN) DBS for reducing gait freezing in PD and also spinal cord stimulation and dual stimulation of STN and substantia nigra (SNr) and VFS of STN for postural instability and gait disorders in Parkinson's disease patients [40]. Nucleus basalis of Meynert stimulation was safe and tolerable but did not improve cognition in a study [4]. For tremor dominant PD or those with very asymmetric symptoms, thalamic ventral intermediate nucleus (VIM) DBS is beneficial [4].

Cerebellar stimulation may improve levodopa-induced dyskinesias and proximal movements in PD patients, though fine motor skills may deteriorate. It has promise as an experimental therapy for PD [47]. DBS-STN has peripheral immunomodulative effect in the rat model of PD [48].

Though, most of the studies confirm the effectiveness of DBS in various genetic forms of Parkinson's disease, however, relative response may differ. However, in this chapter we are focussing on idiopathic Parkinson's disease, per se, and such studies are beyond the scope of this chapter [49].

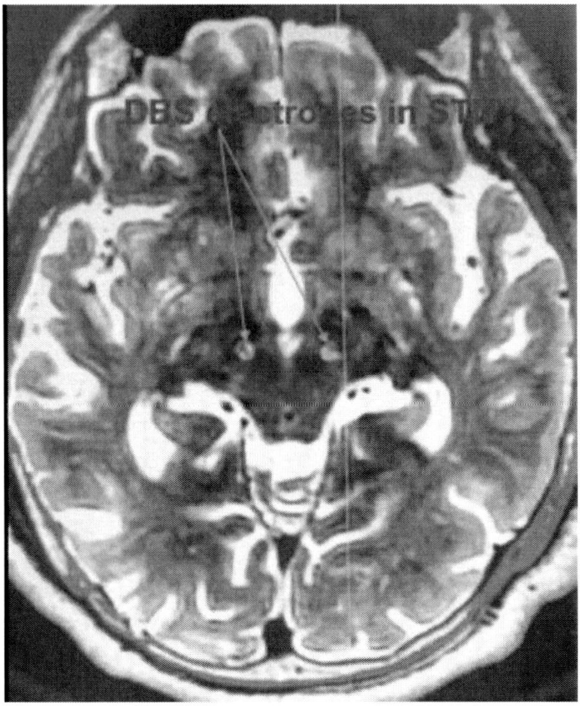

Figure 3. MRI image (T2W sequence) showing the DBS electrodes in bilateral subthalamic nuclei (STN).

Stereotactic Lesions

Recommendations are not for *gamma knife pallidotomy* but those on anticoagulants, with cognitive deficits or with other contraindications to DBS may go for it. Tremor in PD may respond to thalamotomy [50].

Magnetic resonance imaging-guided *high intensity-focused ultrasound (FUS) technique* targets ultrasound waves through the skull to a brain target, thereby creating a lesion. These have a role in PD management. *Unilateral FUS thalamotomy* in tremor-dominant PD reduces tremors. It also reduces dyskinesias and off periods in PD patients with motor fluctuations and dyskinesias [51]. Moderate intensity pulsed FUS may open the blood-brain barrier for delivering substances like proteins, genes, and for cell-based therapy for PD and related disorders [4].

Miscellaneous Treatment Approaches

Among non-invasive approaches, high-frequency *repetitive transcranial magnetic stimulation (rTMS)* to bilateral primary motor cortex improves motor symptoms in Parkinson's disease and high-frequency rTMS to left dorsolateral prefrontal cortex is effective in treating depression in Parkinson's disease [4]. Transcranial static magnetic field stimulation induces dopamine-dependent changes of cortical excitability in PD patients [52]. Also, investigators are analysing the role of rTMS for improving cognition in PD dementia patients [10]. According to researchers, *transcranial direct current stimulation (tDCS)* to dorsolateral prefrontal cortex (DLPFC) may improve dual-task walking [52].

Embedded *home sensors* may assess and possibly prevent falls in PD [8]. Certain genetic factors may predict fall risk like leucine-rich repeat kinase 2 gene mutation confers greater gait variability [8].

A recent concept in PD management is the management of non-motor fluctuations in these patients or fluctuations of symptoms like psychotic symptoms, hypomania/mania, depression, apathy, visual hallucinations, confusion, fatigue, sweating, facial flushing, abdominal bloating and discomfort, urinary frequency and urgency, dyspnoea, blood pressure changes, peripheral oedema, pain, internal tremor, akathisia, numbness and dysesthesia. Most of these symptoms may correspond to the motor fluctuations. Treatment strategies include symptomatic treatment like analgesics and antiepileptic drugs for pain, alpha-blockers for autonomic fluctuations, anxiolytics for neuropsychiatric fluctuations, anticholinesterase inhibitors for cognitive symptoms and high frequency stimulation of STN for non-motor fluctuations [53].

Apart from drug treatment and surgical approaches, there is a *role of exercise* for improving both motor and nonmotor complications of Parkinson's disease and secondary complications arising due to immobility (like cardiovascular and osteoporosis). This may cause neurochemical and neuroplastic changes in the brain. *Targeted exercise intervention* is the need of the hour [8]. Incorporating exercise in games, the so called *exergames,* are a good and interesting alternative to conventional exercises [54]. Exercise may even prevent drug induced dyskinesias in PD patients. *Virtual environment walking* is another approach for improving gait in PD [55]. Biofeedback and cuing devices including smart glasses and videogame rehabilitation programme may help reduce gait freezing and other aspects of PD [56, 57]. Other behavioural therapies like *rhythmic auditory stimulation* are increasingly being used and MEG (Magnetoencephalography) study has endorsed its effects on the lobar functions [58].

Lee Silverman Voice Treatment (LSVT LOUD) may work for swallowing disability in Parkinson's disease patients [4]. Bilinguals may be better protected against cognitive impairment in PD [4]. *Cognitive behavioural therapy* is efficacious in insomnia and bright light therapy and dim-red light therapy is effective in excessive daytime sleepiness [4]. *Polychromatic light therapy* also benefits bradykinesia, rigidity, tremor, altered gait, depression, insomnia, involuntary movements and psychiatric side effects in PD [59]. Cognitive therapy may also help in PD with dementia or minimal cognitive impairment [10]. *Neurofeedback approaches* may enhance cognition in PD [60]. Singing may improve speech of PD patients [61]. Occupational therapy and palliative care also help people with PD [4].

Dystonia

Dystonia comprises sustained muscle contractions, causing twisted and repetitive movements, or abnormal postures [62]. Here, we shall be focusing on the recent advances in the treatment of dystonia. Recently people have classified dystonia as follows:

Classification

CLINICAL	
Age at onset	Infancy (birth to 2 years)
	Childhood (3–12 years)
	Adolescence (13–20 years)
	Early adulthood (21–40 years)
	Late adulthood (>40 years)
Body distribution	Focal
	Segmental
	Multifocal
	Generalized (with or without leg involvement)
	Hemidystonia
Disease course	Static
	Progressive
Variability	Persistent
	Action-specific
	Diurnal
	Paroxysmal

CLINICAL	
Associated features	
Isolated dystonia or combined with another movement disorder	Isolated dystonia
	Combined dystonia
Occurrence of other neurological or systemic manifestations	List of co-occurring neurological manifestations
ETIOLOGY	
Nervous system pathology	Evidence of degeneration
	Evidence of structural (often static) lesions
	No evidence of degeneration or structural lesion
Inherited or acquired	
Inherited	Autosomal dominant
	Autosomal recessive
	X-linked recessive
	Mitochondrial
Acquired	Perinatal brain injury
	Infection
	Drug
	Toxic
	Vascular
	Neoplastic
	Brain injury
	Psychogenic
Idiopathic	Sporadic
	Familial

Recent Advances in Drug Treatment

DYT1-TOR1A and DYT6 (THAP1) were the first two primary generalized dystonia gene mutations discovered. Their discovery paved the way for studies on pathogenesis and pathophysiology of primary dystonia, by comparing physiology of manifesting and non-manifesting carriers, and by studying the structure and interactions of mutant gene products. Gradually researchers found out other gene mutations causing primary dystonia, familial cervical dystonia, dystonia-plus, and paroxysmal dystonia using whole-exome sequencing technology [63]. In the last 10 years, people are discovering newer neurobiological mechanisms of DYT1 dystonia, which may lead to development of newer drugs in future [64]. Recently recognized causes of dystonia include ANO3, GNAL and CIZ1 gene mutations (causing cervical dystonia in adults), ATP1A3 gene mutation and ALS2 gene mutation (causing combined dystonia). Complicated vaginal delivery may be a modifying risk factor in DYT1 [65]. Also, we now recognize dystonic tremor and involvement of thalamus, midbrain, cortex and cerebellum in dystonia, according to translational research [66].

According to recent trials, D1/D2 dopamine receptor agonists like *apomorphine* may treat generalized dystonia [67]. In myoclonus-dystonia due to SGCE, *zonisamide* is a recent addition [68].

Mitochondria and lysosomes may relate to neurodegeneration with brain iron accumulation (NBIA) causing dystonia-parkinsonism and lysosomal storage disorders (LSD), respectively, and Parkinson's disease may be in between these two diseases forming a spectrum [69]. In a recent research paper, iron chelator *deferiprone* decreased brain iron stores in pantothenate kinase–associated neurodegeneration patients and synthetic precursor of coenzyme A is being given to these patients in another clinical trial [69]. In other studies, investigators are trying *ampicillin* for DYT-TOR1A, *cannabis* for paediatric dystonia, *levetiracetam* for cervical or oromandibular dystonia, *perampanel* for cervical dystonia and *sodium oxybate* for laryngeal dystonia [70].

Since, in recent years, people have identified several autoimmune and paraneoplasic syndromes causing dystonia, the use of immunomodulatory therapies and treatment of underlying malignancies for the treatment of dystonia related to these disorders is increasing [71].

Antimuscarinic receptor antagonists by modulating dopamine release, nicotinic receptor agonists, direct or indirect dopamine agonists, mGluR5 negative allosteric modulators, NMDA receptor antagonists, adenosine A2A receptor antagonists, synaptic vesicle protein 2A (SV2A) modulators, eukaryotic initiation factor α (eIF2α) dephosphorylation inhibitor salubrinal, phosphodiesterase inhibitors (PDE10A) and targeting brain derived neurotrophic growth factor (BDNF), are experimental therapies for dystonia [72].

Botulinum neurotoxin (BoNT) works for symptomatic treatment of dystonia. People have recently observed that it may act on sensory terminals as well, so as to reduce pain. Nowadays, neurologists are administering ultrasound guided and EMG (electromyography) guided BoNT injections. Acetyl hexapeptide-8, which is a component of anti-wrinkle creams is also effective in treating blepharospasm along with BoNT [73]. Endplate-targeted BoNT injections, onabotulinumtoxinA plus automatic subdermal injector system, amlodipine along with BoNT are in various phases of trials [73]. Postural component of dystonia may respond better to BoNT, while DBS may be more effective for movements. Dystonia may change phenotype over time and BoNT may work better in such situation [73]. A not so old concept in the treatment of anterocollis-related cervical dystonia is the collum-caput concept and EMG guided selection of muscles for BoNT injection [74]. Dressler et al. in collaboration with IAB-Interdisciplinary Working Group for Movement Disorders have proposed consensus guidelines for botulinum toxin therapy along with dosing tables for dystonia and spasticity, recently [75]. We advise the readers to cast a glance at the cited reference.

TMS (Transcranial Magnetic Stimulation) may work in functional dystonia [66].

Due to the availability of specific and disease modifying treatment nowadays, finding out the cause of dystonia is assuming greater relevance [76]. Early treatment helps in certain disorders like cerebrotendinous xanthomatosis (treated by chenodeoxycholic acid), dystonia/parkinsonism with manganese accumulation (treated by EDTA chelation therapy), Gaucher disease (treated by miglustat), Niemann Pick type C (treated by miglustat), aromatic amino acid decarboxylase deficiency (treated by dopamine agonists, monoamine oxidase inhibitors and pyridoxine), dopa responsive dystonia, episodic ataxia type 2 (treated by 4-aminopyridine and acetazolamide), GLUT1 deficiency (treated by ketogenic diet and triheptanoin), Molybdenum cofactor deficiency (treated by cyclic pyranopterin monophosphate), paroxysmal kinesigenic dyskinesia (treated by carbamazepine and other antiseizure drugs), abetalipoproteinemia (treated by fat restricted diet and vitamins E and A), cerebral creatine deficiency (treated by creatine and/or ornithine and restriction of arginine), glutaric aciduria type 1 (treated by lysine restriction and by L-carnitine), maple syrup urine disease (treated by leucine restricted diet), homocystinuria (treated by pyridoxine and dietary restriction of methionine and betaine), methylmalonic aciduria (treated by dietary protein restriction and L-carnitine), propionic acidemia (treated by dietary protein restriction and L-carnitine), coenzyme Q10 deficiency and pyruvate dehydrogenase complex deficiency (treated by thiamine, ketogenic diet and triheptanoin) [76].

Intrathecal baclofen for spasticity is well-known; however, *intra-ventricular baclofen* is an upcoming treatment for dystonia due to cerebral palsy [77].

Recently, researchers found two VMAT2 (vesicular monoamine transporter type 2) inhibitors to be helpful in tardive dyskinesia, but *clonazepam, Ginkgo biloba, and amantadine* may also help [77, 78]. Role of levetiracetam, piracetam, vitamin B_6, melatonin, baclofen, propranolol, zolpidem, and zonisamide is under trial in tardive dyskinesia [78].

Some dopamine metabolism disorders causing dystonia in children respond to monoamine replacement and enhancement, while in others the response may not be so good warranting research like with pseudoexon-exclusion therapy with antisense morpholino oligonucleotides and gene transfer [79]. Some other experimental therapies for L-dopa–induced dyskinesias include metabotropic glutamate receptor 5 (mGluR5) inhibitors for example *AFQ056 (mavolurant) and ADX48261 (dipraglurant)* and for generalized dystonia include dipraglurant [80].

Neurons derived from induced pluripotent stem cells may be potentially helpful for children with hereditary spastic paraplegias [81].

Neurostimulation

Neurostimulation means altering the function of a neural circuit by applying electric current. Neurostimulation may be invasive or non-invasive [82]. *Non-invasive neurostimulation* includes transcranial magnetic stimulation (TMS). *Invasive neurostimulation* includes deep brain stimulation (DBS), motor cortex stimulation (MCS), responsive neurostimulation (RNS), spinal cord stimulation (SCS), and Vagus nerve stimulation (VNS). Though Food and Drug Administration (FDA) had approved Deep brain stimulation (DBS) of thalamus for refractory essential tremor and it had approved DBS for parkinsonian tremor in 1997, high-frequency stimulation of subthalamic nucleus (STN) and globus pallidus internus (GPi) for refractory PD in 2002 and Humanitarian Device Exemption (HDE) for dystonia in 2003, newer indications for DBS and newer sites in the central nervous system for stimulation and newer innovations in the techniques for DBS keep on emerging. These include rechargeable batteries, smaller impulse generators for small children or thin individuals, personalized long-term neuromodulation systems, high resolution stimulating leads with long-term stimulation and local field potential (LFP) recording, innovative multimodal neuroimaging and electrochemical monitoring techniques, hardware and software engineering advances leading to closed-loop neural control systems with greater efficacy and lesser side effects [69, 82]. Newer MRI techniques causing acquisition of structural image volumes with greater dynamic range, ultra-high-field (like 7-T) MRI, body-transmit MRI in those with implanted stimulators, frameless stereotactic approach (surpassing the need of electrophysiological monitoring during surgery), fMRI and DTI (diffusion tensor imaging), intraoperative electrocorticography sensorimotor cortex recordings, with subcortical LFP recordings, and other techniques are emerging. These technologies enabled recognition of pathological gamma oscillations in the BG–thalamocortical circuitry associated with dyskinesia. They also paved way for so called closed loop DBS systems.

High resolution stimulating leads allow activation of several electrodes at a time, which causes shaping of the electric field and activation of current flow in a particular direction. Directional electrodes deliver current very precisely to their targets and hence, reduce adverse effects due to stimulation of undesired sites. Adaptive stimulation recognizes physiological triggers and delivers current according to needs of the patient. Therefore, it is more effective and saves battery also [69].

Among neuroradiological advances, recently discovered Modified Driven Equilibrium Fourier Transform (MDEFT) MRI sequences may target GPi very well for guiding DBS [83]. DBS with intraoperative image acquisition technology like O-arm may be equally efficacious as post-operative MRI imaging.

In cases of genetically confirmed monogenic dystonia, Burke-Fahn-Marsden Dystonia Rating Scale Motor Score (BFMMS) improves following GPi DBS in DYT-TOR1A, DYT-THAP1 and NBIA/DYT-PANK2 and Burke-Fahn-Marsden Disability Score (BFMDS) improves via GPi DBS in DYT-TOR1A. DYT-TOR1A improves more than DYT-THAP1, NBIA/DYT-PANK2 and CHOR/DYT-ADCY5. Longer the duration and older the age of onset of dystonia in DYT-TOR1A, worse is the motor outcome following DBS. In DYT/PARK-TAF1, longer duration and in DYT-SGCE, younger age at onset of dystonia gives a poor outcome following GPi DBS [84]. Therefore, genetic testing is playing an important role in predicting response to DBS for dystonia as certain syndromes like DYT-TOR1A and *DYT11* (*SCGE*) may respond very well while, some others like DYT-*THAP1* may have an unpredictable response to GPi DBS [66]. KMT2B-related dystonia may improve with DBS [85]. XDP (X-Linked Dystonia-Parkinsonism) involves SINE-VNTR-Alu (SVA)-type retrotransposon insertion inside TAF1 gene and patients have a progressive striatal atrophy. In such patients with both dystonia and parkinsonian features, pallidal DBS improves hyperkinetic movements, although, hypokinetic symptoms may not always improve [86]. For developing a biomarker for adaptive DBS, people have identified low-frequency synchronized oscillations in theta (3–7 Hz) range in the basal ganglia thamalo-cortical circuits corresponding to dystonic movements. There is an evidence for widened somatosensory receptive fields in pallidal neurons in dystonic individuals [87]. These discoveries and recognizing abnormal networks of brain activity to aid adaptive stimulation to normalize abnormal brain network activity are the need of the hour.

Bilateral GPi stimulation is effective in SGCE related myoclonus-dystonia. This disorder may cause GABAergic deficit due to Purkinje cell dysfunction, thereby affecting cerebello-thalamic pathway. Also, it may cause defects in striatal plasticity and serotonin function. New cellular and rodent models may help in finding out the pathogenesis of SGCE related myoclonus-dystonia and thereby assist treatment development [68]. Ventral intermediate (VIM) thalamic nucleus DBS is as efficacious as GPi stimulation for myoclonus in myoclonus dystonia (DYT 11), though dystonia improves more with GPi DBS [73]. In genetic dystonia-ataxias syndromes, like Wilson's disease, ataxia-telangiectasia, spinocerebellar ataxias, episodic ataxia type 2, Cockayne syndrome, PLA2G6-associated neurodegeneration and neurodegeneration with brain iron accumulation type 1 due to mutations in PANK2 gene, response of dystonia to GPi DBS may range from 10-70% (Figure 4). Dystonia with parkinsonism responds better than dystonia with ataxia. Also, response following DBS is independent of age, disease duration, dystonic features at the time of DBS or the severity of dystonia [88]. Therefore, whole exome sequencing is playing a significant role nowadays in the targeted and personalized treatment of dystonia nowadays. Subthalamic DBS is an emerging target for dystonia [66]. Researchers are discovering new pathogenic mechanisms for dystonia like GNAL (responsible for DYT25 causing adult onset cervical dystonia), which encodes the protein Gαolf involved in transducing signals of D1 dopamine receptors downstream in striatonigral projecting gamma aminobutyric acid–ergic neurons and Rhes protein and these could be potential drug targets, similar to TorsinA protein [73]. Since, discussion of several and all of these genetic aspects is beyond the scope of this chapter, interested readers may take a look at the references given at the end of the chapter.

Cerebellar neurostimulation is gaining significance as an experimental therapy for focal dystonia and for posture correction in dystonia [47]. DBS of motor thalamus may be effective in severe dystonic head tremor and thalamic ventral lateral anterior nucleus DBS may be beneficial in people with DYT6 dystonia [73]. For dystonic tremors people are studying Vim DBS and prelemniscal radiation [89].

Gpi DBS works for tardive dystonia according to an RCT. It may be beneficial in status dystonicus and may improve cognition [78]. GPi automated navigation systems for childhood dystonia are underway. Long term 'awake' multi-electrode monitoring in children with acquired combined dystonia has demonstrated that GPi DBS works better in hypertonic components of dystonia, while thalamic DBS may work in the hyperkinetic components of dystonia. Important considerations in DBS for paediatric age group are that we select an appropriate child, choose the best nucleus for placing the electrode and also determine the correct position inside that particular nucleus for optimum results [90].

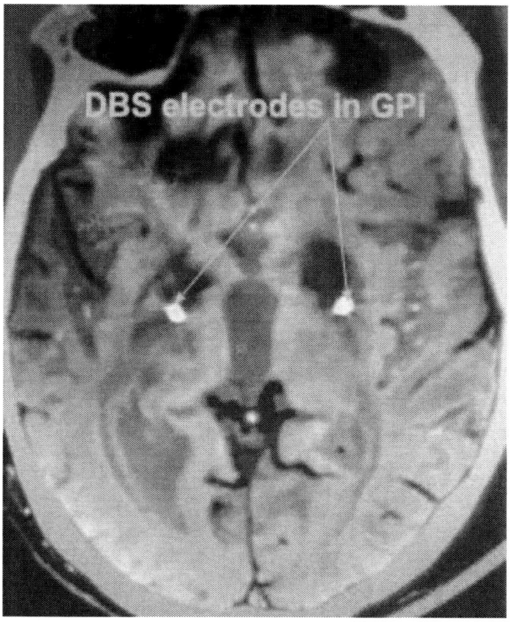

Figure 4. MRI image (SWI sequence) showing the DBS electrodes in bilateral GPi nuclei.

Amongst non-invasive techniques, repetitive transcranial magnetic stimulation (rTMS) may reduce abnormal cortical excitability, hence relieving dystonia. It is effective in focal hand dystonia and axial dystonia and investigators are studying its role in Wilson's disease. rTMS may also help in detecting abnormal gamma frequency facilitation for the diagnosis of dystonia [73].

In a recent study, fine motor movements of musicians with dystonia improved by motor retraining and bi-hemispheric, non-invasive brain stimulation via transcranial direct current stimulation to the motor cortex. Transcranial direct stimulation also enhanced response to rehabilitation in focal hand dystonia and improved dystonia in children. Also, anodal transcranial direct current stimulation to the cerebellum may improve handwriting in patients with writer's cramp. Epidural motor cortex stimulation, may, however not be so fruitful [73].

The response of gamma knife thalamotomy for dystonia takes a long time and is unpredictable and doctor may consider it for people who are not good candidates for DBS [50].

Stereotactic Lesions for the Treatment of Dystonia

A potential treatment for dystonia in future may be applying (MR guided focused ultrasound) MRgFUS to pallidum [66]. It is non-invasive, has real time control over target and temperature, doctor can monitor the response of the patient during procedure; there are no hardware complications and no need for repeated programming [50].

Rhizotomy

A new treatment for dystonic cerebral palsy is emerging, which is ventral and dorsal rhizotomy [70].

Behavioural Therapy

Behavioural therapies may benefit dystonia associated with Tourette's syndrome [91]. Non-motor manifestations in dystonia patients are also gaining focus in managing these patients [92]. Though clinicians infrequently investigate the use of approaches other than surgical and medical, however constraint-induced (CI) therapy, muscle vibration and tactile electric stimulation may also work in musicians with dystonia [93].

A new addition for quantitative diagnosis of cervical dystonia is a wireless wearable hybrid system termed as '*SKINTRONICS*' [94]. These and similar newer approaches involving fields like wireless technology, artificial intelligence, stem cell and gene therapy, neuroimaging including functional neuroimaging, voxel-based morphometry and nanoscience, are ushering in an era of personalized medicine for the management of dystonia in children as well as in adults [95, 96].

Conclusion

Treatment options coming up in the future may help PD as well as dystonia patients in leading a better and independent life and maybe prevent further progression of disease. As personalized medicine becomes increasingly evolved, treatment packages would cater to individual patients rather than diseases or community as a whole.

References

[1] Balestrino R, Schapira AHV. Parkinson disease. *Eur J Neurol.* 2020;27(1):27-42.

[2] Koppel BS. Cannabis in the Treatment of Dystonia, Dyskinesias, and Tics. *Neurotherapeutics.* 2015;12(4):788-92.

[3] Zeuner KE, Schaffer E, Hopfner F, Bruggemann N, Berg D. Progress of Pharmacological Approaches in Parkinson's Disease. *Clin Pharmacol Ther.* 2019;105(5):1106-1120.

[4] Kulisevsky J, Oliveira L, Fox SH. Update in therapeutic strategies for Parkinson's disease. *Curr Opin Neurol.* 2018;31(4):439-447.

[5] Stocchi F. Therapy for Parkinson's disease: what is in the pipeline? *Neurotherapeutics.* 2014;11(1):24-33.

[6] Hung AY, Schwarzschild MA. Treatment of Parkinson's disease: what's in the non-dopaminergic pipeline? *Neurotherapeutics.* 2014;11(1):34-46.

[7] Chen X, Gumina G, Virga KG. Recent Advances in Drug Repurposing for Parkinson's Disease. *Curr Med Chem.* 2019;26(28):5340-5362.

[8] Cacciatore I, Ciulla M, Marinelli L, Eusepi P, Stefano AD. Advances in prodrug design for Parkinson's disease. *Expert Opin Drug Discov.* 2018;13(4):295-305.

[9] Brichta L, Greengard P, Flajolet M. Advances in the pharmacological treatment of Parkinson's disease: targeting neurotransmitter systems. *Trends Neurosci.* 2013;36(9):543-554.

[10] Fasano A, Canning CG, Hausdorff JM, Lord S, Rochester L. Falls in Parkinson's disease: A complex and evolving picture. *Mov Disord.* 2017;32(11):1524-1536.

[11] Goldman JG, Weintraub D. Advances in the treatment of cognitive impairment in Parkinson's disease. *Mov Disord.* 2015;30(11):1471-1489.

[12] Lyons KE, Pahwa R, Hermanowicz N, Davis T, Pagan F, Isaacson S. Changing the treatment paradigm for Parkinson's disease psychosis with pimavanserin. *Expert Rev Clin Pharmacol.* 2019;12(7):681-691.

[13] Paudel YN, Angelopoulou E, Piperi C, Shaikh MF, Othman L. Emerging neuroprotective effect of metformin in Parkinson's disease: A molecular crosstalk. *Pharmacol Res.* 2020;152:104593.

[14] Reed J, Bain S, Kanamarlapudi V. *Recent advances in understanding the role of glucagon-like peptide 1. F1000Res.* 2020 Apr 6;9:F1000 Faculty Rev-239.

[15] Kumar B, Pandey M, Pottoo FH, Fayaz F, Sharma A, Sahoo PK. Liposomes: Novel Drug Delivery Approach for Targeting Parkinson's Disease. *Curr Pharm Des.* 2020;26(37):4721-4737.

[16] Naz S, Beach J, Heckert B, Tummala T, Pashchenko O, Banerjee T, Santra S. Cerium oxide nanoparticles: a 'radical' approach to neurodegenerative disease treatment. *Nanomedicine* (Lond). 2017;12(5):545-553.

[17] Li X, Yu Y, Tu Z. Pyrazole Scaffold Synthesis, Functionalization, and Applications in Alzheimer's Disease and Parkinson's Disease Treatment (2011-2020). *Molecules*. 2021;26(5):1202.

[18] Ishiki HM, Filho JMB, da Silva MS, Scotti MT, Scotti L. Computer-aided Drug Design Applied to Parkinson Targets. *Curr Neuropharmacol.* 2018;16(6):865-880.

[19] Vila M. Neuromelanin, aging, and neuronal vulnerability in Parkinson's disease. *Mov Disord.* 2019;34(10):1440-1451.

[20] Mao Q, Qin WZ, Zhang A, Ye N. Recent advances in dopaminergic strategies for the treatment of Parkinson's disease. *Acta Pharmacol Sin.* 2020;41(4):471-482.

[21] Petersen MV, Lund TE, Sunde N, Frandsen J, Rosendal F, Juul N, Østergaard K. Probabilistic versus deterministic tractography for delineation of the cortico-subthalamic hyperdirect pathway in patients with Parkinson disease selected for deep brain stimulation. *J Neurosurg.* 2017;126(5):1657-1668.

[22] Meles SK, Teune LK, de Jong BM, Dierckx RA, Leenders KL. Metabolic Imaging in Parkinson Disease. *J Nucl Med.* 2017;58(1):23-28.

[23] Nowacki A, Fiechter M, Fichtner J, Debove I, Lachenmayer L, Schüpbach M, Oertel MF, Wiest R, Pollo C. Using MDEFT MRI Sequences to Target the GPi in DBS Surgery. *PLoS One*. 2015;10(9):e0137868.

[24] Shimura H, Hattori N. [Disease-Modifying Therapy for Parkinson's Disease]. *Brain Nerve.* 2017;69(2):159-165.

[25] Ma L, Wei L, Wu F, Hu Z, Liu Z, Yuan W. Advances with microRNAs in Parkinson's disease research. *Drug Des Devel Ther.* 2013;7:1103-1113.

[26] Tofaris GK. A Critical Assessment of Exosomes in the Pathogenesis and Stratification of Parkinson's Disease. *J Parkinsons Dis*. 2017;7(4):569-576.

[27] Huttunen HJ, Saarma M. CDNF Protein Therapy in Parkinson's Disease. *Cell Transplant.* 2019;28(4):349-366.

[28] Stoddard-Bennett T, Pera RR. Treatment of Parkinson's Disease through Personalized Medicine and Induced Pluripotent Stem Cells. *Cells.* 2019;8(1):26.

[29] Safari F, Hatam G, Behbahani AB, Rezaei V, Barekati-Mowahed M, Petramfar P, Khademi F. CRISPR System: A High-throughput Toolbox for Research and Treatment of Parkinson's Disease. *Cell Mol Neurobiol.* 2020;40(4):477-493.

[30] Piotrowski JS, Tardiff DF. From Yeast to Humans: Leveraging New Approaches in Yeast to Accelerate Discovery of Therapeutic Targets for Synucleinopathies. *Methods Mol Biol.* 2019;2049:419-444.

[31] Zhu Z, Yang C, Iyaswamy A, Krishnamoorthi S, Sreenivasmurthy SG, Liu J, Wang Z, Tong BCK, Song J, Lu J, Cheung KH, Li M. Balancing mTOR Signaling and Autophagy in the Treatment of Parkinson's Disease. *Int J Mol Sci.* 2019;20(3):728.

[32] Grunewald A, Kumar KR, Sue CM. New insights into the complex role of mitochondria in Parkinson's disease. *Prog Neurobiol.* 2019;177:73-93.

[33] Jiang X, Ganesan P, Rengarajan T, Choi DK, Arulselvan P. Cellular phenotypes as inflammatory mediators in Parkinson's disease: Interventional targets and role of natural products. *Biomed Pharmacother.* 2018;106:1052-1062.

[34] Carrera I, Cacabelos R. Current Drugs and Potential Future Neuroprotective Compounds for Parkinson's Disease. *Curr Neuropharmacol.* 2019;17(3):295-306.

[35] Bonesi M, Xiao J, Tundis R, Aiello F, Sicari V, Loizzo MR. Advances in the Tyrosinase Inhibitors from Plant Source. *Curr Med Chem.* 2019;26(18):3279-3299.

[36] Mathur D, Goyal K, Koul V, Anand A. The Molecular Links of Re-Emerging Therapy: A Review of Evidence of Brahmi (Bacopa monniera). *Front Pharmacol.* 2016;7:44.

[37] Krishnan S, Pisharady KK, Divya KP, Shetty K, Kishore A. Deep brain stimulation for movement disorders. *Neurol India.* 2018;66(Supplement):S90-S101.

[38] Kuhn AA, Volkmann J. Innovations in deep brain stimulation methodology. *Mov Disord.* 2017;32(1):11-19.

[39] Koeglsperger T, Palleis C, Hell F, Mehrkens JH, Botzel K. Deep Brain Stimulation Programming for Movement Disorders: Current Concepts and Evidence-Based Strategies. *Front Neurol.* 2019;10:410.

[40] Lee DJ, Lozano CS, Dallapiazza RF, Lozano AM. Current and future directions of deep brain stimulation for neurological and psychiatric disorders. *J Neurosurg.* 2019;131(2):333-342.

[41] Wong JK, Middlebrooks EH, Grewal SS, Almeida L, Hess CW, Okun MS. A Comprehensive Review of Brain Connectomics and Imaging to Improve Deep Brain Stimulation Outcomes. *Mov Disord.* 2020;35(5):741-751.

[42] de Almeida Marcelino AL, Horn A, Krause P, Kuhn AA, Neumann WJ. Subthalamic neuromodulation improves short-term motor learning in Parkinson's disease. *Brain.* 2019;142(8):2198-2206.

[43] Palleis C, Gehmeyr M, Mehrkens JH, Botzel K, Koeglsperger T. Establishment of a Visual Analog Scale for DBS Programming (VISUAL-STIM Trial). *Front Neurol.* 2020;11:561323.

[44] Jia F, Zhang J, Wang H, Liang Z, Liu W, Wang X, Liu Y, Guo Y, Ling Z, Cai X, Wu X, Wu J, Lv W, Xu X, Zhang W, Li L. Variable- versus constant-frequency deep-brain stimulation in patients with advanced Parkinson's disease: study protocol for a randomized controlled trial. *Trials.* 2019;20(1):749.

[45] Habets JGV, Heijmans M, Kuijf ML, Janssen MLF, Temel Y, Kubben PL. An update on adaptive deep brain stimulation in Parkinson's disease. *Mov Disord.* 2018;33(12):1834-1843.

[46] Moran CH, Pietrzyk M, Sarangmat N, Gerard CS, Barua N, Ashida R, Whone A, Szewczyk-Krolikowski K, Mooney L, Gill SS. Clinical Outcome of "Asleep" Deep Brain Stimulation for Parkinson Disease Using Robot-Assisted Delivery and Anatomic Targeting of the Subthalamic Nucleus: A Series of 152 Patients. *Neurosurgery.* 2020;88(1):165-173.

[47] Miterko LN, Baker KB, Beckinghausen J, Bradnam LY, Cheng MY, Cooperrider J, DeLong MR, Gornati SV, Hallett M, Heck DH, Hoebeek FE, Kouzani AZ, Kuo SH, Louis ED, Machado A, Manto M, McCambridge AB, Nitsche MA, Taib NOB, Popa T, Tanaka M, Timmann D, Steinberg GK, Wang EH, Wichmann T, Xie T,

Sillitoe RV. Consensus Paper: Experimental Neurostimulation of the Cerebellum. *Cerebellum.* 2019;18(6):1064-1097.

[48] Grembecka B, Glac W, Listowska M, Jerzemowska G, Plucińska K, Majkutewicz I, Badtke P, Wrona D. Subthalamic Deep Brain Stimulation Affects Plasma Corticosterone Concentration and Peripheral Immunity Changes in Rat Model of Parkinson's Disease. *J Neuroimmune Pharmacol.* 2020 Jul 9. doi: 10.1007/s11481-020-09934-7. Epub ahead of print.

[49] Rizzone MG, Martone T, Balestrino R, Lopiano L. Genetic background and outcome of Deep Brain Stimulation in Parkinson's disease. *Parkinsonism Relat Disord.* 2019;64:8-19.

[50] Cahan LD, Young RF, Li F. Radiosurgical Pallidotomy for Parkinson's Disease. *Prog Neurol Surg.* 2018;33:149-157.

[51] Fishman PS, Frenkel V. Treatment of Movement Disorders With Focused Ultrasound. *J Cent Nerv Syst Dis.* 2017;9:1179573517705670.

[52] Mishra RK, Thrasher AT. Transcranial direct current stimulation of dorsolateral prefrontal cortex improves dual-task gait performance in patients with Parkinson's disease: A double blind, sham-controlled study. *Gait Posture.* 2021;84:11-16.

[53] Brun L, Lefaucheur R, Fetter D, Derrey S, Borden A, Wallon D, Bourre B, Maltete D. Non-motor fluctuations in Parkinson's disease: prevalence, characteristics and management in a large cohort of parkinsonian outpatients. *Clin Neurol Neurosurg.* 2014;127:93-96.

[54] Garcia-Agundez A, Folkerts AK, Konrad R, Caserman P, Tregel T, Goosses M, Gobel S, Kalbe E. Recent advances in rehabilitation for Parkinson's Disease with Exergames: A Systematic Review. *J Neuroeng Rehabil.* 2019;16(1):17.

[55] Kim A, Darakjian N, Finley JM. Walking in fully immersive virtual environments: an evaluation of potential adverse effects in older adults and individuals with Parkinson's disease. *J Neuroeng Rehabil.* 2017;14(1):16.

[56] Zhao Y, Heida T, van Wegen EEH, Bloem BR, van Wezel RJA. E-health Support in People with Parkinson's Disease with Smart Glasses: A Survey of User Requirements and Expectations in the Netherlands. *J Parkinsons Dis.* 2015;5(2):369-378.

[57] Nuic D, Vinti M, Karachi C, Foulon P, Hamme AV, Welter ML. The feasibility and positive effects of a customised videogame rehabilitation programme for freezing of gait and falls in Parkinson's disease patients: a pilot study. *J Neuroeng Rehabil.* 2018;15(1):31.

[58] Buard I, Dewispelaere WB, Teale P, Rojas DC, Kronberg E, Thaut MH, Kluger BM. Auditory entrainment of motor responses in older adults with and without Parkinson's disease: An MEG study. *Neurosci Lett.* 2019;708:134331.

[59] Willis GL, Boda J, Freelance CB. Polychromatic Light Exposure as a Therapeutic in the Treatment and Management of Parkinson's Disease: A Controlled Exploratory Trial. *Front Neurol.* 2018;9:741.

[60] Lavermicocca V, Dellomonaco AR, Tedesco A, Notarnicola M, Fede RD, Battaglini PP. [Neurofeedback in Parkinson's disease: technologies in speech and language therapy]. *Recenti Prog Med.* 2018;109(2):130-132.

[61] Barnish J, Atkinson RA, Barran SM, Barnish MS. Potential Benefit of Singing for People with Parkinson's Disease: A Systematic Review. *J Parkinsons Dis.* 2016;6(3):473-484.

[62] Albanese A, Bhatia K, Bressman SB, DeLong MR, Fahn S, Fung VSC, Hallett M, J6nkovic J, Jinnah HA, Klein C, Lang AE, Mink JW, Teller JK. Phenomenology and classification of dystonia: a consensus update. *Mov Disord.* 2013;28(7):863-873.

[63] Skogseid IM. Dystonia-new advances in classification, genetics, pathophysiology and treatment. *Acta Neurol Scand Suppl.* 2014;(198):13-9.

[64] Gonzalez-Alegre P. Advances in molecular and cell biology of dystonia: Focus on torsinA. *Neurobiol Dis.* 2019;127:233-241.

[65] Balint B, Bhatia KP. Dystonia: an update on phenomenology, classification, pathogenesis and treatment. *Curr Opin Neurol.* 2014;27(4):468-476.

[66] Jinnah HA, Neychev V, Hess EJ. The Anatomical Basis for Dystonia: The Motor Network Model. *Tremor Other Hyperkinet Mov* (N Y). 2017;7:506.

[67] Fan X, Donsante Y, Jinnah HA, Hess EJ. Dopamine Receptor Agonist Treatment of Idiopathic Dystonia: A Reappraisal in Humans and Mice. *J Pharmacol Exp Ther.* 2018;365(1):20-26.

[68] Roze E, Lang AE, Vidailhet M. Myoclonus-dystonia: classification, phenomenology, pathogenesis, and treatment. *Curr Opin Neurol.* 2018;31(4):484-490.

[69] Kara E, Hardy J, Houlden H. The pallidopyramidal syndromes: nosology, aetiology and pathogenesis. *Curr Opin Neurol.* 2013;26(4):381-394.

[70] Jinnah HA. Medical and Surgical Treatments for Dystonia. *Neurol Clin.* 2020;38(2):325-348.

[71] Sioufi F, Sioufi K. Autoimmune dystonia-a group of patients responsive to immunotherapy (P2.2-046). *Neurology.* 2019;92(15Supplement):P2.2-046.

[72] Downs AM, Roman KM, Campbell SA, Pisani A, Hess EJ, Bonsi P. The neurobiological basis for novel experimental therapeutics in dystonia. *Neurobiol Dis.* 2019;130:104526.

[73] Albanese A, Romito LM, Calandrella D. Therapeutic advances in dystonia. *Mov Disord.* 2015;30(11):1547-1556.

[74] Finsterer J, Maeztu C, Revuelta GJ, Reichel G, Truong D. Collum-caput (COL-CAP) concept for conceptual anterocollis, anterocaput, and forward sagittal shift. *J Neurol Sci.* 2015;355(1-2):37-43.

[75] Dressler D, Altavista MC, Altenmueller E, Bhidayasiri R, Bohlega S, Chana P, Chung TM, Colosimo C, Fheodoroff K, Garcia-Ruiz PJ, Jeon B, Jin L, Kanovsky P, Milanov I, Micheli F, Orlova O, Pandey S, Pirtosek Z, Relja M, Rosales R, Sagastegui-Rodriguez JA, Shahidi GA, Timerbaeva S, Wan X, Walter U, Saberi FA.Consensus guidelines for botulinum toxin therapy: general algorithms and dosing tables for dystonia and spasticity. *J Neural Transm* (Vienna). 2021;128(3):321–335.

[76] Jinnah HA, Albanese A, Bhatia KP, Cardoso F, Da Prat G, de Koning TJ, Espay AJ, Fung V, Garcia-Ruiz PJ, Gershanik O, Jankovic J, Kaji R, Kotschet K, Marras C, Miyasaki JM, Morgante F, Munchau A, Pal PK, Rodriguez Oroz MC,

Rodriguez-Violante M, Schols L, Stamelou M, Tijssen M, Uribe Roca C, de la Cerda A, Gatto EM; International Parkinson's Disease Movement Disorders Society Task Force on Rare Movement Disorders. Treatable inherited rare movement disorders. *Mov Disord.* 2018;33(1):21-35.

[77] Nahm NJ, Graham HK, Gormley ME, Georgiadis AG. Management of hypertonia in cerebral palsy. *Curr Opin Pediatr.* 2018;30(1):57-64.

[78] Factor SA. Management of Tardive Syndrome: Medications and Surgical Treatments. *Neurotherapeutics.* 2020;17(4):1694-1712.

[79] Marecos C, Ng J, Kurian MA. What is new for monoamine neurotransmitter disorders? *J Inherit Metab Dis.* 2014;37(4):619-626.

[80] Jankovic J. Medical treatment of dystonia. *Mov Disord.* 2013;28(7):1001-1012.

[81] Lallemant-Dudek P, Darios F, Durr A. Recent advances in understanding hereditary spastic paraplegias and emerging therapies. *Fac Rev.* 2021;10:27.

[82] Edwards CA, Kouzani A, Lee KH, Ross EK. Neurostimulation Devices for the Treatment of Neurologic Disorders. *Mayo Clin Proc.* 2017;92(9):1427-1444.

[83] Nowacki A, Fiechter M, Fichtner J, Debove I, Lachenmayer L, Schupbach M, Oertel MF, Wiest R, Pollo C. Using MDEFT MRI Sequences to Target the GPi in DBS Surgery. *PloS One.* 2015;10(9):e0137868.

[84] Artusi CA, Dwivedi A, Romagnolo A, Bortolani S, Marsili L, Imbalzano G, Sturchio A, Keeling EG, Zibetti M, Contarino MF, Fasano A, Tagliati M, Okun MS, Espay AJ, Lopiano L, Merola A. Differential response to pallidal deep brain stimulation among monogenic dystonias: systematic review and meta-analysis. *J Neurol Neurosurg Psychiatry.* 2020;91(4):426-433.

[85] Li XY, Dai LF, Wan XH, Guo Y, Dai Y, Li SL, Fang F, Wang XH, Zhang WH, Liu TH, Xie ZH, Fang T, Wang L, Ding CH. Clinical phenotypes, genotypes and treatment in Chinese dystonia patients with KMT2B variants. *Parkinsonism Relat Disord.* 2020;77:76-82.

[86] Bragg DC, Sharma N, Ozelius LJ. X-Linked Dystonia-Parkinsonism: recent advances. *Curr Opin Neurol.* 2019;32(4):604-609.

[87] Iwamuro H. Electrophysiological evidences of organization of cortical motor information in the Basal Ganglia. *J Mov Disord.* 2011;4(1):8-12.

[88] Rossi M, Balint B, Vernetti PM, Bhatia KP, Merello M. Genetic Dystonia-ataxia Syndromes: Clinical Spectrum, Diagnostic Approach, and Treatment Options. *Mov Disord Clin Pract.* 2018;5(4):373-382.

[89] Elble R, Deuschl G. Milestones in tremor research. *Mov Disord.* 2011;26(6):1096-1105.

[90] Lumsden DE, Kaminska M, Ashkan K, Selway R, Lin JP. Deep brain stimulation for childhood dystonia: Is 'where' as important as in 'whom'? *Eur J Paediatr Neurol.* 2017;21(1):176-184.

[91] Silveira-Moriyama L, Lin JP.A field guide to current advances in paediatric movement disorders. *Curr Opin Neurol.* 2015;28(4):437-446.

[92] Junker J, Berman BD, Hall J, Wahba DW, Brandt V, Perlmutter JS, Jankovic J, Malaty IA, Shukla AW, Reich SG, Espay AJ, Duque KR, Patel N, Roze E, Vidailhet M, Jinnah HA, Bruggemann N. Quality of life in isolated dystonia: non-

motor manifestations matter. *J Neurol Neurosurg Psychiatry.* 2021;jnnp-2020-325193.

[93] Furuya S, Altenmuller E. Acquisition and reacquisition of motor coordination in musicians. *Ann N Y Acad Sci.* 2015;1337:118-124.

[94] Kwon YT, Lee Y, Berkmen GK, Lim HR, Scorr L, Jinnah HA, Yeo WH. Soft Material-Enabled, Active Wireless, Thin-Film Bioelectronics for Quantitative Diagnostics of Cervical Dystonia. *Adv Mater Technol.* 2019;4(10):1900458.

[95] Lin JP. Advances in pharmacotherapies for movement disorders in children: current limitations and future progress. *Curr Opin Pediatr.* 2017;29(6):652-664.

[96] Rowland NC, Sammartino F, Lozano AM. Advances in surgery for movement disorders. *Mov Disord.* 2017;32(1):5-10.

Chapter 20

Neurorehabilitation in the Treatment of Brain Tumors

Ved Prakash Maurya, Amanjot Singh Boparai, Abhishek Kumar Thakur, Sudhir Sasapardhi, Rana Pratap Singh and Kuntal Kanti Das
Department of Neurosurgery, Sanjay Gandhi Postgraduate Institute of Medical Sciences, Lucknow, India

Abstract

The development in diagnostic as well as therapeutic modalities have resulted in increased incidence of brain tumors in the modern society. These tumors after undergoing proper clinico radiological work-up are subjected to Neoadjuvant and Adjuvant therapy with or without surgical decompression depending upon the size, histopathological characteristics as well as residual disease. These patients often suffer the impact of disease even after surgery as well as adjuvant therapy. The importance of rehabilitation after surgery for brain tumors was a less explored area and has gained popularity during the last couple of decades. The onco-neurosurgical fraternity including the psychiatrist have underscored the survival rate due to anticipated low overall survival rates. In the latter half of twentieth century, Lehmann et al., first advocated the importance of rehabilitation in patients suffering from malignancy. Following their landmark initiative, several studies were conducted which focused primarily on the recovery of patients after brain tumor surgery. It was believed for a long time that there exists significant resemblance in the symptomatology between stroke and brain tumor patients. The rehabilitative measures resulted in similar short-term benefits between both the group, but the long-term survival was not well established. The

In: Advances in Neurosurgery Research
Editors: Amit Agrawal, Pradeep Chouksey, Adesh Shrivastava et al.
ISBN: 978-1-68507-859-1

cognitive deficits arising due to brain tumor or their treatment results in significant impairment in the quality of life of the patient as well as the care givers. In the present chapter, we focus on the neurorehabilitation deemed necessary for the management of patients with brain tumor.

Introduction

Malignancy of the brain contributes about 2% of the total incidence of tumor. These tumors can occur without any age barriers but the incidence at the advanced age is more frequent. Meningioma, Schwannoma, Primary CNS Lymphoma and Gliomas (particularly Glioblastoma, Anaplastic astrocytoma, and benign lesions such as low-grade astrocytoma as well as Oligodendroglioma). WHO grade 3 and 4 comprises of high grade glioma, and these contribute most common primary brain tumor in adult patient population (Louis et al., 2007; Louis et al., 2014). Glioblastoma tops the list due to its most common occurrence but with worst outcome. The median overall survival in glioblastoma patients remains poor even with best available care. This duration ranges from 15 months for newly diagnosed glioblastoma and up to 7 months for the recurrent glioblastoma. The gender wise incidence of brain tumor is nearly equal in both males and females. The relative benign pathologies such as meningioma and schwannoma are more frequent in females while glioblastoma tends to occur more commonly in males (Stupp et al., 2005). Keeping in view the poor prognosis of most of the brain tumors, the primary goal of management is to preserve or restore the neurological functions as well as to decrease the morbidity, if not possible to avoid totally. The treatment with this intention delivers the potential to perform their daily activities for a longer duration following surgical intervention.

The presence of brain tumor itself and their management are well known to affect the cognitive function of an individual across multiple domains. This in turn has significant impact on the quality of life (QOL) of any individual. The impairment in cognitive function is noticed frequently in patients with brain tumor. These cognitive deficits may be caused due to the presence of tumor itself, seizures induced due to tumor itself, the psychological discomfort arising due to presence of tumor. The impairment in cognitive function also occurred due to treatment itself, which include a wide spectrum of surgery, radiotherapy, antiepileptics, steroids as well as chemotherapy (Bergo et al., 2019). In a study conducted by Tucha et al., in over 139 patients of brain tumor, they concluded that there was impairment in at least one area of cognition. It included impaired executive function in nearly 78% of patient populations and problems associated with attention as well as memory were noticed in more than 60% of patients (Tucha et al., 2000).

Another study conducted by Zucchella et al., revealed that more than half of the patient population (54.4%) with brain tumor showed impairment in cognitive functions. Out of these patients with cognitive impairment, multimodal impairment was most common followed by cognitive deficits which were limited to language, memory, attention, carrying out logical-executive functions along with impaired visuospatial ability (Zucchella et al., 2013). Gehrke et al., conducted an extensive review of the existing literature where they concluded that the commonest cognitive disturbances are impaired working memory, executive functions as well as general attention. These effects are noticed without any limitations of age, gender as well as level of educational qualification (Gehrke et al., 2013).

Efforts in the field of cognitive rehabilitation have turned out to be effective in patients suffering from Stroke as well as in Alzheimer's disease (Sitzer et al., 2006). Till date very limited study have reviewed the potential advantages of rehabilitation measures for the patients suffering from primitive brain tumor. There have been significant scarcity of studies analysing the impact of cognitive rehabilitation in an individual's life. Study on cognitive rehabilitation in patients with Glioma may turn out to be a pivotal step towards better neurocognitive functions as well as improved quality of life following treatment (Bergo et al., 2019). There has been a recent surge in the studies dealing with the outcome of cognitive rehabilitation in patients suffering with brain tumors.

Principles of Cognitive Rehabilitation

The neuronal plasticity of the brain forms the basic principle of cognitive remediation/rehabilitation therapy. This modality of rehabilitation leads to exercises targeted at continuous betterment of varied cognitive domains such as attention, memory, language as well as executive functions. The optimum outcome is a positive impact on the functional deficits which affects the day-to-day living. These therapies are definitely intended to increase the professional as well as social integration amongst the patients undergoing treatment. Cognitive rehabilitation employs two main types of exercises to attain the treatment goals. These are: compensation and retraining. In compensation technique the individual is trained to work with the preserved cognitive functions. Here the individuals are encouraged to develop alternative methods in order to attain the pre-determined targets.

In case of retraining exercise, we used to retrain the functions of the brain with regular and repeated exercises keeping in focus a deficient aspect of cognitive function. This repeated training leads to restoration of the deficient function up to significant extent. The use of planners, memory notebooks as well as checklists are the newer strategies to enhance the process of cognitive rehabilitation. These two modalities of training go hand-in-hand. The restorative phenomenon enhances the development of compensatory process and vice versa. The ultimate aim is to enhance the overall functionality as well as well-being of the individual (Dirette et al., 1999).

Impact of Brain Tumor on the Society

The tumors of the CNS may involve brain as well as the spinal cord. These tumors may be further categorized into either primary or secondary/ metastatic in origin. The impact of these tumors significantly affects the degree of independence as a result of injury to the neuronal structures. These structures which are involved in the pathological process of neuronal injury result in impairment of motor, sensory, cognitive or speech functions of an individual. These gradually evolving pathology carries a huge impact not only in the life of an individual as well as the family and the society. Every year, more than 15,000 cases of primary brain tumor as well as 4,000 cases of tumor of the spinal cord are diagnosed (American Cancer Society, 1990). The impact of brain tumor can be estimated by the fact that it contributes about 2% of all cancer deaths, accounting about 11,000 mortality per year (American Cancer Society 1990).

The metastatic lesions of the brain contribute about 20% to 40% of all the brain tumors and produce a combination of neurological symptoms in about 85,000 individuals annually. In order to combat these lesions of the brain, patients are subjected to surgery, chemotherapy and/or radiotherapy depending upon the histological characteristic of the tumor. Significant neurological signs may be detected before a patient comes into clinical attention. These includes impaired cognition (77%), unilateral weakness (66%), sensory loss (27%), difficulty in walking (24%), and aphasia (19%) (Caraceni and Martini, 1999a). In addition to these complaints, common complications of brain tumor and their management include: dysphagia, bladder and bowel complaints, psychological issues, generalised fatigue, endocrine abnormalities, sexual dysfunction as well as psychiatric disturbances (Caraceni and Martini, 1999a).

The main goal of rehabilitation services is to restore and maximize the independence of an individual with minimum dependence on the care givers. With the progression of the brain tumor, a decline in functional skills is noticed. At this point, rehabilitation plays a supportive role with modified goals according to anatomic and physiological limitations. At the end-stage of disease, palliative rehabilitation provides comfort as well as maintains the quality of life until end of life. A rehabilitation team providing holistic care comprised of Physiatrist, Primary physician, Nurse, Physical therapist, Occupational therapist, Speech-language therapist, Recreational therapist, Social worker, Case manager, Dietician as well as Chaplain depending upon the social customs being practiced (Garden and Gillis, 1996).

Rehabilitation in Accordance to Nature of Malignancy, Benign vs Malignant

The impact of brain tumor depends not only on its size but also on its nature, benign versus malignant, as well as its vicinity to the eloquent areas of the brain. It should be understood before commencement of management that lesions adjacent to the brainstem may lead to significant deficit of cranial nerves, motor and sensory functions as well as impaired coordination. Gliomas constitutes more than 90% of the primary adult brain tumors, and majority of them are having malignant potential. Amongst the gliomas, glioblastoma carries the worst outcome while low grade astrocytomas are associated with better prognosis. Depending upon their location these gliomas manifests most commonly as seizure disorder, cognitive impairment, sensory motor deficits, impairment of speech as well as visual distribution (Bondy and Wrensch, 1993; Black, 1991).

Lesions of the Pituitary gland manifests most commonly as headache, bilateral impairment of vision as well as hormonal disturbances with widespread systemic manifestations.

The lesions of the cerebellopontine angle (most commonly Vestibular Schwannoma) manifest as hearing loss, vertigo as well as difficulty in deglutition and phonation due to involvement of the lower cranial nerves. Associated with these tumors are facial nerve palsy and features of raised intracranial pressure leading to headache and visual impairment. Impaired growth pattern is noticed in children suffering from craniopharyngioma while visual disturbances and sexual disturbances are present in adults with such tumors (Black, 1991).

Most common source of primary for the brain metastatic lesion are lung, breast followed by carcinoma of the gastrointestinal tract, kidney as well as malignant melanoma. These tumors beside their local infiltration are highly destructive due to the phenomenon of cerebral edema as well as leptomeningeal involvement.

Common Principles of Rehabilitation for Brain Tumor Patients

The nature of the disease must be taken into account and discussed with the patient beforehand in view of the severity and guarded outcome. The interventions must be tailored in accordance with the tumor behaviour, neurological status of the patient and the ongoing clinical course.

In case of severe cognitive impairment with limited possibility of recovery, the priority of rehabilitation must focus on caregivers' education and adaptation towards patient's environment. In case the expected survival is not more than 2 months, the primary focus should be towards injury prevention and patient's hygiene.

Area Wise Effect of Tumors

The lesions specific to particular territory of the brain carries a significant spectrum of clinical presentation. These symptom complex in turn directs the rehabilitative measures essential in the care of such patients. The tumor of the temporal lobe leads to difficulty in speech, defective hearing as well as memory impairment. The parietal lobe lesion leads to vision loss, impaired spatial orientation, dressing apraxia along with proprioceptive agnosia.

Behavioural anomalies are the most prominent feature of frontal lobe lesions, which includes personality and change in libido, impulsive behaviour as well as emotional liability. Some of the metabolic changes associated with the physiologic effects of brain tumor include SIADH (syndrome of inappropriate anti diuretic hormone secretion) manifesting as hyponatremia which in turn leads to mental status changes (Nelson et al., 1993). After radiotherapy, a significant change in appetite, behaviour, endocrine dysfunction as well as fatigue are noticed (Bondy and Wrensch, 1993). The process of rehabilitation therapy becomes complicated once steroid psychosis adds to the existing problems.

Patients who are bedridden for prolonged period requires regular position changes in order to avoid pressure sores as well as deep vein thrombosis. The position needs to be changed every hourly in order to avoid in bed sores. Range of movement of all joints are mandatory to avoid joint contracture and maintain essential proprioceptive and stretch responses. Sensory stimulation, regular exposure to sunlight in order to maintain day-night orientation and socialization are all essential components of rehabilitation. Prolonged usage of steroids to mitigate peritumoral cerebral edema leads to myopathy reflecting in the form of proximal muscular weakness in addition to weakness arising due to prolonged immobility. Exercise and muscle strengthening therapy must be initiated once steroids are initiated for brain tumor patients.

Autonomic system involvement manifests mostly in the form of alterations in bladder and bowel habits. Urinary incontinence manifests due to lack of the cortical control. Patients with impaired cognition requires behavioural training leading to progressive control of bladder contractility in the form of increased inter-voiding interval. This interval is increased every 10 to 15 minutes for a period of 4-5 days to attain a reasonable interval between two voiding episodes. Other modalities of treatment include anticholinergic and antispasmodic medications, use of external catheters as well as diapers to avoid urinary incontinence. These diapers are changed every 2 hours to avoid skin breakdown. Patients who are immobile or bedridden for a longer duration develop decreased mobility of bowel and requires high intake of fluid, stool softeners, enemas or digital evacuation of faecoliths, if not dealt on a timely fashion.

In order to avoid these problems, early ambulation is a rule in the rehabilitative measures of brain tumor patients. Orthotic devices, in order to support a joint or limb and assistive devices such as a walker as well as walking sticks are encouraged. Wheelchair ambulation are recommended for those having significant coordination and imbalance problems. Physical and occupational therapist are engaged early in the rehabilitation process to encourage about activities of daily living (ADL), ambulation and stretching exercises. Speech therapists play a vital role in the cognition assessment, assistance in the linguistic and communication deficits. These specialists identify the problems associated with swallowing and suggests the compensatory manoeuvres, provide the therapeutic exercise as well as modify the consistency of the diet.

The presence of seizure disorder and hydrocephalus manifests as complications of brain tumor and plays a negative impact in rehabilitation in the form of decreasing functional performance. The presence of these two features results in declining neurological status and may preclude participation in rehabilitation program. These components need to be evaluated with the help of computed tomography scan (CT), lumbar puncture for CSF analysis and measures to divert the CSF in order to decrease the raised intracranial pressure.

Cranial Nerve Deficits

In brain tumor patients cranial nerve functions must be assessed judiciously in order to greatly improve the functional status of an individual. Vision, hearing impairment with facial palsy are notice frequently in meningioma, vestibular schwannoma as well as pituitary adenomas (Rowland 1995). The rehabilitation of visual deficits includes ophthalmological consultation to detect the degree of visual impairment. The patients are trained to utilize the compensatory techniques in order to improve visual spatial awareness. Clear instructions must be mentioned regarding guidelines for driving a vehicle and clear instructions about next visits in order to avoid unnecessary delay in delivery of health care services. Those patients with double vision needs to undergo alternate - eye patching technique. The complaint of facial pain is one of the major debilitating symptoms and are encountered in a number of intracranial space occupying lesions. It involves the lesion located at the cerebellopontine angle, Meckel's cave proper and anomalies of cavernous sinus in variable combination. The distressing facial pain arising from these structures involved in these areas may be managed with the help of Tricyclic antidepressants, antiepileptics, analgesics as well as narcotic medications in several combinations. The paralysis involving the eyelids as well as the face requires an intervention from the plastic surgeon for cosmetic reasons and corneal protection. The involvement of the hearing apparatus needs timely intervention and evaluation in order to differentiate sensorineural from conductive hearing loss. These work-up will help the physicians to seek consultation from the speech therapist in order to adopt a timely rehabilitative measure for communication. There exists a crucial role of dietician as well as the nutritionist who are actively involved in the enteral and parenteral nutrition in those who are not able to carry out deglutition of the foods after lower cranial nerve involvement. The paralysis of hypoglossal nerve in addition to lower cranial nerve presents an additional challenge for chest infection and repeated aspiration episodes. The present of chest infection in such cases leads to a guarded outcome. Adequate rehabilitative measures play a crucial role in the early recovery and increased overall survival of these patients.

Rehabilitation of Speech/Cognitive Deficits

The basic etiology of cognitive impairment arises due to the structural impairment caused by the lesion itself, during surgical resection of the tumor and the effects arising after adjuvant therapy, mainly radiation therapy. The medications used to control the seizures and the radiotherapy have been well documented to impair the cognitive functions of the patient undergoing treatment. The underlying medical conditions such as hypothyroidism becomes obvious during the period of stress and must be treated to overcome the depression and anxiety. Cognitive impairments are seen mostly involving the areas of memory, attention, drive as well as psychomotor retardation. The initial intervention in order to overcome the impairment in memory include visual imagery and memory aids. Adaptive strategies and compensatory techniques are taught with the help of cognitive remediation programs (Silberfarb 1983).

Attention and distractibility are ameliorated with the use of Dopamine agonists and antidepressants. The problem of aphasia and dysarthria are not uncommon and are noticed to adversely affect the language and articulation. The aphasic patients possess significant challenges in the communication and the differential for this situation includes visual constructive difficulties and apraxia (Gualtieri et al., 1989).

The Abnormalities of Balance

The information about balance of human body from various receptors are integrated and processed in brainstem and cerebellum which involve the visual, vestibular as well as the somatosensory systems. The abnormality in the proprioception, muscle strength, vertigo, unsteadiness and dizziness lead to anomalies of human balance. The neuroanatomical structures which are severed, such as spinal cord, parasagittal or sensory cortex of the brain, results into balance difficulties. The availability of a Balance Meter System is used to quantify the degree of balance disorder as well as actively involved in the treatment of balance disorders. The vestibular and visual complaints would be isolated with the help of device's environment. An individualised exercise program based on the existing deficits helps to overcome the determined deficits. A controlled mobility and gradual increase in the range of motion as well as trunk strength helps to overcome the proprioceptive responses. A number of pharmacological measures were employed to mitigate the problem of balance disorder such as, meclizine and dimenhydrinate.

Conclusion

The rehabilitation of patients suffering with brain tumor requires a multidisciplinary team for the holistic management of their symptoms as well as side effects following treatment. A convincing description regarding benefits in the motor, sensory as well as cognitive functions is still lacking but the care givers and family members expressed a great amount of satisfaction in those cases who underwent rehabilitation therapy.

References

American Cancer Society. *"Cancer Facts and Figures."* New York: American Cancer Society (1990).

Bergo, E., G. Lombardi, I. Guglieri, E. Capovilla, Ardi Pambuku, and V. Zagone. "Neurocognitive functions and health-related quality of life in glioblastoma patients: a concise review of the literature." *European journal of cancer care* 28, no. 1 (2019): e12410.

Black, P. M. "Brain tumors. Part 1 and part 2." *N Engl J* Med 324 (1991): 1471-1476, 1555-1564.

Bondy, M. L., and M. Wrensch. "Update on brain cancer epidemiology." Cancer Bulletin-Houston- 45 (1993): 365-369.

Caraceni, A., Martini, C. "Neurological problems. In: Doyle D., Hanks G. W. C., MacDonald N. (eds)." *Oxford Textbook of Palliative Medicine,* 2nd ed. New York: Oxford University Press, (1999a): 727-749.

Dirette, D. K., Jim Hinojosa, and George J. Carnevale. "Comparison of remedial and compensatory interventions for adults with acquired brain injuries." *The Journal of Head Trauma Rehabilitation* 14, no. 6 (1999): 595-601.

Garden, F. H., Gillis, T. A. "Principles of cancer rehabilitation. In: Braddom RL (ed)." *Physical Medicine and Rehabilitation,* 1st ed. Philadelphia: WB Saunders, (1996): 1199-1214.

Gehrke, A. K., Margaret C. Baisley, Alexander L. B. Sonck, Samantha L. Wronski, and Michael Feuerstein. "Neurocognitive deficits following primary brain tumor treatment: systematic review of a decade of comparative studies." *Journal of neuro-oncology* 115, no. 2 (2013): 135-142.

Gualtieri, T., Mark Chandler, Tena B. Coons, and Lloyd T. Brown. "Amantadine: a new clinical profile for traumatic brain injury." *Clinical neuropharmacology* 12, no. 4 (1989): 258-270.

Louis, D. N., A. Perry, P. Burger, D. W. Ellison, G. Reifenberger, A. von Deimling, K. Aldape et al., "International Society of Neuropathology-Haarlem: International Society of Neuropathology-Haarlem consensus guidelines for nervous system tumor classification and grading." *Brain Pathol* 24, no. 5 (2014): 429-435.

Louis, D. N., Hiroko Ohgaki, Otmar D. Wiestler, Webster K. Cavenee, Peter C. Burger, Anne Jouvet, Bernd W. Scheithauer, and Paul Kleihues. "The 2007 WHO classification of tumours of the central nervous system." *Acta neuropathologica* 114, no. 2 (2007): 97-109.

Nelson, D. F., McDonald, J. V., Lapham, L. W., Qazi, R., and Rubin, P. "Central Nervous System Tumors. In McDonald, J., Qazi, R., and Rubin, P. (Eds.)" *Clinical Oncology: A Multidisciplinary Approach for Physicians and Students*. Seventh edition. Philadelphia: W.B. Saunders Co. (1993): 617–644.

Rowland, L. P. 1995. *"Merritt's Textbook of Neurology, 9th ed. Baltimore":* Williams & Wilkins. (1995): 1058.

Silberfarb, P. M. "Chemotherapy and cognitive defects in cancer patients." *Annual review of medicine* 34, no. 1 (1983): 35-46.

Sitzer, D. I., Elizabeth W. Twamley, and D. V. Jeste. "Cognitive training in Alzheimer's disease: a meta-analysis of the literature." *Acta Psychiatrica Scandinavica* 114, no. 2 (2006): 75-90.

Stupp, R., Warren P. Mason, Martin J. van den Bent, Michael Weller, Barbara Fisher, Martin J. B. Taphoorn, Karl Belanger, et al., "Radiotherapy plus Concomitant and Adjuvant Temozolomide for Glioblastoma." *New England Journal of Medicine* 352, no. 10 (March 10, 2005): 987-996.

Tucha, O., Christian Smely, Michael Preier, and Klaus W. Lange. "Cognitive deficits before treatment among patients with brain tumors." *Neurosurgery* 47, no. 2 (2000): 324-334.

Zucchella, C., Michelangelo Bartolo, Cherubino Di Lorenzo, Veronica Villani, and Andrea Pace. "Cognitive impairment in primary brain tumors outpatients: a prospective cross-sectional survey." *Journal of Neuro-Oncology* 112, no. 3 (2013): 455-460.

Chapter 21

Innovation in Neurosurgical Education and Safety

Hernán David Vergara-Burgos, María Alejandra Aguilar-Vergara and Ivan David Lozada-Martínez*

School of Medicine, Universidad de Cartagena, Cartagena, Colombia and
Colombian Clinical Research Group in Neurocritical Care,
Latin American Council in Neurocritical Care, Cartagena, Colombia

Abstract

Over time the application of scientific knowledge has allowed the advancement of medicine. Neurosurgery has evolved rapidly through the development of various innovations in surgical techniques, diagnostic methods and treatment, which goes hand in hand with the advent of the Internet and the use of e-learning resources that have promoted a change in the medical and surgical training of residents and students in order to overcome the limitations posed by previous educational models. Historically, neurosurgical education has relied on traditional sources of training, the availability of which was limited and expensive, such as books, articles, courses and surgical practices on cadaver, in order to acquire the necessary clinical knowledge and surgical skills. However, modern advances and accessibility to digital tools have enabled the development of academic resources that can be used by students worldwide regardless of the wealth of their country, thus improving their learning process, visual-spatial skills and understanding of anatomy, along with establishing supportive relationships and knowledge

* Corresponding Author's Email: ilozadam@unicartagena.edu.co.

In: Advances in Neurosurgery Research
Editors: Amit Agrawal, Pradeep Chouksey, Adesh Shrivastava et al.
ISBN: 978-1-68507-859-1

exchange between students and surgeons worldwide. It also allows the evaluation and rehearsal of specific surgical training of any procedure to be performed with the ultimate goal of reducing the associated risks to the patient. This chapter will review strategies and interventions that have drastically improved neurosurgical education.

Introduction

Neurological disorders including congenital disorders, traumatic brain injuries, and degenerative diseases affect up to one billion people and collectively cause more than 6.8 million deaths a year, regardless of age, sex, educational level or income [1]. However, surgical care, especially neurosurgery due to its high costs, has not been considered a priority regarding healthcare in many low-income countries, which is evidenced by the scarcity of facilities and basic equipment necessary for surgical procedures, this accompanied by the lack of adequate training for medical professionals. Therefore, although the obtaining of modern equipment and the progress of the infrastructure will generate a significant advance in the short term, it is established that the improvement of the training of neurosurgery residents will do so in the long term [2].

The main objective of neurosurgical education is to teach the clinical knowledge, surgical skills and the principles of the scientific method that are necessary to become a neurosurgeon [3], allowing students to understand their role within the health care system by demonstrating their abilities and skills during teamwork by making decisions focused on each patient [4], since, as we know, the performance of neurosurgical procedures, even when they allow the possibility of offering a considerable benefit, require large amounts of knowledge accompanied by impeccable technical skill due to the proximity of their surgical instruments to critical neural structures and fragile cerebral blood vessels susceptible to permanent damage [5], for which surgical training, either through observation or practice in and out of the operating room is essential, in order to achieve the dexterity which is an essential trait of every neurosurgical resident [6].

In recent decades, thanks to medical research, new prophylactic, diagnostic, and therapeutic procedures have been proposed and evaluated through clinical practice to establish their efficacy and safety [7]. In the field of neurosurgery as a result of important technological innovations there has been a rapid evolution in diagnostic modalities, minimally invasive techniques and adjuvant therapies [8], generating significant adjustments in both medical work and patient care, which in turn has influenced medical education, and in particular the training of residents by seeking to improve neurosurgical education in order to increase and better patient outcomes with the greatest possible efficiency and safety [9].

As we know, medical-surgical education has traditionally been characterized by following the "see one, do one, teach one" principle that worked well for more than a century [10], based on repeated exposure and the opportunity to achieve practice through experience. However, for specialties requiring high precision and acute perception, such as neurosurgery, there is a requirement that should be met especially in teaching hospitals, it is to have the means and strategies to improve surgical training while reducing the associated risk to the patient [11], by being subjected to inexperienced surgical trainees with a higher probability of error who have developed much of their technical surgical training in the operating room assisting more experienced surgeons or in the cadaver laboratory complemented by clinical knowledge acquired by reading books or lectures [12, 13]. Therefore, it is imperative to develop innovative technologies to promote a change in current medical and surgical education that will allow residents to receive adequate training within established standards of knowledge and work [14, 15].

Visits Based Model

Historically, strategies to improve international neurosurgical care have been promoted by organizations such as the World Federation of Neurological Surgeons (WFNS) and the Foundation for International Education in Neurological Surgery (FIENS) they are based on international conferences and visits by international surgeons to regions of low- and middle-income countries in need of these interventions. These activities have served to establish contact between colleagues and have allowed the development of knowledge from experience in areas of training in which the local or regional team has not previously been present, while benefiting the patients that is being operated during the visits. However, this approach has several limitations that affect its suitability as a long-term neurosurgical training model. Currently, international surgical training depends on the initiative of international surgeons to allocate the time and financial resources to reach particular regions, so visits are often episodic, making it difficult to obtain a continuous educational experience. It may also lead to disruptions in the local clinical environment as medical staff may reduce their scheduled responsibilities to participate in neurosurgical training activities [2, 16]. Hence, the use of structured and methodical online education is proposed as appropriate to decrease educational inequality [17].

Online Electronic Learning (E-Learning) Model

In an increasingly complex and competitive professional environment, it is necessary to improve methods for training neurosurgical residents, ensuring high quality patient care [18]. With the emergence and development of computer technology and the internet as a global communication tool along with the popularity of e-learning resources has promoted a change in medical-surgical education establishing new approaches for information exchange and communication [14, 18]. E-learning is a teaching approach that relies on the use of electronic media and devices as utensils to enhance access to training and interaction [4, 19], increasingly fulfilling a growing need in the field of medical education and becoming a self-sustaining and cost-effective substitute for face-to-face learning based on the visit model, which is estimated to spend more than $250 million each year and relies on the presence of visiting neurosurgeons to conduct the training process [2, 17]. If used properly, e-learning could help to improve and standardize neurosurgical training and care. However, this theoretical training is not enough, and requires the accompaniment of educational techniques that contribute to the development of inherent technical skills [20, 21]. It should also be mentioned that the quality of the different e-learning tools depends both on their content and the way in which they are structured and their adaptation to the needs of the participating public, taking into account the advantages and disadvantages of each one [17, 18, 22].

Some of the advantages of e-learning include the standardization of learning objectives across a wider group of participants with neurosurgical training interests, the limited infrastructure required, the scheduling of study time according to the learner's availability since the training material is available 24 hours a day with built-in feedback systems that ensure regular evaluation. However, there are still limitations to this method of learning, such as the lack of computers and stable Internet connections and the difficulties in offering practical courses to complement the theoretical modules in some regions with fewer resources. In addition, there are problems in the availability of high quality, free or affordable resources, coupled with the fact that most of the information is in English and not all learners who wish to access it have sufficient knowledge of the language. Additional barriers to consider are cultural differences such as ethical, moral, and religious thoughts that may arise [17, 18].

The advantages and disadvantages of each e-learning tool are presented below.

Listservs

Listservs are e-mail lists that allow a defined group of people to discuss topics or concepts relevant to the group of members. Listservs have the lowest level of structure of all educational formats and are essentially an online forum for teachers, learners, and interested individuals to discuss interesting cases or request help with complicated diagnoses, depending solely on the knowledge, experience, and motivation of the list members. Generally, there are no formal methods of evaluation and they are entirely self-taught, and may have low participation rates, low levels of moderation, and the possibility of unrelated information being posted [17, 18].

Blogs

Blogs are frequently offered by major neurosurgical journals to distribute recent abstracts to the subscribing neurosurgical community who can sometimes comment on the subject matter, allowing for a direct exchange of information and dynamic discussion [18].

Social Media Platforms

Social networks were originally developed to promote interpersonal exchange, but have been recognized as useful for professional networking, as for joining neurosurgical community groups, commenting relevant news or concepts that can be shared with others. However, discussion of individual cases cannot take place because of the lack of confidentiality [18, 23].

Smartphone Applications

Apps can provide step by step instructions on various medical procedures with the help of videos and high-resolution images. These can contain information on basic neuroanatomy, relevant scoring systems, interpretation of plain radiographs, computed tomography or magnetic resonance imaging, and help on drug dosing and interactions, thus aiding in evidence-based decision making [18, 24].

Online Libraries

Online libraries are the most traditional and possibly the most widely utilized form of e-learning because of their ease of use, thus enhancing access to learning resources by medical personnel worldwide for the purpose of writing articles or searching for specific information [25]. During the early efforts to establish this initiative, the methods chosen were the conversion of physical textbooks into electronic textbooks by scanning them and the distribution of information through notes, slides and additional material [13]. However, the effectiveness of online libraries is limited by the total reliance on self-directed learning by searching for relevant information in a large amount of associated material, which can lead to difficulties, and the open approach does not allow the generation of defined learning objectives [17, 18].

Modular Courses and Webinars

Modular courses and webinars are structured modules that are based on a topic for the delivery of information and can be part of a larger set of courses, allowing for a continuous learning experience based on objectives. Courses may be followed by a quiz to check whether learning objectives have been achieved and there is usually no direct interaction between students and faculty, so there is no formal supervision or mentoring [17, 18, 26].

Structured Online Courses

Structured online courses deliver instruction directly and interactively, using the advantages of the Internet to simulate a face-to-face classroom with a pre-established curriculum, defined faculty and students, as well as training start and end dates. This eliminates geographical barriers and replaces physical classrooms with virtual classrooms using sophisticated course management systems [17, 18].

Physical Learning Models

The educational algorithms and paradigms to be followed during the implementation of a neurosurgical training program were established based on learning protocols followed by our ancestors, which contributed to the development of educational objectives defined in each program but not of a formative standardization [9]. Additionally, thanks to the reduction of the working day of physicians in training, especially in the USA and Europe, in order to improve the working conditions of residents and patient safety, it is necessary to implement a high quality and time-efficient training that guarantees the autonomy of the student without affecting patient care, defining then the appropriate preparation not in terms of time of service but by the development of specific skills and knowledge [3, 26, 27]. Therefore, simulation has been postulated as a possible solution to this problem, providing adequate training in less time and contributing to the development of surgical performance of residents in a safe and realistic learning environment [27]. Simulation-based medical education with safe operating room practice has even been proposed as a better training method, compared to traditional clinical education in which a technical error can lead to devastating patient outcomes [27, 28].

The mentioned time limitations and the need to maximize learning have led to a reduction in the teaching time of anatomy and laboratory with samples of human cadavers in medical schools, with textbooks and two-dimensional images as the main complementary material [29]. Therefore, the multimodal teaching method offered by new technologies for cognitive and practical development, based on senses such as sight, hearing and tactile sensation used simultaneously, has been proposed as a solution, achieving the development of constant educational experiences. Added to the fact that the complexity of the anatomy of the central nervous system has traditionally been taught in two-dimensional space, so these relationships must be translated into three-dimensional through complex mental reconstructions that can impair neuroanatomical learning in beginning residents, overloading them cognitively and reducing their training performance, thus increasing both the time required per procedure as well as the risk of error during the procedure [6, 9, 29].

Simulation models, being complex computerized equipment, are awfully expensive and not very accessible in certain regions. However, they have certain advantages over other educational models, since they allow practice at the student's convenience, learning and improving their skills more quickly in a specifically manufactured and controlled environment, regardless of the available capacity of cadavers or patients [6]. Moreover, such an artificial environment allows the student to develop in difficult clinical situations that often simulate a crisis by acquiring indispensable technical and non-technical skills such as communication, leadership, and teamwork, without posing a direct risk to potential patients [9, 27, 30]. However, the ideal scenario to decrease surgical risk is to achieve simulations of complex procedures using real patient data, rather than computer-generated topographies or generic brain reconstructions, allowing the development of particular surgical strategies for each patient [11].

Visualization technology in the operating room allows neurosurgeons to gather the necessary information in a timely manner to create a complete mental image improving surgical accuracy. These visualization modalities include: digital stereomicroscopy, surgical planning, augmented reality (AR) and virtual reality (VR).

Digital Stereoscopic Visualization

Digital stereoscopic visualization executes the integration of various forms of multimedia such as videos, interactive anatomy and computer rendered animations, allowing for the accurate recreation of anatomy and neurosurgical approaches. (HENN) The use of a stereoscopic digital microscope contributes to the neurosurgeon's ability to create 3D mental images during surgery, especially in microsurgical procedures such as anastomosis, aneurysms, arteriovenous malformations, bypasses, and spinal or cranial surgery. This image is captured by a camera and displayed on external stereoscopic monitors, helping the surgeon to guide his instruments, visualize the target and avoid any neuronal or vessel damage. Currently, the quality of the visual image and light is being improved through the use of computer technologies that allow it to be integrated with other data, such as the radiological image, thus increasing the perception of reality [6, 31].

Surgical Planning and Assistance

Surgical planning allows precise analysis of the procedure to be performed using a computer and then transferring the information for review. However, it can display limitations, for example, neurosurgeons are forced to develop a complex hand and unnatural eye coordination as they must constantly look up at the two-dimensional navigation monitor located in the operating room and down into the surgical field to manipulate the surgical instruments, basing their movements on the information provided by the navigation system. This affects the surgical work and extends the time per procedure [6].

Likewise, neurosurgeons need to mentally interpret two-dimensional images to imagine the relationship between the patient's complex anatomy and the surgical instruments during the procedure, based on the two-dimensional information provided by the surgical navigation system, thus increasing the surgeon's stress level and the risk of human error [6].

Neuronavigation

Visualization technologies in neurosurgery become relevant, especially in the surgical act because they contribute positively to the outcome of the procedure performed [6]. The use of neuronavigation systems in neurosurgery is essential because it allows improving the vision of the neurological anatomy and localizing complex lesions in the central nervous system. The equipment calibrates the preoperative images with the patient's intraoperative coordinate system using a transformation matrix that creates a link between the preoperative images and the anatomical structures, giving surgeons a three-dimensional orientation of the position of the region of interest [32].

The main modalities are intraoperative ultrasound (iUS), intraoperative magnetic resonance imaging (iMRI) and intraoperative computed tomography (iCT), the first one being the most widely used due to its cost, high availability, and real-time image production, particularly in resource-limited countries [33]. The most important clinical utilities in neurosurgery include localization of small intracranial lesions, skull base surgery, intracerebral biopsies, intracranial endoscopy, functional neurosurgery, and spinal navigation [34].

Recent advances have yielded promising results with iUS using shear waves instead of longitudinal waves, which has been shown to be useful in localizing deep vascular lesions. However, iUS images are of low quality and depend on user interpretation, so it is not widely used. iMRI is considered the gold standard imaging modality for soft-tissue lesions. A prospective randomized controlled trial used iMRI to increase the extent of resection of tumors demonstrating that it increases progression-free survival. Likewise, iCT is most commonly used in spine surgeries [32].

Some limitations of this method include the assumption that the brain and skull are rigid structures, however, during surgery there is distortion of the brain tissue, manipulation of the anatomy, tissue inflammation and loss of cerebrospinal fluid, causing the images of the navigation system to be inaccurate, which can cause damage in functional areas of the brain adjacent to the lesions. In addition, it requires a lot of time and calculations to obtain an adequate image and contributes little to the improvement and learning of spatial reasoning as a skill. Therefore, it is advisable to rely on other visualization systems or more recent tools such as stereomicroscopy, augmented reality and virtual reality [6, 32, 34].

Virtual Reality (VR)

Virtual reality (VR) is a computerized environment where the user navigates and interacts by generating real-time simulations to his or her senses, providing a sensory experience [35]. It is also defined as a human-computer interface that facilitates highly interactive visualization and control of three-dimensional images generated by computers and similar components whose quality, detail and speed evoke life-like experiences [6]. A key element of VR is the high level of user immersion and high level of fidelity of structures, as well as user interaction with them [36]. High-resolution images, sound quality, haptic input, and feedback devices are the parameters for creating a virtual reality environment. In addition, organ and tissue structures should be of high fidelity, and the change in their shape, size, and viewing angle should fully correspond to the user's movements and manipulations [37].

This method of visualization encompasses learners of all educational levels: surgeons, residents, medical students, nurses and allied health professionals. VR can strengthen skills from basic knowledge and thought processes to techniques employed in neurosurgical procedures. In addition, it can serve as a useful tool for educators to objectively examine assessments, observe the learning process, and track the learner's improvement [26].

VR simulators bring multiple benefits to education, but their dissemination is limited because their efficacy and validity have not been clarified and their impact on patient outcome and results has not been studied [38].

Studies concluded that VR simulators allow access to better training opportunities for surgeons and trainees because it strengthens medical skills in terms of speed and accuracy for residents and even results in improvement patient attention and limits concerns and risks in the delivery of medical care [39, 40].

VR simulators offer near to unlimited training opportunities, increasing the frequency with which trainees could perform educational exercises and reducing the resources used, thus avoiding the need for patient or cadaver availability. Associated with VR, 3D printing allows us to create reproducible models that can undergo real-world manipulation [26, 38]. In contrast, cadavers, because of the preparation required, the cost, and the ethical and health implications they may represent, pose a challenge for their use in education or training. Similarly, the cost of traditional synthetic models that are not reusable is a limitation compared to VR simulators, which are more cost-effective to access and allow the use of real tools and instruments for the resident to become accustomed to their usage. VR training can be variable depending on the subject's capabilities and competencies, adjusting to them, and providing a more objective and efficient assessment with more truthful performance measures. The above in turn provides the opportunity to certify trainees and compare their results [38].

VR provides the ability to train interprofessional teams to intervene in complex scenarios, train surgical procedures, plan surgery in patient-specific conditions allowing for superior preparation of surgeons and providing the opportunity to study different surgical strategies virtually without the risk of affecting patients. The cases presented do not suffer from the problem of repetition as they are digital programs [41]. Due to the programming and lack of graphical limitations, virtual reality models can mimic a wide range of anatomic and physical variations, making it an advantageous aspect compared to physical models that generally do not present any pathologic alterations [26].

Studies propose that VR simulation in neuroanatomy education offers learners the opportunity to quickly conceptualize anatomical structures in 3D. This technology is increasingly being incorporated into medical training and its adoption is likely to become coarser and more widespread over time. It is now used in the training of medical students and surgical residents and even among surgeons for preoperative planning and anticipating response to potential complications, all this contributing with the establishment as a system as effective as traditional methods in terms of student performance, but superior in engagement with the content learned, utility and learner motivation [37, 42].

Augmented Reality

Augmented reality (AR) is an immersive environment whose principle consists of the projection of virtual objects onto real-world entities, thus allowing data from the real environment to be merged with virtual information and vice versa [39]. In the context of surgical navigation, AR complements traditional neuronavigation. AR systems provide a real-time updated 3D virtual model of anatomical details of interest by superimposing CT and MRI images on the actual surgical field [41, 44]. The augmented image can be visualized through various means: a screen mounted on the surgeon's head, monitors, semitransparent surfaces, by projecting images on the surgical microscope or even on the patient's body [44, 45]. In neurosurgery, there is a special need for AR to improve the perception of the surgical environment, which tends to be small and limited, to guide the surgeon during the procedure, trying to avoid unnecessary manipulations or inadvertent injuries. This becomes even more important with the introduction of minimally invasive neurosurgery, which requires limited access in search of benefits for patients, although at the same time it represents a surgical challenge [41, 44]. AR is useful because it solves the problem of manipulating the instruments while looking at a screen separate from the surgical field and at the same time transferring the movements to the operative site, which is why AR allows the surgeon to interact in a much more effective way with the tissues [41, 46]. Although AR is a relevant advance for neurosurgery, its clinical experience is limited.

Studies have reported that the most frequent intraoperative uses of augmented reality include surgeries for meningiomas, gliomas, pituitary tumors, cerebral cavernomas and arteriovenous malformations [44]. Some of these studies evaluated the use of AR in aneurysm surgery, in this one they agreed that AR optimizes the patient's position and consequently improves the surgical trajectory; it allowed the planning of the craniotomy, contributed to intraoperative orientation and finally the projection of the aneurysm and adjacent vessels, reminding the surgeon of the vascular structure while performing the procedure and thus contributing to the confirmation of the clipping, refining the results.

Surgeons using the virtual interactive presence and augmented reality (VIPAR) system reported that it allows a remote surgeon to communicate real-time visual and verbal information to a local surgeon performing a procedure in a safer manner. In the educational setting, it is believed that this system can complement standard neurosurgical training by allowing mentoring without the physical presence of the experienced surgeon [43].

Among its current applications in the different fields of neurosurgery, we have:

- Cranial surgery: the utility of virtual simulations involves intracranial and skull base procedures whose visualization is limited.
- Vascular neurosurgery: the clinical application of virtual reality contributes to the way vascular diseases are diagnosed and managed because they are highly dependent on imaging techniques. It is currently used during invasive angiography and in training for mechanical thrombectomy in the context of acute stroke.
- Peripheral nerve surgery: are common in all forms of extremity trauma, including lacerations, fractures, dislocations, ligamentous tears, and crushing or amputation injuries. Therefore, most common surgeries are microsurgeries [39].

Training in Middle to Low-Income Countries

Universally the gold standard for neurosurgical education is a solid theoretical foundation supported by vastly improved digital technologies and must be accompanied by intense practice that can be obtained in the operating room, cadaver laboratory or through physical simulation models. Training programs in neurosurgery may differ significantly between countries as they are established on the basis of local epidemiology, available funds, distribution of health care facilities and internal organization [19]. Nevertheless, the gap in the standards of neurosurgical education between different countries has been a constant concern for all those engaged worldwide in the training of new neurosurgeons, who posit that some digital tools that demonstrate neurosurgical practice or simulate surgical scenarios may provide an accessible way to reduce the gap in training between surgeons from different countries and create a standardized curriculum [17, 19]. However, technological advances have been used mainly in developed countries, while middle- to low-income countries have not fully benefited from these tools, due to lack of access to a stable internet or certain technological devices, problems in language comprehension and certain cultural differences that can present as a major barrier to online training, causing lack of interest or feeling of excessive burden for students participating in the course [17, 25].

Accordingly, long-term sustainable improvement in resource lacking settings depends on a collaborative approach, in which locally accessible education and hands-on training initiatives such as model visits by international trainers are complemented by online curriculum and interaction, that would contribute to the continuous improvement of their neurosurgical knowledge and would similarly help international neurosurgeons to become familiar with the clinical and sociocultural challenges of the region and investigate available resources prior to visiting, which would allow timely addressing of locally identified needs and timely support of local surgical capacity, while working to make technologies and internet access in these regions more stable and with greater accessibility [2].

Conclusion

Historically, the training of neurosurgery residents has been guided by traditional pedagogical models based on obtaining knowledge and surgical skills by reading books, attending conferences, practicing on human cadavers, support in the operating room and visits from international surgeons. However, thanks to the development of information technologies and the availability of informatics tools, the limits of education posed by previous pedagogical methods have been enhanced and expanded, allowing globalization and access to academic material that was previously in the hands of a privileged few. The most notorious advances that have reduced the problems raised are under the categories of e-learning, physical models and simulators that have contributed to the improvement of medical education and especially neurosurgical education, thanks to a cognitive and practical training in a safe and realistic learning environment that will increase surgical performance and therefore benefit the patient. Yet, the implementation of such pedagogical conditions requires the availability of an adequate physical and technological infrastructure to take full advantage of them, which are not available for residents in certain middle to low-income countries where their training method will be guided by a collaborative approach between the visit-based model and new technologies. Future directions for the widespread application of these methods in clinical practice, together with research to estimate the contribution to patient surgical outcomes, are needed to effectively evaluate these training methods and establish possible future improvements.

References

[1] Kea, X, Saksenaa, P, Hollyb, A.: The determinants of health expenditure: a country-level panel data analysis. *World Health Organization* 1: 1-28, 2011.

[2] Liang, K. E., Bernstein, I., Kato, Y., Kawase, T., & Hodaie, M. (2016). Enhancing Neurosurgical Education in Low- and Middle-income Countries: Current Methods and New Advances. *Neurologia Medico-Chirurgica,* 56(11), 709-715. doi: https:// 10.2176/nmc.ra.2016-0092.

[3] Kim, D. H., Dacey, R. G., Zipfel, G. J., Berger, M. S., McDermott, M., Barbaro, N. M., Day, A. L. (2017). Neurosurgical Education in a Changing Healthcare and Regulatory Environment: A Consensus Statement from 6 Programs. *Neurosurgery,* 80(4S), S75-S82. doi: https://10.1093/neuros/nyw146.

[4] Carbonaro, M., King, S., Taylor, E., Satzinger, F., Snart, F., & Drummond, J. (2008). Integration of e-learning technologies in an interprofessional health science course. *Medical Teacher,* 30(1), 25-33. doi: https://10.1080/01421590701753450.

[5] Pelargos, P. E., Nagasawa, D. T., Lagman, C., Tenn, S., Demos, J. V., Lee, S. J., Yang, I. (2017). Utilizing virtual and augmented reality for educational and clinical enhancements in neurosurgery. *Journal of Clinical Neuroscience*, 35, 1-4. doi: https://10.1016/j.jocn.2016.09.002.

[6] Bernardo, A. (2017). Virtual Reality and Simulation in Neurosurgical Training. *World Neurosurgery,* 106, 1015-1029. doi: https://10.1016/j.wneu.2017.06.140.

[7] Bernstein, M., & Bampoe, J. (2004). Surgical innovation or surgical evolution: an ethical and practical guide to handling novel neurosurgical procedures. *Journal of Neurosurgery,* 100(1), 2-7. doi: https://10.3171/jns.2004.100.1.0002.

[8] Kato, Y., Liew, B. S., Sufianov, A. A., Rasulic, L., Arnautovic, K. I., Dong, V. H., … Germano, I. M. (2020). Review of global neurosurgery education: Horizon of Neurosurgery in the Developing Countries. *Chinese Neurosurgical Journal,* 6(1). doi: https://10.1186/s41016-020-00194-1.

[9] Harrop, J., Lobel, D. A., Bendok, B., Sharan, A., & Rezai, A. R. (2013). Developing a Neurosurgical Simulation-Based Educational Curriculum. *Neurosurgery,* 73, S25-S29. doi: https://10.1227/neu.0000000000000101.

[10] Singh, H., Kalani, M., Acosta-Torres, S., El Ahmadieh, T. Y., Loya, J., & Ganju, A. (2013). History of Simulation in Medicine. *Neurosurgery,* 73, S9-S14. doi: https://10.1227/neu.0000000000000093.

[11] Clarke, D. B., D'Arcy, R. C. N., Delorme, S., Laroche, D., Godin, G., Hajra, S. G., … DiRaddo, R. (2012). Virtual Reality Simulator. *Surgical Innovation,* 20(2), 190-197. doi: https://10.1177/1553350612451354.

[12] Kelz, R. R., & Morris, J. B. (2009). Patient Safety and Surgical Training. *Annals of Surgery,* 249(6), 877-878. doi: https://10.1097/sla.0b013e3181a7be96.

[13] Larvin, M. (2009). E-Learning in surgical education and training. *ANZ Journal of Surgery,* 79(3), 133-137. doi: https://10.1111/j.1445-2197.2008.04828.x.

[14] Teton, Z. E., Freedman, R. S., Tomlinson, S. B., Linzey, J. R., Onyewuenyi, A., Khahera, A. S., Hendricks, B. K., & Cohen-Gadol, A. A. (2020). The Neurosurgical Atlas: advancing neurosurgical education in the digital age, *Neurosurgical Focus FOC*, 48(3), E17. doi: https://10.3171/2019.12.FOCUS19820.

[15] Trelease, R. B. (2016). From chalkboard, slides, and paper to e-learning: How computing technologies have transformed anatomical sciences education. *Anatomical Sciences Education,* 9(6), 583-602. doi: https://10.1002/ase.1620.

[16] Shrime, M. G., Sleemi, A., & Ravilla, T. D. (2014). Charitable Platforms in Global Surgery: A Systematic Review of their Effectiveness, Cost-Effectiveness, Sustainability, and Role Training. *World Journal of Surgery,* 39(1), 10-20. doi: https://10.1007/s00268-014-2516-0.

[17] Blankstein, U., Dakurah, T., Bagan, M., & Hodaie, M. (2011). Structured Online Neurosurgical Education as a Novel Method of Education Delivery in the Developing World. *World Neurosurgery,* 76(3-4), 224-230. doi: https://10.1016/j.wneu.2011.02.041.

[18] Stienen, M. N., Schaller, K., Cock, H., Lisnic, V., Regli, L., & Thomson, S. (2016). eLearning resources to supplement postgraduate neurosurgery training. *Acta Neurochirurgica,* 159(2), 325-337. doi: https://10.1007/s00701-016-3042-7.

[19] Nicolosi, F., Rossini, Z., Zaed, I., Kolias, A. G., Fornari, M., & Servadei, F. (2018). Neurosurgical digital teaching in low-middle income countries: beyond the frontiers of traditional education. *Neurosurgical Focus,* 45(4), E17. doi: https://10.3171/2018.7.focus18288.

[20] Stienen, M. N., Netuka, D., Demetriades, A. K., Ringel, F., Gautschi, O. P., Gempt, J., … Schaller, K. (2016). Residency program trainee-satisfaction correlate with results of the European board examination in neurosurgery. *Acta Neurochirurgica,* 158(10), 1823-1830. doi: https://10.1007/s00701-016-2917-y.

[21] Robison, R. A., Liu, C. Y., & Apuzzo, M. L. J. (2011). Man, Mind, and Machine: The Past and Future of Virtual Reality Simulation in Neurologic Surgery. *World Neurosurgery,* 76(5), 419-430. doi: https://10.1016/j.wneu.2011.07.008.

[22] Cook, D. A. (2006). Where are we with Web-based learning in medical education? *Medical Teacher,* 28(7), 594-598. doi: https://10.1080/01421590601028854.

[23] Barbosa Pereira, J. L., Kubben P. L., de Albuquerque L. A., et al., E-learning for neurosurgeons: Getting the most from the new web tools. *Asian Journal of Neurosurgery.* 2015 Jan-Mar;10(1):48. doi: https://10.4103/1793-5482.151514.

[24] Hughes, M. A., & Brennan, P. M. (2011). The Internet for neurosurgeons: current resources and future challenges. *British Journal of Neurosurgery,* 25(3), 347-351. doi: https://10.3109/02688697.2011.554582.

[25] Derbew, M., Beveridge, M., Howard, A., & Byrne, N. (2006). Building Surgical Research Capacity in Africa: The Ptolemy Project. *PLoS Medicine,* 3(7), e305. doi: https://10.1371/journal.pmed.0030305.

[26] Konakondla, S., Fong, R., & Schirmer, C. M. (2017). Simulation training in neurosurgery: advances in education and practice. *Advances in Medical Education and Practice, Volume 8,* 465-473. doi: https://10.2147/amep.s113565.

[27] Kirkman, M. A., Ahmed, M., Albert, A. F., Wilson, M. H., Nandi, D., & Sevdalis, N. (2014). The use of simulation in neurosurgical education and training. *Journal of Neurosurgery,* 121(2), 228-246. doi: https://10.3171/2014.5.jns131766.

[28] McGaghie, W. C., Issenberg, S. B., Cohen, E. R., Barsuk, J. H., Wayne, D. B. Does simulation-based 8 medical education with deliberate practice yield better results than traditional clinical 9 education? A meta-analytic comparative review of the evidence. *Acad Med.* 2011;86(6): 706-10 711. https://doi.org/10.1097/ACM. 0b013e318217e119.

[29] Ekstrand, C., Jamal, A., Nguyen, R., Kudryk, A., Mann, J., & Mendez, I. (2018). Immersive and interactive virtual reality to improve learning and retention of neuroanatomy in medical students: a randomized controlled study. *CMAJ Open,* 6(1), E103-E109. doi: https://10.9778/cmajo.20170110.

[30] Hull, L., Arora, S., Aggarwal, R., Darzi, A., Vincent, C., & Sevdalis, N. (2012). The Impact of Nontechnical Skills on Technical Performance in Surgery: A Systematic Review. *Journal of the American College of Surgeons,* 214(2), 214-230. doi: https://10.1016/j.jamcollsurg.2011.10.016.

[31] Henn, J. S., Lemole, G. M., Jr., Ferreira, M. A. T., González, L. F., Schornak, M., Preul, MC y Spetzler, RF (2002). Realidad virtual estereoscópica interactiva: una nueva herramienta para la educación neuroquirúrgica, *Journal of Neurosurgery,* 96 (1), 144-149. https://doi.org/10.3171/jns.2002.96.1.0144.

[32] Ashraf, M., Choudhary, N., Hussain, S. S., Kamboh, U. A., & Ashraf, N. (2020). Role of intraoperative computed tomography scanner in modern neurosurgery - An early experience. *Surgical neurology international,* 11, 247. https://doi.org/10. 25259/SNI_303_2020.

[33] Kaale, A. J., Rutabasibwa, N., Mchome, L. L., Lillehei, K. O., Honce, J. M., Kahamba, J., & Ormond, D. R. (2021). The use of intraoperative neurosurgical ultrasound for surgical navigation in low- and middle-income countries: the initial experience in Tanzania, *Journal of Neurosurgery JNS,* 134(2), 630-637. Retrieved Jun 21, 2021, from https://thejns.org/view/journals/j-neurosurg/134/2/article-p630. xml.

[34] Khoshnevisan, A., & Allahabadi, N. S. (2012). Neuronavigation: principles, clinical applications and potential pitfalls. *Iranian Journal of Psychiatry,* 7(2), 97-103.

[35] Flavián, C., Ibáñez-Sánchez, S., & Orús, C. (2018). The impact of virtual, augmented and mixed reality technologies on the customer experience. *Journal of Business Research.* doi: https://10.1016/j.jbusres.2018.10.050.

[36] Pantelidis, P., Chorti, A., Papagiouvanni, I., Paparoidamis, G., Drosos, C., Panagiotakopoulos, T., … Sideris, M. (2018). Virtual and Augmented Reality in Medical Education. *Medical and Surgical Education - Past, Present and Future.* doi: https://10.5772/intechopen.71963.

[37] Barsom, E. Z., Graafland, M., & Schijven, M. P. (2016). Systematic review on the effectiveness of augmented reality applications in medical training. *Surgical Endoscopy,* 30(10), 4174-4183. doi: https://10.1007/s00464-016-4800-6.

[38] Pfandler, M., Lazarovici, M., Stefan, P., Wucherer, P., & Weigl, M. (2017). Virtual reality-based simulators for spine surgery: a systematic review. *The Spine Journal,* 17(9), 1352-1363. doi: https://10.1016/j.spinee.2017.05.016.

[39] Fiani, B., De Stefano, F., Kondilis, A., Covarrubias, C., Reier, L., Sarhadi, K. Virtual Reality in Neurosurgery: "Can You See It?"-A Review of the Current Applications and Future Potential. *World Neurosurg.* 2020 Sep;141:291-298. doi: https://10.1016/j.wneu.2020.06.066. Epub 2020 Jun 17. PMID: 32561486.

[40] Schutte, N. S., & Stilinović, E. J. (2017). Facilitating empathy through virtual reality. *Motivation and Emotion,* 41(6), 708-712. doi: https://10.1007/s11031-017-9641-7.

[41] Meola, A., Cutolo, F., Carbone, M., Cagnazzo, F., Ferrari, M., & Ferrari, V. (2016). Augmented reality in neurosurgery: a systematic review. *Neurosurgical Review,* 40(4), 537-548. doi: https://10.1007/s10143-016-0732-9.

[42] Stepan, K., Zeiger, J., Hanchuk, S., Del Signore, A., Shrivastava, R., Govindaraj, S., & Iloreta, A. (2017). Immersive virtual reality as a teaching tool for neuroanatomy. *International Forum of Allergy & Rhinology,* 7(10), 1006-1013. doi: https://10.1002/alr.21986.

[43] Cho, J., Rahimpour, S., Cutler, A., Goodwin, C. R., Lad, S. P., & Codd, P. (2020). Enhancing Reality: A Systematic Review of Augmented Reality in Neuronavigation and Education. *World Neurosurgery.* doi: https://10.1016/j.wneu.2020.04.043.

[44] Cabrilo, I., Bijlenga, P., & Schaller, K. (2014). Augmented Reality in the Surgery of Cerebral Aneurysms. *Neurosurgery,* 10, 252-261. doi: https://10.1227/neu.00000 00000000328.

[45] Lee, C., & Wong, G. K. C. (2019). Virtual reality and augmented reality in the management of intracranial tumors: A review. *Journal of Clinical Neuroscience.* doi: https://10.1016/j.jocn.2018.12.036.

[46] Guha, D., Alotaibi, N. M., Nguyen, N., Gupta, S., McFaul, C., & Yang, V. X. D. (2017). Augmented Reality in Neurosurgery: A Review of Current Concepts and Emerging Applications. *Canadian Journal of Neurological Sciences/Journal Canadien Des Sciences Neurologiques,* 44(03), 235-245. doi: https://10.1017/cjn.2016.443.

Editors' Contact Information

Dr. Amit Agrawal
(MCh): Department of Neurosurgery,
All India Institute of Medical Sciences,
Saket Nagar, Bhopal 462020,
Madhya Pradesh, India

Dr. Pradeep Chouksey
(MCh): Department of Neurosurgery,
All India Institute of Medical Sciences,
Saket Nagar, Bhopal 462020,
Madhya Pradesh, India

Dr. Adesh Shrivastava
(MCh): Department of Neurosurgery,
All India Institute of Medical Sciences,
Saket Nagar, Bhopal 462020, Madhya Pradesh, India

Dr. Sumit Raj
(MCh): Department of Neurosurgery,
All India Institute of Medical Sciences,
Saket Nagar, Bhopal 462020,
Madhya Pradesh, India

Dr. Rakesh Mishra
(M.Ch): Assistant Professor, Department of Neurosurgery,
Institute of Medical Sciences,
Banaras Hindu University,
Varanasi, Uttar Pradesh-221005, India

Index

E

F

G

L

M

T

U

V